中医经典译丛
Chinese-English Translation of Traditional Chinese Medicine Classics

本草崇原
Reverence for the Origin of Materia Medica
（汉英对照）

原　著　〔清〕张志聪
主　译　孙　慧
副主译　赵　栋　周　茜
译　者　姚秋慧　王丽君　邱　冬
　　　　周　茜　赵　栋　孙　慧

本书为山东中医药大学"中医英译及中医文化对外传播研究"科研创新团队项目资助成果、山东中医药大学英语专业学科建设资助成果。

U0396075

苏州大学出版社

图书在版编目(CIP)数据

本草崇原:汉英对照 / (清)张志聪原著；孙慧主
译. —苏州：苏州大学出版社，2021.8
（中医经典译丛）
书名原文：Reverence for the Origin of Materia
Medica
ISBN 978-7-5672-3560-1

Ⅰ.①本… Ⅱ.①张… ②孙… Ⅲ.①《神农本草经》
—注释—汉、英 Ⅳ.①R281.2

中国版本图书馆 CIP 数据核字(2021)第 108822 号

书　　名：本草崇原 BEN CAO CHONG YUAN
　　　　　Reverence for the Origin of Materia Medica
　　　　　（汉英对照）
原　　著：〔清〕张志聪
主　　译：孙　慧
责任编辑：汤定军
策划编辑：汤定军
装帧设计：刘　俊

出版发行：苏州大学出版社（Soochow University Press）
社　　址：苏州市十梓街 1 号　邮编：215006
印　　装：广东虎彩云印刷有限公司
网　　址：www. sudapress. com
邮　　箱：sdcbs@ suda. edu. cn
邮购热线：0512-67480030
销售热线：0512-67481020

开　　本：700 mm×1 000 mm　1/16　印张：27.75　字数：412 千
版　　次：2021 年 8 月第 1 版
印　　次：2021 年 8 月第 1 次印刷
书　　号：ISBN 978-7-5672-3560-1
定　　价：98.00 元

凡购本社图书发现印装错误，请与本社联系调换。服务热线：0512-67481020

翻译说明

1. 本次所译的《本草崇原》以清末 1896 年刊印的《医林指月》所辑集的版本内容为基础,并参考了已有的《本草崇原》通行本。

2. 本书是汉英对照版本,每个汉语条目对应英语译文进行编排。

3. 本草名称的翻译采取"四保险"的翻译方法,即每个本草名称均按拼音、汉字、英语和拉丁语的方式进行翻译,如"柏子仁"译为 Baiziren [柏子仁,Chinese Arborvitae Kernel,Semen Platycladi]。个别中药名经多方考证仍无法确定其拉丁名称,采取 Materia Medica 加音译的方法,如"桑寄生实"译为 Materia Medica Sangjisheng Shi。

4. 本草名称如果是三个字及以下,其音译合并在一起,如"赤茯苓"音译为 Chifuling;如果是四个字及以上,根据文义将其音译分开,便于阅读,如"桑上寄生"音译为 Sangshang Jisheng。

5. 古籍名称采用音译的方法翻译,每个字独立音译,括号中附以中文和英文翻译。例如,《黄帝内经》译为 *Huang Di Nei Jing* [《黄帝内经》,*Huangdi's Internal Classic*]。

6. 原《本草崇原》卷中条目有动物制品入药,根据《中华人民共和国野生动物保护法》,其中涉及的珍稀野生动物及制品本版不予保留,共删除犀角、羚羊角、羖羊角三个条目。

7. 书中出现的繁体字、异体字根据现行出版规范改为简体字、通行字。中文版原文中有些语言文字与现行出版编辑规范要求不一致的地方,遵从原文。书中涉及的计量单位名称采用音译方法,基本形式和公制换算如下。

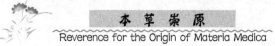
传统计量单位	公制换算	音译形式
尺	0.33 米	Chi
寸	0.03 米	Cun
丈	3.33 米	Zhang
匕	2~3 克	Bi
合	0.1 升	Ge

Translation Specification

1. The translation of *Reverence for the Origin of Materia Medica* is based on the content of the version in *Collection of Twelve Medical Books* published by Shanghai Publishing House in 1896 in the late Qing Dynasty, and refers to several current editions.

2. This book is a Chinese-English version, and each Chinese entry is followed by its corresponding English translation.

3. As to the translation of herbal names, the "Four Assurance Method" is adopted, namely, every herbal name is translated in the sequence of Pinyin, Chinese characters, English and Latin. For instance, "柏子仁" is translated as Baiziren [柏子仁, Chinese Arborvitae Kernel, Semen Platycladi]. If textual researches can not locate the Latin equivalent, it is presented as "Materia Medica" plus Pinyin. For instance, the Latin translation of "桑寄生实" is Materia Medica Sangjisheng Shi.

4. If a herbal name has three or less than three Chinese characters, its transliteration of Pinyin is put together, for instance, "赤茯苓" is transliterated as "Chifuling"; if it has four or more than four Chinese characters, its transliteration of Pinyin is divided into two parts according to its literal meaning for the convenience of easy reading. For instance, "桑上寄生" is transliterated as "SangshangJisheng".

5. The names of ancient works are transliterated with their Chinese names and English versions in brackets, each Chinese character being transliterated separately. For instance, 《黄帝内经》is translated as *Huang Di Nei Jing* [《黄帝内经》, *Huangdi's Internal Classic*].

6. According to the *Law of the People's Republic of China on the*

Protection of Wildlife, rare wild animal parts and their related products involved in the Chinese version of the original text are not retained in this Chinese-English edition. Totally three entries of rhino horn, antelope horn and male goat horn are canceled.

7. The traditional Chinese characters and variant Chinese characters in the Chinese version of the original text are changed into the simplified and current characters in this Chinese-English edition according to the current publication specifications. The style of the original text is retained for some expressions in the Chinese version of the original text that are inconsistent with the requirements of the current publishing and editing. The unit of measurement involved in this edition is transliterated by Pinyin. Examples are shown in the table below.

Traditional Unit	Metric Unit	Pinyin
尺	0.33 meters	Chi
寸	0.03 meters	Cun
丈	3.33 meters	Zhang
匕	2~3 grams	Bi
合	0.1 litres	Ge

目　录

Contents

Volume 1 Top Grade Medicinals

Contents

Contents

Volume 2   Medium-Grade Medicinals

Contents

Volume 3   Low-Grade Medicinals

Contents

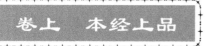

Volume 1 Top Grade Medicinals

1. 人 参

人参 气味甘,微寒,无毒。主补五脏,安精神,定魂魄,止惊悸,除邪气,明目,开心,益智,久服轻身延年。

人参,一名神草,一名地精。春秋运斗枢云,瑶光星散,而为人参。生上党山谷、辽东幽冀诸州,地土最厚处,故有地精之名。相传未掘取时,其茎叶夜中隐隐有光。其年发深久者,根结成人形,头面四肢毕具,谓之孩儿参,故又有神草之名。

人参气味甘美,甘中稍苦,故曰微寒。凡属上品,俱系无毒。独人参禀天宿之光华,钟地土之广厚,久久而成人形,三才具备,故主补人之五脏。脏者藏也。肾藏精,心藏神,肝藏魂,肺藏魄,脾藏智。安精神,定魂魄,则补心肾肺肝之真气矣。夫真气充足,则内外调和,故止惊悸之内动,除邪气之外侵。明目者,五脏之精上注于目也。开心者,五脏之神皆主于心也。又曰益智者,所以补脾也,上品之药,皆可久服,兼治病者,补正气也,故人参久服,则轻身延年。

1. Renshen〔人参, ginseng, Radix Ginseng〕

It is sweet in taste, slightly cold and non-toxic in property, and it is mainly used to tonify the five-zang organs, quiet the spirit, tranquilize the ethereal soul and corporeal soul, cease fright and palpitation, eliminate pathogenic qi, improve vision, soothe the heart and promote wisdom. Long-term taking of it will keep healthy and prolong life.

It is also called Shencao (神草) or Dijing (地精). *Chun Qiu Yun Dou Shu* 〔《春秋运斗枢》, *The Key to Astrology of All Year Round*〕 says that Renshen (ginseng) transforms from the brilliance of the Yaoguang Star scattering on the ground. It grows in the valley of Shangdang (上党) and in areas of Liaodong

（辽东）and Youji（幽冀）where the soil is very fertile, so it is also called Dijing（地精）. It is said that its stems and leaves gleam at night when not dug out. Those growing over years have human-like roots with face and limbs, and then are called Hai'ershen［孩儿参, pseudostellaria, Pseudostellariae Radix］, also called Shencao（神草）.

Renshen（ginseng）is sweet with a little bitterness in taste and slightly cold in property. Those pertaining to the top grade are non-toxic in property. It is the only medicinal herb that receives the brilliance of stars, takes in the essence of soil and becomes a human-like plant after a long time. It possesses the three talents（heaven, humankind, and earth）, so it can tonify the five zang-organs. The function of the zang-organs is to store. The kidney stores the essence; the heart stores the spirit; the liver stores the ethereal soul; the lung stores the corporeal soul; the spleen stores the wisdom. It can quiet the spirit, tranquilize the ethereal soul and the corporeal soul, and accordingly tonify the genuine qi of the heart, kidney, lung and liver. Both the interior and the exterior will be harmonized with sufficient genuine qi. Thus, the interior fright and palpitation will be ceased, and the invasion of the exterior pathogenic qi will be eliminated. It improves vision, because it can make the essence of the five zang-organs move upward into the eyes; it soothes the heart, because the heart governs the spirit of the five zang-organs; it can tonify the spleen, because it promotes wisdom. All top-grade drugs can be taken for a long time, some of which can replenish the healthy qi to treat diseases as well. So long-term taking of it will keep healthy and prolong life.

2. 甘 草

甘草 气味甘平，无毒。主五脏六腑寒热邪气，坚筋骨，长肌肉，倍气力，金疮尰，解毒，久服轻身延年。

甘草始出河西川谷、积沙山，及上郡，今陕西河东州郡皆有之。一名国老，又名灵通。根长三四尺、粗细不定、皮色紫赤，上有横梁，梁下皆细根也，以坚实断理者为佳。调和脏腑，通贯四旁，故有国老、灵通之名。

甘草味甘，气得其平，故曰甘平。《本经》凡言平者，皆谓气得其平也。主治五脏六腑之寒热邪气者，五脏为阴，六腑为阳。寒病为阴，热病为阳。甘草味甘,调和脏腑,通贯阴阳,故治理脏腑阴阳之正气,以除寒热阴阳之邪气也。坚筋骨,长肌肉,倍气力者,坚肝主之筋,肾主之骨,长脾主之肉,倍肺主之气,心主之力。五脏充足,则六腑自和矣。金疮乃刀斧所伤,因金伤而成疮。金疮㾴,乃因金疮而高㾴也。解毒者,解高㾴无名之毒,土性柔和,如以毒物埋土中,久则无毒矣。脏腑阴阳之气皆归土中,久服则土气有余,故轻身延年。

2. Gancao〔甘草, licorice root, Radix Glycyrrhizae〕

It is sweet in taste, mild and non-toxic in property, and it is mainly used to treat the diseases caused by the pathogenic cold qi and the heat qi in the five zang-organs and the six fu-organs, strengthen the sinews and bones, promote the growth of the muscles, replenish qi, increase strength, treat the swollen foot caused by the incised wound and remove toxin. Long-term taking of it will keep healthy and prolong life.

Firstly recorded to be growing in the river valley and a mountain with sands in Hexi (河西) and Shangjun (上郡), now it grows everywhere in Hedong (河东) of Shaanxi (陕西) Province. It is also called Guolao (国老) or Lingtong (灵通). With purple-red peel and transverse creases, its root is three or four Chi long varying with thickness, below which there are fine roots. The roots which are firm and can be broken completely are of good quality. It is used to harmonize the zang-fu organs and connect the parts next to them. Therefore, it is also called Guolao (国老) or Lingtong (灵通).

It is sweet in taste and mild in property, thus it is also called Ganping (甘平, sweet and mild). The meaning of being mild mentioned in *Shen Nong Ben Cao Jing* 〔《神农本草经》, *Shennong's Classic of Materia Medica*〕 refers to being mild in property. It can mainly treat the diseases caused by the pathogenic cold qi and the heat qi in the five zang-organs and the six fu-organs, because the five zang-organs pertain to yin and the six fu-organs pertain to yang while cold diseases pertain to yin and heat diseases pertain to yang. It is sweet in taste and can be used to harmonize the zang-fu organs and connect yin and yang. Therefore, it can be used to regulate the healthy qi of yin and yang in the zang-fu organs and eliminate pathogenic cold qi and heat qi, and pathogenic yin qi and yang qi. It can be used to strengthen the sinews and bones, promote the growth of the muscles, replenish qi and increase strength, i. e., it can strengthen the sinews governed by the liver, nourish the bones governed by the kidney, promote the growth of the muscles governed by the spleen, replenish qi governed by the lung and increase strength governed by the heart. The sixfu-organs will be harmonized if the qi of the five-zang organs are sufficient. The incised wound, the wound made by the knife or axe, can cause swollen foot. In terms of detoxification, it can resolve the unknown toxin of swollen foot. Earth is mild in property, and the toxic substances will be non-toxic after they are buried in the earth for a long time. Both yin qi and yang qi in the zang-fu organs can return to the spleen earth. Long-term taking of it will have abundant earth qi, thus it will keep healthy and prolong life.

3. 黄 芪

黄芪 气味甘,微温,无毒。主痈疽,久败疮,排脓止痛,大风癞疾,五痔鼠瘘,补虚,小儿百病。

黄芪生于西北,得水泽之精,其色黄白,紧实如箭竿,折之柔韧如绵,以出山西之绵上者为良,故世俗谓之绵黄芪,或者只以坚韧如绵解之,非是。

黄芪色黄,味甘,微温。禀火土相生之气化。土主肌肉,火主经脉,故主治肌肉之痈,经脉之疽也。痈疽日久,正气衰微,致三焦之气不温肌肉,则为久败疮。黄芪助三焦出气,以温肌肉,故可治也。痈疽未溃,化血为脓,痛不可忍,黄芪补气助阳,阳气化血而排脓,脓排则痛止。大风癞疾,谓之疬疡,乃风寒客于脉而不去,鼻柱坏而色败,皮肤溃癞者是也。五痔者,牡痔、牝痔、肠痔、脉痔、血痔,是热邪淫于下也;鼠瘘者,肾脏水毒,上淫于脉,致颈项溃肿,或空或凸,是寒邪客于上也。夫癞疾、五痔、鼠瘘,乃邪在经脉,而证见于肌肉皮肤。黄芪内资经脉,外资肌肉,是以三证咸宜。又曰补虚者,乃补正气之虚,而经脉调和,肌肉充足也。小儿经脉未盛,肌肉未盈,血气皆微,故治小儿百病。

3. Huangqi〔黄芪, milkvetch root, Radix Astragaliseu Hedysari〕

It is sweet in taste, slightly warm and non-toxic in property, and it is mainly used to treat welling-abscesses and chronic severe sores, expel pus, relieve pain, treat leprosy, resolve five kinds of hemorrhoids and scrofula, tonify deficiency and treat various kinds of infantile diseases.

Growing in Northwest China, Huangqi (milkvetch root) is nourished by the essence of water. Yellow and white in color, it is as tight as an arrow pole and as flexible as silk floss. Those growing in Mianshang (绵上) of Shanxi (山西) Province are of good quality, so it is popularly called Mianhuangqi (绵黄芪). It is a false idea that it obtains such a name just because it is as flexible as silk floss.

Yellow in color, sweet in taste and slightly warm in property, it receives the qi transformation of mutual generation of fire and earth. Earth governs the muscles, and fire governs the meridians. Therefore, it can be used to treat the carbuncle in the muscles and the abscess in the meridians. Chronic welling-abscesses will lead to the debilitation of healthy qi and failure to warm the muscles with the qi of the triple energizer, resulting in chronic severe sores. It can help the triple energizer promote qi to warm the muscles, thus it can treat chronic severe sores. The blood in welling-abscesses will turn into pus before they rupture, resulting in severe pain. It can replenish qi and assist yang. Yang qi can resolve blood to expel pus, which can therefore relieve pain. Leprosy, also known as Liyang (疬疡), is caused by the invasion of wind cold into the meridians, which leads to the damage of the nasal bridge, distorted countenance, ulcer and leprosy in the skin. Five kinds of hemorrhoids are male hemorrhoid, female hemorrhoid, intestine hemorrhoid, anal fissure hemorrhoid and blood hemorrhoid, which are caused by excessive pathogenic heat affecting the lower part of the body. Scrofula is caused by excessive water toxin in the kidney affecting the upper meridians, leading to ulcer, swelling, pits and prominence in the neck. The above is caused by the invasion of pathogenic cold into the upper part of the body. Leprosy, five kinds of hemorrhoids and scrofula are caused by the invasion of pathogen into the meridians, with the syndromes manifested in the muscles and the skin. Huangqi (milkvetch root) can be used both to nourish the meridians internally and to strengthen the muscles externally. Therefore, it is suitable to treat the three kinds of diseases mentioned above. To tonify the deficiency is to tonify deficiency of healthy qi, thus to harmonize the meridians and strengthen the muscles. Children usually have not-fully-developed meridians and muscles as well as weak blood and qi. Therefore, it can be used to treat various kinds of infantile diseases.

4. 白 术

白术 气味甘温，无毒。治风寒湿痹、死肌、痉、疸，止汗、除热、消食，作煎饵。久服，轻身延年不饥。

术始出南郑山谷，今处处有之，以嵩山、茅山及野生者为胜。其根皮黄，肉白，老则苍赤，质多膏液，有赤白二种。《本经》未分，而汉时仲祖汤方始有赤术、白术之分，二术性有和暴之殊，用有缓急之别。

按：《本经》单言曰术，确是白术一种，苍术固不可以混也，试取二术之苗、叶、根、茎、性、味察之，种种各异。白术近根之叶，每叶三岐，略似半夏，其上叶绝似棠梨叶，色淡绿不光。苍术近根之叶，作三五叉，其上叶则狭而长，色青光润。白术茎绿，苍术茎紫。白术根如人指，亦有大如拳者，皮褐色，肉白色，老则微红。苍术根如老姜状，皮色苍褐，肉色黄，老则有朱砂点。白术味始甘，次微辛，后乃有苦。苍术始甘，次苦，辛味特胜。白术性和而不烈，苍术性燥而烈，并非一种可知。后人以其同有术名，同主脾胃，其治风寒湿痹之功亦相近，遂谓《本经》兼二术言之，盖未尝深辩耳。观《本经》所云止汗二字，唯白术有此功，用苍术反是写得相混耶。白术之味，《本经》云苦，陶弘景云甘，甄权云甘辛，张果云味苦而甘，今取浙中所产白术尝之，实兼甘辛苦三味。夏采者，辛多甘少，冬采者，甘多辛少，而后皆归于苦。是知诸说各举其偏，而未及乎全也。隐庵于《本经》原文定苦字为甘字，爰以白术为调和脾土之品，甘是正味，苦乃兼味，故采弘景之说，以订正之耳。

白术气味甘温，质多脂液，乃调和脾土之药也。主治风寒湿痹者，《素问·痹论》云：风寒湿三气杂至，合而为痹。白术味甘，性温，补益脾土，土气运行，则肌肉之气外通皮肤，内通经脉，故风寒湿之痹证皆可治也。夫脾主肌肉，治死肌者，助脾气也。又脾主四肢，痉者，四肢强而不和。脾主黄色，疸者，身目黄而土虚。白术补脾，则痉疸可治也。止汗者，土能胜湿也。除热者，除脾土之虚热也。消食者，助脾土之转运也。作煎饵者，言白术多脂，又治脾土之燥，作煎则味甘温而质滋润，土气和平矣。故久服则轻身延年不饥。

愚按：太阴主湿土而属脾，为阴中之至阴，喜燥恶湿，喜温恶寒。然土有湿气，始能灌溉四旁，如地得雨露，始能发生万物。若过于炎燥，则止而不行，为便难脾约之证。白术作煎饵，则燥而能润，温而能和，此先圣教人之苦心，学人所当体会者也。

4. Baizhu [白术, white atractylodes rhizome, Rhizoma Atractylodis Macrocephalae]

It is sweet in taste, warm and non-toxic in property, and it is used to treat the impediment due to wind, cold and dampness, the numbness of the muscles, convulsion and jaundice, stop sweating, eliminate heat and promote digestion. It should be decocted and made into cakes for taking to treat diseases. Long-term taking of it will keep healthy, prolong life and tolerate hunger.

Firstly recorded to be growing in the valley of Nanzheng (南郑), now it grows everywhere. Those growing in Mount Song (嵩山), Maoshan Mountain (茅山) and in the wild are of much better quality. The bark of its root is yellow in color, and the flesh is white in color. Its flesh turns greenishred when the root is old. It is high-fat and juicy. There are two herbs of this kind. One is Baizhu (white atractylodes rhizome), and the other is Cangzhu [苍术, atractylodes rhizome, Rhizoma Atractylodis]. The differences between them were not told in *Shen Nong Ben Cao Jing* [《神农本草经》, *Shennong's Classic of Materia Medica*]. It was not until in the decoction formula written by Zhang Zhongjing (张仲景) of the Han Dynasty that the two were differentiated. One is mild in property, and the other is violent. One is slow in effect, and the other is drastic.

Note by Gao Shishi (高世栻): Only Baizhu (white atractylodes rhizome) is mentioned in *Shen Nong Ben Cao Jing* [《神农本草经》, *Shennong's Classic of Materia Medica*], which should not be confused with Cangzhu (atractylodes rhizome). Examined carefully, the two kinds have different seedlings, leaves, roots, stems, properties and tastes. Each leaf growing near the root of Baizhu (white atractylodes rhizome) is divided into three small leaves, which are slightly similar to those of Banxia [半夏, pinellia tuber, Rhizoma Pinelliae]. Its upper leaves are very much like those of Tangli [棠梨, birchleaf pear, Pyrus betulaefolia] and are light green in color, looking opaque. Each leaf growing near the roots of Cangzhu (atractylodes rhizome) has three or five lobes. Its upper leaves are narrow and long, and are blue-green in color, looking glassy.

The stems of Baizhu (white atractylodes rhizome) are green in color while the stems of Cangzhu (atractylodes rhizome) are purple in color. The roots of Baizhu (white atractylodes rhizome) are like human fingers while some are as big as fists. Its bark is brown, and its flesh is white, which will be slightly red when turning old. The root of Cangzhu (atractylodes rhizome) is like an old ginger. Its bark is greenish-brown, and its flesh is yellow in color, which will have cinnabar-like spots when turning old. Baizhu (white atractylodes rhizome) tastes sweet at first, then slightly pungent and finally bitter in the end. Cangzhu (atractylodes rhizome) tastes sweet at first and then bitter with strong pungency. Baizhu (white atractylodes rhizome) is mild and not violent in property while Cangzhu (atractylodes rhizome) is dry and violent in property. So they are now known as two different kinds. People later on thought that both of them had the character "Zhu" (术) in their names, could treat the diseases of the spleen and stomach, and had the similar effects for resolving the impediment due to wind, cold and dampness, so they took it for granted to regard them as one herb in *Shen Nong Ben Cao Jing* [《神农本草经》, *Shennong's Classic of Materia Medica*], which was actually because they did not distinguish between them carefully. In *Shen Nong Ben Cao Jing* [《神农本草经》, *Shennong's Classic of Materia Medica*], only Baizhu (white atractylodes rhizome) was recorded to have the effect of stopping sweating. There must be confusion if Cangzhu (atractylodes rhizome) was recorded to have the effect because Cangzhu (atractylodes rhizome) only has the effect of inducing sweating. The taste of Baizhu (white atractylodes rhizome) is bitter according to *Shen Nong Ben Cao Jing* [《神农本草经》, *Shennong's Classic of Materia Medica*], sweet according to Tao Hongjing (陶弘景), sweet and pungent according to Zhen Quan (甄权), and bitter and sweet according to Zhang Gao (张杲). Those growing in Zhezhong (浙中) are sweet, pungent and bitter in taste. Those collected in summer are more pungent and less sweet in taste, and those collected in winter are sweeter and less pungent in taste. However, Baizhu (white atractylodes rhizome) tastes bitter in the end regardless of the season. Therefore, every point of view presented is partially right, and none of them is completely right. I changed "bitter" in *Shen Nong Ben Cao Jing* [《神农本草

经》, *Shennong's Classic of Materia Medica*] into "sweet", because Baizhu (white atractylodes rhizome) is a herb used to harmonize spleen earth. Thus the main taste of it should be sweet with some bitterness. Therefore, I adopted what Tao Hongjing (陶弘景) said to make corrections here.

Sweet in taste and warm in property, it is rich in fat and juice, which is used to harmonize spleen earth. It can mainly treat the impediment due to wind, cold and dampness. *Su Wen · Bi Lun* [《素问·痹论》, *Plain Questions · Discussion on Bi Syndrome*] says, "The interaction of wind, cold and dampness causes Bi (impediment)." Sweet in taste and warm in property, it can tonify spleen earth and move earth qi. Then the qi of the muscles will connect the skin externally and the meridians internally. Therefore, the impediment due to wind, cold and dampness can be treated. The spleen governs the muscles, and treating the numbness of the muscles will need to assist spleen qi. The spleen also governs the limbs, and the convulsion is the stiffness of the limbs. The spleen governs the yellow color, and jaundice is manifested as yellow in the body and eyes as well as the deficiency of the earth. It can tonify the spleen, thus to treat convulsion and jaundice. It can stop sweating, because earth can predominate dampness. Eliminating heat is to eliminate the deficiency heat of spleen earth. Promoting digestion is to help spleen earth move. It is rich in fat and it can also overcome the dryness of spleen earth, so it can be decocted and made into cakes for taking, which will be sweet in taste and warm and moist in property, thus to harmonize earth qi. So long-term taking of it will keep healthy, prolong life and tolerate hunger.

Note by Zhang Zhicong (张志聪): Greater yin governs wet earth and pertains to the spleen which is the beginning of yin of all yin. Greater yin likes dryness and is averse to dampness, and also likes warmth and is averse to cold. However, only with damp qi can earth irrigate the surroundings, which is similar to that everything cannot grow under natural earth unless rain and dew hits the ground. If earth is too hot and dry, it will stop moving, leading to constipation and spleen constrained syndromes. The decocted cakes of Baizhu (white atractylodes rhizome) can moisten despite its dryness and harmonize with its warmth. This is how ancient sages taught people with great pains, and later scholars should understand this.

5. 苍 术 ^附

苍术 ^附　气味苦温,无毒。主治风寒湿痹、死肌、痉疸,除热,消食,作煎饵。久服轻身延年不饥。

白术性优,苍术性劣,凡欲补脾,则用白术,凡欲运脾,则用苍术,欲补运相兼,则相兼而用。如补多运少,则白术多而苍术少。运多补少,则苍术多而白术少。品虽有二,实则一也。

《本经》未分苍白,而仲祖《伤寒》方中,皆用白术,《金匮》方中,又用赤术,至陶弘景《别录》,则分而为二,须知赤白之分,始于仲祖,非弘景始分之也。赤术,即是苍术,其功用与白术略同,故仍以《本经》术之主治为本,但白术味甘,苍术兼苦,白术止汗,苍术发汗,故止汗二字,节去不录。后人谓:苍术之味苦,其实苍术之味,甘而微苦。

5. Cangzhu〔苍术, atractylodes rhizome, Rhizoma Atractylodis〕 *supplement*

It is bitter in taste, warm and non-toxic in property, and it is mainly used to treat the impediment due to wind, cold and dampness, numbness of muscles, convulsion and jaundice, eliminate heat and promote digestion. It should be decocted and made into cakes for taking. Long-term taking of it will keep healthy, prolong life and tolerate hunger.

Baizhu〔白术, white atractylodes rhizome, Rhizoma Atractylodis Macrocephalae〕is better than Cangzhu (atractylodes rhizome) in terms of medicinal effect. To tonify the spleen, use Baizhu (white atractylodes rhizome); to move the spleen, use Cangzhu (atractylodes rhizome); to tonify and move the spleen, use both. If intending to achieve the result of more tonificaion and less movement of the spleen, use more Baizhu (white atractylodes rhizome) and less Cangzhu (atractylodes rhizome); if intending to achieve the result of more movement and less tonification of the spleen, use more Cangzhu (atractylodes rhizome) and less Baizhu (white atractylodes rhizome). They are two different herbs, but actually they pertain to the same kind.

The differences between Baizhu (white atractylodes rhizome) and Cangzhu (atractylodes rhizome) were not distinguished in *Shen Nong Ben Cao Jing* [《神农本草经》, *Shennong's Classic of Materia Medica*]. Baizhu (white atractylodes rhizome) was used in all formulas of *Shang Han Lun* [《伤寒论》, *Treatise on Cold Damage Diseases*] written by Zhang Zhongjing (张仲景) while Cangzhu (atractylodes rhizome) was used in the formulas of *Jin Gui Yao Lüe* [《金匮要略》, *Synopsis of the Golden Chamber*]. It was not until in *Ming Yi Bie Lu* [《名医别录》, *Miscellaneous Records of Famous Physicians*] written by Tao Hongjing (陶弘景) that they were distinguished as two different herbs. It must be noted that it was Zhang Zhongjing (张仲景) not Tao Hongjing (陶弘景) who firstly classified them as two different herbs. Cangzhu (atractylodes rhizome), whose effect is slightly similar to that of Baizhu (white atractylodes rhizome), is also called Chishu (赤术). Therefore, its actions are recorded on the basis of those of Baizhu (white atractylodes rhizome) recorded in *Shen Nong Ben Cao Jing* [《神农本草经》, *Shennong's Classic of Materia Medica*]. However, Baizhu (white atractylodes rhizome) is sweet in taste while Cangzhu (atractylodes rhizome) is both sweet and bitter in taste. Baizhu (white atractylodes rhizome) is used to stop sweating while Cangzhu (atractylodes rhizome) is used to induce sweating, and the two words "stop sweating" are omitted when describing the effect of Cangzhu (atractylodes rhizome). People later on said that Cangzhu (atractylodes rhizome) is bitter, but actually sweet with slight bitterness in taste.

6. 薯蓣

薯蓣 气味甘平,无毒。主伤中,补虚羸,除寒热邪气,补中,益气力,长肌肉,强阴。久服耳目聪明,轻身不饥,延年。

薯蓣即今山药,因唐代宗名预,避讳改为薯药,又因宋英宗名署,避讳改为山药。始出嵩高山谷,今处处有之,入药野生者为胜。种薯蓣法,以杵打穴,截块投于杵穴之中,随所杵之窍而成形,如预备署,所因名薯蓣也,今时但知山药,不知薯蓣矣。

山药气味甘平,始出中岳,得中土之专精,乃补太阴脾土之药,故主治之功皆在中土。治伤中者,益中土也。补虚羸者,益肌肉也。除寒热邪气者,中土调和，肌肉充足，则寒热邪气自除矣。夫治伤中，则可以补中而益气力。补虚羸，则可以长肌肉而强阴。阴强，则耳目聪明。气力益，则身体轻健，土气有余，则不饥而延年。

凡柔滑之物，损即腐坏，山药切块，投于土中，百合分瓣种之，如种蒜法，地黄以根节多者，寸断埋土中，皆能生长。所以然者，百合得太阴之天气，山药、地黄得太阴之地气也。

6. Shuyu〔薯蓣，dioscorea，Rhizoma Dioscoreae〕

It is sweet in taste, mild and non-toxic in property, and it is mainly used to treat internal damage, improve deficiency and emaciation, eliminate pathogenic cold qi and heat qi, tonify the middle, replenish qi and energy, promote the growth of the muscles and strengthen yin. Long-term taking of it will improve hearing and vision, keep healthy, tolerate hunger and prolong life.

Shuyu (dioscorea) is also called Shanyao (山药) nowadays. There was a taboo in ancient China on using the personal names of emperors. For this reason, Shuyu (dioscorea) was renamed Shuyao (薯药) in the Tang Dynasty since Emperor Daizong of Tang was called Liyu (李豫). For the same reason, it was renamed Shanyao (山药) in the Song Dynasty since Emperor Yingzong of Song was called Zhaoshu (赵署). Firstly recorded to be growing in the valley of Mount Song (嵩山), now it grows everywhere. Those growing in the wild are better to be used as medicinal. The method of planting it is to dig a hole with a pestle, cut it into parts and drop one part into the hole, which will grow into the shape in accordance with the hole. The hole is like a Yubeishu (预备署, a prepared place). That is why it is called Shuyu (薯蓣). However, now people only know that it is called Shanyao (山药) instead of Shuyu (薯蓣).

Sweet in taste and mild in property, it was firstly recorded to be growing in Zhongyue (Mount Song) and it receives the essence of center earth. It is a medicinal to tonify spleen earth from greater yin. Therefore, all its actions are related to center earth. Treating internal damage will benefit center earth. Improving deficiency and emaciation will benefit the muscles. Eliminating pathogenic cold qi and heat qi means that center earth is harmonized and the muscles are strengthened, thus pathogenic cold qi and heat qi will be eliminated naturally. Treating internal damage will tonify the middle and replenish qi and energy. Improving deficiency and emaciation will promote the growth of the muscles and strengthen yin. If yin is strengthened, then the hearing and vision are improved. If qi and energy are replenished, then health will be kept and earth qi will be abundant, which will be effective in tolerating hunger and prolonging life.

Everything that is soft and slippery will rot if damaged. The way of planting Shuyu (dioscorea) is to cut it into parts and put them into the soil. The way of planting Baihe〔百合, lily bulb, Bulbus Lilii〕is the same as that of Suan〔蒜, garlic, Allii Sativi Bulbus〕, which is to plant their scale leaves. The way of planting Dihuang〔地黄, rehmannia, Radix Rehmanniae〕is to cut the one with more nodes into parts of one Cun long and bury them into the soil, and they will grow. Planting them in different ways is because Baihe (lily bulb) obtains the heaven qi from greater yin while Shuyu (dioscorea) and Dihuang (rehmannia) obtain the earth qi from greater yin.

7. 石 斛

石斛 气味甘平,无毒。主伤中,除痹,下气,补五脏虚劳羸瘦,强阴益精。久服,厚肠胃。

石斛始出六安山谷水旁石上,今荆襄、汉中、庐州、台州、温州诸处皆有。一种形如金钗,谓之钗石斛,为俗所尚,不若川地产者,其形修洁,茎长一二尺,气味清疏,黄白而实,入药最良。其外更有木斛,长而中虚,不若川石斛之中实也。又有麦斛,形如大麦,累累相连,头生一叶,其性微冷。又有竹叶斛,形如竹,节间生叶。又有雀髀斛,茎大如雀之髀,叶在茎头,性皆苦寒,不堪用之。石斛丛生石上,其根纠结,茎叶生皆青翠。干则黄白而软,折之悬挂屋下,时灌以水,经年不死,俗呼为千年润。

愚按:今之石斛,其味皆苦,无有甘者,须知《本经》诸味,皆新出土时味也,干则稍变矣。善读圣经,当以意会之。

石斛生于石上,得水长生,是禀水石之专精而补肾。味甘色黄,不假土力,是夺中土之气化而补脾。斛乃量名,主出主入,治伤中者,运行其中土也。除痹者,除皮脉肉筋骨五脏外合之痹证也。夫治伤中则下气,言中气调和,则邪气自下矣。除痹则补五脏虚劳羸瘦,言邪气散除,则正气强盛矣,脾为阴中之至阴,故曰强阴。肾主藏精,故曰益精。久服则土气运行,水精四布,故厚肠胃。

《本经》上品,多主除痹,不曰风寒湿,而但曰痹者,乃五脏外合之痹也。盖皮者,肺之合。脉者,心之合。肉者,脾之合。筋者,肝之合。骨者,肾之合。故除痹即所以治五脏之虚劳羸瘦,是攻邪之中而有补益之妙用。治伤中即所以下气,是补益之中而有攻邪之神理云。

7. Shihu〔石斛, dendrobium, Herba Dendrobii〕

It is sweet in taste, mild and non-toxic in property, and it is mainly used to treat internal damage, eliminate impediment, descend qi, tonify the five zang-organs to treat the deficiency due to overstrain and emaciation, strengthen yin and replenish essence. Long-term taking of it will invigorate the intestines and stomach.

Firstly recorded to be growing on the rock near water in Lu'an（六安）valley, now it grows everywhere in Jingxiang（荆襄）, Hanzhong（汉中）, Luzhou（庐州）, Taizhou（台州）and Wenzhou（温州）. There is one kind like the golden hairpin in shape, known as Chaishihu（钗石斛, hairpin dendrobium）, which is valued among people. Unlike those growing in Sichuan（四川）, it is neat and clean, and its stalk is one or two Chi tall. Yellow-white in color, it is solid with light smell, and it is the best kind to be used as medicinal. Besides, there is Muhu（木斛）which is long and hollow and not as solid as the one growing in Sichuan（四川）. There is also Maihu（麦斛）like barley in shape, with one fruit connecting with the other. With one leaf growing on the top, it is slightly cold in property. There is also Zhuyehu（竹叶斛）like the bamboo in shape, having leaves between nodes. There is also Quebihu（雀髀斛）whose stalk is as big as the bird's thigh, with leaves growing on the top of its stalk. Both its stalk and leaves are bitter in taste and cold in property, which cannot be used as medicinal. Shihu（dendrobium）grows in clusters on the rock, with its roots intertwining. Both its stalk and leaves are green in color when raw, and they will be yellow-white and soft when dried. Collect one Shihu（dendrobium）, hang it under the eave, irrigate it regularly with water, and it will not wither even after years. Therefore, it is called Qiannianrun (千年润).

Note by Gao Shishi (高世栻): Shihu (dendrobiume) collected nowadays is bitter in taste, and those that are sweet in taste cannot be found. It should be kept in mind that the tastes of herbs mentioned in *Shen Nong Ben Cao Jing* [《神农本草经》, *Shennong's Classic of Materia Medica*] are all those of the herbs when just dug out from the earth. The tastes will be slightly different when the herbs are dried. The practitioners of TCM should be good at reading classic works related to the materia medica to have an insightful understanding of them.

Shihu (dendrobiume), growing on the rock and surviving with water, receives the essence of water and rock to tonify the kidney. Sweet in taste and yellow in color, without the help of earth, it can tonify the spleen by obtaining the qi transformation of center earth. Hu (斛), a kind of measuring vessel, governs exiting and entering. To treat internal damage is to move center earth. To eliminate impediment is to eliminate impediment syndromes which are externally in accordance with the skin, meridians, muscles, sinews, bones and five-zang organs. Treating internal damage will descend qi. That is to say, when center qi is harmonized, pathogenic qi will be eliminated naturally. Eliminating impediment will tonify the five zang-organs to treat the deficiency due to overstrain and emaciation. That is to say, eliminating pathogenic qi will strengthen healthy qi. The spleen is the beginning of yin of all yin, so to tonify the spleen is to strengthen yin. The kidney governs the storage of essence, so to tonify the kidney is to replenish essence. Long-term taking of it will make earth qi move and make the body full of water essence. Therefore, it can invigorate the intestines and stomach.

The top-grade medicinals in *Shen Nong Ben Cao Jing* [《神农本草经》, *Shennong's Classic of Materia Medica*] are mostly used to eliminate impediment rather than the impediment due to wind, cold and dampness. However, the impediment is the one in accordance with the five-zang organs externally, because the skin is in accordance with the lung. The meridians are in accordance with the heart; the muscles are in accordance with the spleen; the sinews are in accordance with the liver and the bones are in accordance with the kidney. Therefore, eliminating impediment will tonify the five zang-organs to treat the deficiency due to overstrain and emaciation, because it has the magical effect of tonifying while attacking pathogen. Treating internal damage will descend qi, because it has the magical action of attacking pathogen while tonifying.

8. 酸枣仁

酸枣仁 气味酸平，无毒。主治心腹寒热，邪结气聚，四肢酸痛，湿痹。久服安五脏，轻身延年。

酸枣始出河东川泽，今近汴洛及西北州郡皆有之。一名山枣，《尔雅》名樲，孟子曰：养其樲棘是也。其树枝有刺，实形似枣而圆小，其味酸，其色红紫。八月采实，只取核中之仁。仁皮赤，仁肉黄白。

按：酸枣肉味酸，其仁味甘而不酸。今既云酸枣仁，又云气味酸平，讹也，当改正。

枣肉味酸，肝之果也。得东方木味，能达肝气上行，食之主能醒睡。枣仁形园色赤，禀火土之气化。火归中土，则神气内藏，食之主能瘳寐。《本经》不言用仁，而今时多用之。心腹寒热，邪结气聚者，言心腹不和，为寒为热，则邪结气聚。枣仁色赤象心，能导心气以下交，肉黄象土，能助脾气以上达，故心腹之寒热邪结之气聚可治也。土气不达于四肢，则四肢酸痛。火气不温于肌肉，则周身湿痹。枣仁禀火土之气化，故四肢酸痛，周身湿痹可治也。久服安五脏，轻身延年。言不但心腹和平，且安五脏也。五脏既安，则气血日益，故又可轻身延年。

8. Suanzaoren [酸枣仁, spine date seed, Semen Ziziphi Spinosae]

It is sour in taste, mild and non-toxic in property, and it is mainly used to treat the cold and heat in the heart and abdomen, pathogen binding and qi accumulation, the aching pain of the four limbs and dampness impediment. Long-term taking of it will harmonize the five zang-organs, keep healthy and prolong life.

Firstly recorded to be growing in the rivers and lakes of Hedong（河东），now Suanzao [酸枣, crataegus, Crataegi Fructus] grows everywhere near Bianluo（汴洛）and in Northwest China. It is also called Shanzhao（山枣）. It is mentioned as Er（樲）in *Er Ya* [《尔雅》, *On Elegance*]. Mencius said, "A horticulturist cultivates his Suanzao（crataegus）trees." Its branches have thorns. Like smaller Zao［枣, Chinese date, Fructus Jujubae］, the fruit is round. Red and purple in color, it is sour in taste. Pick it in the eighth lunar month and only keep the kernel in its pit. The peel of its kernel is red in color, and the flesh of its kernel is yellow-white in color.

Note by Gao Shishi（高世栻）: Its flesh is sour in taste, but the kernel is sweet rather than sour in taste. Nowadays, it is stated that Suanzaoren（spine date seed）is sour in taste and mild in property, which is a false idea and should be corrected.

The flesh of Suanzao（crataegus）is sour in taste, which pertains to the fruit of liver. It obtains the taste of wood in the east and makes liver qi move upward. Eating it can treat insomnia. Round in shape and red in color, Suanzaoren（spine date seed）receives the qi transformation of fire and earth. Besides, fire pertains to center earth, thus Suanzaoren（spine date seed）can store spirit qi inside. So eating it can also treat insomnia. *Shen Nong Ben Cao Jing*［《神农本草经》, *Shennong's Classic of Materia Medica*］says that the kernel cannot be used as medicinal, but now it is widely used. The cold and heat in the heart and abdomen, pathogen binding and qi accumulation mean that when the heart and abdomen are not in harmony, it will result in the cold and heat in the heart and abdomen, which leads to pathogen binding and qi accumulation. Red in color, the kernel is like the heart and can guide heart qi to move downward to interact with kidney qi. Yellow in color, the flesh is like the earth and can aid spleen qi to move upward to the lung. Thus, the cold and heat in the heart and abdomen, pathogen binding and qi accumulation can be treated. If earth qi cannot reach the four limbs, then there will be pain in the four limbs. If fire qi cannot warm the muscles, then there will be dampness impediment in the whole body. The kernel receives the qi transformation of fire and earth, so the pain of the four limbs and the dampness impediment of the whole body can be treated. Long-term taking of it will harmonize the five zang-organs, keep healthy and prolong life. It is stated that it can not only calm the heart and abdomen, but also can harmonize the five zang-organs. If they are harmonized, qi and blood will accordingly be boosted day by day. Therefore, it can also keep healthy and prolong life.

9. 大　枣

大枣　气味甘平，无毒。主心腹邪气，安中，养脾气，平胃气，通九窍，助十二经，补少气，少津液，身中不足，大惊，四肢重，和百药。久服轻身延年。《本经》。

　　枣始出河东平泽，今近北州郡及江南皆有，唯青州、晋州所生者肥大甘美。五月开白花，八九月果熟黄赤色，烘曝则黑，入药为良。其南方所产者，谓之南枣，北方所产不肥大者，谓之小枣，烘曝不黑者，谓之红枣，只充果食，俱不入药。

　　大枣气味甘平，脾之果也。开小白花，生青熟黄，熟极则赤，烘曝则黑，禀土气之专精，具五行之色性。《经》云：脾为孤脏，中央土，以灌四旁。主治心腹邪气，安中者，谓大枣安中，凡邪气上干于心，下干于腹，皆可治也。养脾气，平胃气，通九窍，助十二经者，谓大枣养脾则胃气自平，从脾胃而行于上下，则通九窍。从脾胃而行于内外，则助十二经。补少气、少津液、身中不足者，谓大枣补身中之不足，故补少气而助无形，补少津液而资有形。大惊、四肢重、和百药者，谓大枣味甘多脂，调和百药，故大惊而心主之神气虚于内，四肢重而心主之神气虚于外，皆可治也。四肢者，两手两足，皆机关之室，神气之所畅达者也。久服则五脏调和，血气充足，故轻身延年。

9. Dazao［大枣，Chinese date，Fructus Jujubae］

It is sweet in taste, mild and non-toxic in property, and it is mainly used to relieve the pathogenic qi in the heart and abdomen, harmonize the middle, nourish spleen qi, pacify stomach qi, relieve the nine orifices, assist the twelve meridians, tonify the insufficiency of qi, fluid and energy in the body, resolve the severe fright disorder and heaviness of the four limbs, and harmonize all medicinals. Long-term taking of it will keep healthy and prolong life. Recorded in *Shen Nong Ben Cao Jing*［《神农本草经》，*Shennong's Classic of Materia Medica*］.

　　Firstly recorded to be growing in the lakes and swamps of Hedong（河东）, now it grows everywhere near Beizhou（北州）and in Jiangnan（江南）, but only those growing in Qingzhou（青州）and Jinzhou（晋州）are big in shape and sweet and delicious in taste. It blossoms with white flowers in the fifth lunar month. Yellow and red in color, its fruit gets ripe in the eighth and ninth lunar month. The fruit turns black after it is baked and exposed to the sun, and it is good to be used as medicinal. Those growing in the south are called Nanzao (南枣). Those growing in the north which are thin and small in shape are called Xiaozao (小枣). Those which do not turn black after they are baked and exposed to the sun are called Hongzao (红枣). All of those three can only be used as fruits instead of medicinal.

Dazao (Chinese date), sweet in taste and mild in property, is a fruit pertaining to the spleen. It blossoms with little white flowers. It is green in color when unripe, while it turns yellow in color when ripe. When getting extremely ripe, it turns red. When baked and exposed to the sun, it turns black. It receives the essence of earth qi and has the colors and properties of the five elements. In *Huang Di Nei Jing* [《黄帝内经》, *Huangdi's Internal Classic*] it is said that the spleen is a solitary organ locating in the center, pertains to earth and irrigates the other four organs. It can mainly relieve the pathogenic qi in the heart and abdomen and harmonize the middle. That is to say, it can harmonize the middle to treat the diseases caused by the pathogenic qi which moves upward to disturb the heart and downward to disturb the abdomen. It can be used to nourish spleen qi, pacify stomach qi, relieve the nine orifices and assist the twelve meridians. That is, it can nourish the spleen, and result in pacifying stomach qi which moves upward and downward from the spleen and stomach thus to relieve the nine orifices. Stomach qi moves from the interior to the exterior out of the spleen and stomach, and results in assisting the twelve meridians. Dazao can tonify the deficiency of the body, then it can tonify the insufficiency of qi, fluid and energy. That is, it can tonify the insufficiency of qi with assisting the intangible, and it can tonify the insufficiency of fluid with strengthening the tangible. It can be used to resolve the severe fright and heaviness of the four limbs, and harmonize all medicinals. That is to say, it is sweet in taste and rich in fat, and it can harmonize all medicinals. Therefore, both the internal weak spirit qi governed by the heart caused by severe fright and the external weak spirit qi governed by the heart caused by heaviness of the four limbs can be treated. The four limbs refer to the two legs and two arms which are all pivots, the places to which spirit qi can have easy access. Long-term taking of it will harmonize the five-zang organs and have sufficient blood and qi thus to keep healthy and prolong life.

10. 芡 实

芡实 气味甘平涩,无毒。主湿痹,腰脊膝痛,补中,除暴疾,益精气,强志,令耳目聪明,久服轻身不饥,耐老神仙。

芡始出雷池池泽,今处处有之,武林者最胜。三月生叶贴水,似荷而大,皱纹如谷,蹙衄如沸,面青背紫,茎叶皆有刺。五六月开花,紫色,花必向日,结苞处有青刺,如猬刺及栗球之形,花在苞顶,正如鸡喙,苞内有子,壳黄肉白,南楚谓之鸡头者,青徐、淮泗谓之芡。

芡实气味甘平,子黄仁白,生于水中,花开向日,乃阳引而上,阴引而下,故字从欠,得阳明少阴之精气。主治湿痹者,阳明之上,燥气治之也。治腰脊膝痛者,少阴主骨,外合腰膝也。补中者,阳明居中土也。除暴疾者,精气神三虚相搏,则为暴疾。芡实生于水而向日,得水之精,火之神。茎刺肉白,又禀秋金收敛之气,故治三虚之暴疾。益精气,强志,令耳目聪明者,言精气充益,则肾志强。肾志强则耳目聪明。盖心肾开窍于耳,精神共注于目也。久服则积精全神,故轻身不饥,耐老神仙。

10. Qianshi [芡实, gordon euryale seed, Semen Euryale]

It is sweet and astringent in taste, mild and non-toxic in property, and it is mainly used to treat dampness impediment and the pain of the waist, spine and knees, tonify the middle, eliminate severe diseases, replenish essential qi, strengthen memory and improve hearing and vision. Long-term taking of it will keep healthy, tolerate hunger and prevent aging like immortals.

Firstly recorded to be growing in the lakes and pools of Leichi (雷池), now it grows everywhere, and those growing in Wulin (武林) are of the best quality. It grows leaves which float on the water in the third lunar month. Like bigger lotus leaves, its leaves have folds which are like valleys. The small bumps on the leaves are like being scalded by boiling water. The surface of its leaves is green in color, and the back is purple in color. Both its stalks and leaves have thorns. It blossoms in the fifth or sixth lunar month with purple flowers which are absolutely sunward. There are green thorns around the bud which look like the thorns on a hedgehog and those on the chestnut's fruit. The flower is on the top of the bud, which is like a chicken's beak. The bud has seeds inside, whose shell is yellow in color and whose flesh is white in color. People in Nanchu（南楚）call it Jitou（鸡头）, and people in Qingxu（青徐）and Huaisi（淮泗）call it Qian（芡）.

Qianshi（gordon euryale seed）is sweet in taste and mild in property. Its seeds are yellow in color, and its kernels are white in color. It grows in water with flowers sunward, because yang can conduct upward and yin can conduct downward. Therefore, its Chinese name has the character "欠"（Qian）. It receives the essential qi from yang brightness and lesser yin. It can mainly treat dampness impediment, because the upper part of yang brightness is governed by dry qi. It can mainly treat the pain of the waist, spine and knees, because lesser yin governs the bones and corresponds with the waist and knees externally. It is used to tonify the middle, because yang brightness stays in center earth. It can also be used to eliminate severe diseases. Three deficiency—essence, qi and spirit contends with each other, resulting in severe diseases. It grows in water, is sunward and receives the essence of water and the spirit of fire. Its stalk has thorns, its flesh is white in color, and it receives the astringent qi of autumn metal. Therefore, it can treat the severe diseases caused by the contention of three deficiency. It can replenish essential qi, strengthen memory and improve hearing and vision. That is to say, sufficient essential qi will strengthen the kidney will. If the kidney will is strengthened, the hearing and vision will be improved, because the heart and kidney open the two orifices at ears and both essence and spirit will pour into the eyes. Long-term taking of it will accumulate essence and strengthen spirit, thus to keep healthy, tolerate hunger and prevent aging like immortals.

11. 莲 实

莲实　气味甘平, 无毒。主补中, 养神、益气力、除百疾。久服轻身耐老, 不饥延年。

莲始出汝南池泽,今所在池泽皆有。初夏其叶出水,渐长如扇。六七月间开花,有红、白、粉红三色,香艳可爱。花心有黄须,花褪房成,房外青内白,子在房中,如蜂子在窠之状。六七月采嫩者,生食鲜美,至秋房枯子黑、壳坚而硬,谓之石莲子。今药肆中一种石莲子形长味苦,肉内无心,生于树上,系苦珠之类,不堪入药,宜于建莲子中拣带壳而黑色者,用之为真。

莲生水中,茎直色青,具风木之象,花红,须黄,房白,子黑,得五运相生之气化,气味甘平。主补中,得中土之精气也。养神,得水火之精气也。益气力,得金木之精气也。百疾之生,不离五运,莲禀五运之气化,故除百疾。久服且轻身不饥延年。

11. Lianshi〔莲实, lotus fruit/seed, Nelumbinis Semen〕

It is sweet in taste, mild and non-toxic in property, and it is mainly used to tonify the middle, nourish the spirit, replenish qi and energy and eliminate all diseases. Long-term taking of it will keep healthy, prevent aging, tolerate hunger and prolong life.

Firstly recorded to be growing in the lakes and pools of Runan (汝南), now Lian〔莲, lotus, Nelumbo Adans〕grows in any lake or pool. Its leaves grow above the water in early summer and gradually grow as big as fans. It blossoms in the sixth and seventh lunar month with red, white and pink flowers, which are fragrant, beautiful and lovely. There are yellow lotus stamens in the center of the flower. There will be a lotus receptacle when the flowers fall, which is green outside and white inside. There are seeds in the receptacle, which are like bees in the hive. The tender seeds picked in the sixth and seventh lunar month are delicious when eaten raw. In autumn the seeds become black, and the shell of the receptacle becomes strong when the receptacle withers. The seeds at that time are called Shilianzi (石莲子). Drug stores nowadays sell the so-called Shilianzi (石莲子) which is long in shape and bitter in taste with no plumule in the flesh. Growing on the trees, it is actually a kind of Kuzhu〔苦珠, Chinese castanopsis seed, Castanopsidis Chinensis Semen〕, which cannot be used as medicinal. Shelled and black lotus seeds growing in Fujian (福建) are the genuine ones.

Growing in water, Lian (lotus) has a straight stalk and is green in color. It has red flowers, yellow stamens, white receptacles and black seeds, representing the sign of wind and wood. It receives qi transformation from the mutual generation of five circuits. Sweet in taste and mild in property, it can mainly tonify the middle, because it receives the essential qi of center earth. It can nourish the spirit, because it receives the essential qi of water and fire. It can replenish qi and energy, because it receives the essential qi of metal and wood. All diseases result from five circuits. Lian (lotus) receives the qi transformation of five circuits, thus it can eliminate all diseases. Long-term taking of it will keep healthy, tolerate hunger and prolong life.

12. 莲 花 附

莲花 附 气味苦甘温,无毒。主镇心、益色、驻颜、身轻。《日华本草》

12. Lianhua [莲花, lotus flower, Nelumbinis Flos] *supplement*

It is bitter and sweet in taste, warm and non-toxic in property, and it is mainly used to settle the heart, luster complexion, retain youthful appearances and keep healthy. Recorded in *Ri Hua Ben Cao* [《日华本草》, *Rihuazi's Materia Medica*]

13. 莲蕊须 附

莲蕊须 附 气味甘涩温,无毒。主清心,通肾,固精气,乌须发,悦颜色,益血,止血崩、吐血。《本草纲目》附。

13. Lianruixu [莲蕊须, lotus stamen, Nelumbinis Stamen] *supplement*

It is sweet and astringent in taste, warm and non-toxic in property, and it is mainly used to clear the heart, dredge the kidney, secure essential qi, blacken the beard and hair, luster complexion, boost blood, stop metrorrhagia and hematemesis. Supplemented in *Ben Cao Gang Mu* [《本草纲目》, *Compendium of Materia Medica*].

14. 莲 房 附

莲房 附 气味苦涩温,无毒。主破血《食疗本草》,治血胀腹痛,及产后胎衣不下。解野菌毒《本草拾遗》附。

莲房即莲蓬壳,陈久者良。

14. Lianfang〔莲房, lotus receptacle, Nelumbinis Receptaculum〕 *supplement*

It is bitter and astringent in taste, warm and non-toxic in property, and it is mainly used to break blood. Recorded in *Shi Liao Ben Cao*〔《食疗本草》, *Materia Medica for Dietotherapy*〕. It is used to treat blood distention, abdominal pain and the postpartum retention of the placenta. It is also used to remove the toxin of wild mushrooms. Supplemented in *Ben Cao Shi Yi*〔《本草拾遗》, *Supplement to Materia Medica*〕.

In fact, Lianfang (lotus receptacle) is the lotus shell, and those stored for a long time are of good quality.

15. 莲 薏 附

莲薏 附 气味苦寒,无毒。主治血渴、产后渴《食性本草》,止霍乱《日华本草》,清心去热《本草纲目》附。

莲薏即莲子中青心。

15. Lianyi〔莲薏, lotus plumule, Nelumbinis Plumula〕 *supplement*

It is bitter in taste, cold and non-toxic in property, and it is mainly used to treat blood thirst and postpartumthirst. Recorded in *Shi Xing Ben Cao*〔《食性本草》, *Materia Medica on Diet Habits*〕. It is used to check cholera. Recorded in *Ri Hua Ben Cao*〔《日华本草》, *Rihuazi's Materia Medica*〕. It is also used to clear the heart and eliminate heat. Supplemented in *Ben Cao Gang Mu*〔《本草纲目》, *Compendium of Materia Medica*〕.

In fact, Lianyi (lotus plumule) is the young leaf and radicle in the lotus seed.

16. 荷 叶 附

荷叶 附　气味苦平,无毒。主治血胀腹痛、产后胎衣不下,酒煮服之《本草拾遗》。治吐血、衄血、血崩、血痢、脱肛、赤游火丹、遍身风疬、阳水浮肿、脚膝浮肿、痘疮倒靥《新增》附。

16. Heye〔荷叶, lotus leaf, Nelumbinis Folium〕*supplement*

It is bitter in taste, mild and non-toxic in property, and it is mainly used to treat blood distention, abdominal pain and the retention of the placenta, and should be taken after it is decocted with liquor. Supplemented in *Ben Cao Shi Yi*〔《本草拾遗》, *Supplement to Materia Medica*〕. It is also used to treat hematemesis, epistaxis, metrorrhagia, blood dysentery, the prolapse of rectum, red wandering cinnabar toxin, generalized wind pestilence, yang edema, the edema in the feet and knees as well as smallpox failing to crust. Supplemented in *Xin Zeng*〔《新增》, *New Supplement to Materia Medica*〕.

17. 荷 鼻 附

荷鼻 附　气味苦平,无毒。主安胎,去恶血,留好血,止血痢,杀菌蕈毒,并水煮服《本草拾遗》附。

　　荷鼻,荷叶蒂也。

17. Hebi〔荷鼻, lotus leaf base, Nelumbinis Basis Folii〕*supplement*

It is bitter in taste, mild and non-toxic in property, and it is mainly used to prevent abortion, eliminate malign blood, retain healthy blood, resolve blood dysentery and eliminate mushroom toxin, and should be taken after it is decocted with water. Supplemented in *Ben Cao Shi Yi*〔《本草拾遗》, *Supplement to Materia Medica*〕.

In fact, Hebi (lotus leaf base) is the base of the lotus leaf.

18. 薏苡仁

薏苡仁　气味甘,微寒,无毒。主筋急拘挛,不可屈伸,久风湿痹,下气。久服轻身益气。

薏苡其形似米,故俗名米仁。始出真定平泽及田野,今处处有之。春生苗叶如黍。五六月结实,至秋则老。其仁白色如珠,可煮粥,同米酿酒。

薏苡仁,米谷之属,夏长秋成,味甘色白,其性微寒,禀阳明金土之精。主治筋急拘挛,不可屈伸者,阳明主润宗筋,宗筋主束骨而利机关,盖宗筋润,则诸筋自和。机关利,则屈伸自如。又,金能制风,土能胜湿,故治久风湿痹。肺属金而主气,薏苡禀阳明之金气,故主下气。治久风湿痹,故久服轻身,下气而又益气。

18. Yiyiren [薏苡仁, coix seed, Semen Coicis]

It is sweet in taste, slightly cold and non-toxic in property, and it is mainly used to treat spasm and the hypertonicity of the sinews, the inability to bend and stretch, and the chronic wind-dampness impediment, and it descends qi. Long-term taking of it will keep healthy and replenish qi.

Yiyiren (coix seed) is in a rice-like shape, so it is called Miren (米仁). Firstly recorded to be growing in the lakes and fields of Zhending (真定), now it grows everywhere. It grows seedlings and leaves in spring which are like those of Shu [黍, broomcorn millet, Panici Miliacei Semen]. It bears seeds in the fifth and sixth lunar months which will be ripe in autumn. Its kernels, as white as a pearl, can be used to cook porridge and make liquor with rice.

Yiyiren (coix seed), pertaining to the category of rice and grain, grows in summer and gets ripe in autumn. Sweet in taste, white in color, slightly cold in property, it receives the essence of metal and earth from yang brightness. It can mainly treat spasm and the hypertonicity of the sinews, and the inability to bend and stretch, because yang brightness is responsible for moistening all tendons that control the bones and lubricate the joints. If all tendons get moistened, then all the sinews will be harmonized naturally. If the joints get lubricated, then people are free to bend and stretch. Besides, metal controls wind, and earth predominates dampness. Therefore, the chronic wind-dampness impediment can be treated. The lung pertains to metal and governs qi, and Yiyiren (coix seed) receives the metal qi from yang brightness. Therefore, it can descend qi. It can be used to treat the chronic wind-dampness impediment, so long-term taking of it will keep healthy, descend qi and replenish qi.

19. 大麻仁

大麻仁 气味甘平,无毒。主补中、益气。久服肥健,不老神仙。

大麻即火麻,俗名黄麻。始出泰山川谷,今处处种之,其利颇饶。叶狭茎长,五六月开细黄花成穗,随结子可取油。《齐民要术》曰:麻有雌雄,于放花时拔出雄者,若未花先拔,则不结子。

大麻放花结实于五六月之交,乃阳明太阴主气之时。《经》云:阳明者,午也。五月盛阳之阴也。又,长夏属太阴主气,夫太阴、阳明,雌雄相合,麻仁禀太阴、阳明之气,故气味甘平。主补中者,补中土也。益气者,益脾胃之气也。夫脾胃气和则两土相为资益,阳明燥土得太阴湿气以相资,太阴湿土得阳明燥气以相益,故久服肥健,不老神仙。

19. Damaren〔大麻仁, cannabis fruit, Cannabis Fructus〕

It is sweet in taste, mild and non-toxic in property, and it is mainly used to tonify the middle and replenish qi. Long-term taking of it will fortify the body and prolong life like immortals.

Dama〔大麻, hemp, Cannabis Sativa L.〕 is also called Huoma (火麻) and popularly called Huangma (黄麻). Firstly recorded to be growing in the river valley of Mount Tai (泰山), now it is planted everywhere, and it is profitable. It has narrow leaves and long stalks. It blossoms in the fifth and sixth lunar months with little yellow flowers which will grow into the spikes of flowers. Its seeds, growing from the spikes, can be used to extract oil. *Qi Min Yao Shu*〔《齐民要术》, *Arts of People*〕 says, "There are male and female Dama (hemp). Remove the male one when it starts to blossom. If removing the male one before it starts to blossom, then it will not bear seeds.

Dama (hemp) blossoms and bears fruits between the fifth and sixth lunar months, the time when yang brightness and greater yin govern qi. *Huang Di Nei Jing* [《黄帝内经》, *Huangdi's Internal Classic*] says that yang brightness is the noon of the day, and the fifth lunar month is the yin of great yang. Moreover, the long summer pertains to greater yin governing qi, and greater yin and yang brightness are the combination of male and female. Damaren (cannabis fruit) receives the qi of greater yin and yang brightness, so it is sweet in taste and mild in property. To tonify the middle is to tonify center earth. To replenish qi is to replenish the qi of the spleen and abdomen. If spleen qi and abdomen qi are harmonized, then the two kinds of earth, i.e., the dry earth from yang brightness and the damp earth from greater yin, will assist and strengthen each other. The dry earth from yang brightness is assisted by the damp qi from greater yin while the damp earth from greater yin is strengthened by the dry qi from yang brightness. Therefore, long-term taking of it will fortify the body and prolong life like immortals.

20. 巨胜子

巨胜子 气味甘平,无毒。主治伤中虚羸,补五内,益气力,长肌肉,填髓脑。久服轻身不老。

巨胜一名胡麻,一名狗虱。本出胡地,故名胡麻。巨,大也。本生胡地大宛,故又名巨胜。八谷之中,唯此为良。寇宗奭曰:胡麻正是今之大脂麻,独胡地所产者肥大,因名胡麻,又名巨胜。今市肆中一种形如小茴,有壳无仁,其味极苦,伪充巨胜。夫巨胜即胡麻,是属谷类,刘阮深入天台,仙女饲以胡麻饭,若有壳无仁,其味且苦,何堪作饭。须知市肆中巨胜系野生狗虱,故有壁虱胡麻之名。壁虱、狗虱不堪入药。如无胡麻,当于脂麻中捡色赤而肥大者用之,庶乎不误。

麻乃五谷之首,禀厥阴春生之气。夫五运始于木,而递相资生。主治伤中虚羸者,气味甘平,补中土也。补五内,益气力,所以治伤中也。长肌肉,填髓脑,所以治虚羸也。补五内,益气力之无形,长肌肉,填髓脑之有形,则内外充足,故久服轻身不老。

20. Jushengzi〔巨胜子, black sesame, Sesami Semen Nigrum〕

It is sweet in taste, mild and non-toxic in property, and it is mainly used to resolve internal damage and emaciation and weakness, tonify the five zang-organs, replenish qi and energy, promote the growth of the muscles, and enrich the brain. Long-term taking of it will keep healthy and prevent aging.

Jushengzi (black sesame) has another two names. One is Huma (胡麻), and the other is Goushi (狗虱). It was firstly recorded to be growing in Hu (胡) land, so it is called Huma (胡麻). Ju (巨) means big. It was firstly recorded to be growing in Dayuan (大宛) of Hu (胡) land, so it is also called Jusheng (巨胜). Among the eight cereals, it is the best one. Kou Zongshi (寇宗奭) said, "Huma (胡麻) is today's big Zhima〔脂麻, sesame, Sesami Semen〕. Those growing in Hu (胡) land are plump and big, so it is called Huma (胡麻) or Jusheng (巨胜)." There is one kind of so-called Jusheng (巨胜) sold in the market nowadays, which is like Xiaohui〔小茴, fennel, Foeniculi Fructus〕with shells outside, but with no kernels inside. It is severely bitter in taste, and it is used to fake genuine Jusheng (black sesame). Jusheng (black sesame), in fact, is Huma (胡麻) which pertains to the category of cereals. Liu Ruan (刘阮) went to the fairyland in heaven, and the fairies fed him Huma (胡麻) rice. If Huma (胡麻) only has the shell but no kernels and is bitter in taste, then how could it be used for cooking rice? One should know that the so-called Jusheng (巨胜) sold in the market is actually wild Goushi (狗虱), so it is also called Bishi (壁虱) or Huma (胡麻). Bishi (壁虱) and Goushi (狗虱) cannot be used as medicinal. If there is no Huma (胡麻), then pick the red and big Zhima (sesame) to be used as medicinal, which almost has the same effect as Huma (胡麻).

Dama〔大麻, hemp, Cannabis sativa L.〕is the head of five cereals and receives the qi of reverting yin and spring resuscitation. The five circuits begin with wood and promote each other. It can mainly resolve internal damage and emaciation and weakness, for it can tonify center earth with its sweet taste and mild property. It can be used to tonify the five zang-organs and replenish qi and energy, so internal damage can be resolved. It can be used to promote the growth of the muscles and enrich the brain, so emaciation and weakness can be resolved. Tonifying the five zang-organs and replenishing qi and energy are intangible while promoting the growth of the muscles and enriching the brain are tangible, thus the interior and the exterior will be strengthened. Therefore, long-term taking of it will keep healthy and prevent aging.

21. 赤 箭

赤箭 气味辛温,无毒。主杀鬼精物,蛊毒恶气。久服益气力,长阴,肥健。

《本经》名赤箭苗也。宋《开宝本草》名天麻根也。《本经》主治,根苗并论。今则但用天麻,不用赤箭矣。始出陈仓川谷、雍州,及太山少室。春生苗,中抽一茎直上如箭竿,色正赤,贴茎梢之半,微有小红叶,远看如箭之有羽,有风不动,无风自摇,故有神草之名。根形如王瓜,皮色黄白,晒干则黑,去根三五寸,有游子环列如卫,皆有细根如白发,气相通而实不相连,故根又有离母之名。

赤箭气味辛温,其根名天麻者,气味甘平。盖赤箭辛温属金,金能制风,而有弧矢之威,故主治杀鬼精物。天麻甘平属土,土能胜湿,而居五运之中,故治蛊毒恶气。天麻形如芋魁,有游子十二枚,周环之,以仿十二辰。十二子在外,应六气之司天,天麻如皇极之居中,得气运之全,故功同五芝,力倍五参,为仙家服食之上品。是以久服,益气力,长阴,肥健。

李时珍曰:补益上药,天麻为第一。世人只用之治风,良可惜也。

21. Chijian [赤箭, gastrodia, Gastrodiae Rhizoma]

It is pungent in taste, warm and non-toxic in property, and it is mainly used to eliminate strange pathogenic factors like ghosts and resolve worm toxin and malign qi. Long-term taking of it will replenish qi and energy, nourish yin and fortify the body.

Chijian (gastrodia) is mentioned as Chijianmiao [赤箭苗, Chijian shoot] in *Shen Nong Ben Cao Jing* [《神农本草经》, *Shennong's Classic of Materia Medica*] and is mentioned as Tianmagen [天麻根, Tianma root] in *Kai Bao*

Ben Cao [《开宝本草》, *Materia Medica of the Kaibao Reign*] of the Song Dynasty. Actions in *Shen Nong Ben Cao Jing* [《神农本草经》, *Shennong's Classic of Materia Medica*] are recorded in terms of both Gen [根, root] and Miao [苗, shoot]. Nowadays, people only use Tianma [天麻, tall gastrodia tuber, Rhizoma Gastrodiae] rather than Chijian (gastrodia) to treat diseases. It was firstly recorded to be growing in the river valleys of Chencang (陈仓) as well as in Yongzhou (雍州), Shaoshi Mountain (少室山) and Taishan Mountain (太山). It sprouts in spring with one stalk towering from the center like an arrow pole. The stalk is red in color, and there are a few little red leaves around the middle of the stalk tip. The stalk, which looks like an arrow with feathers over a long distance, never moves when there is wind, but spontaneously moves when there is no wind. So it has the name of Shencao [神草, divine grass]. Its root, whose shape is like Wanggua [王瓜, cucumber gourd, Trichosanthis Cucumeroidis Fructus], has yellow-white peel. The peel becomes black when the root is dried in the sun. When the root is cut off three or five Cun, there will be halimasch circling like guards on it. Its seeds all have small roots like white hair. Qi among roots interacts with each other, but the roots themselves do not. So the root is also called Limu (离母).

Chijian (gastrodia) is pungent in taste and warm in property. Its root, called Tianma (tall gastrodiatuber), is sweet in taste and mild in property. Chijian (gastrodia) pertains to metal as it is pungent in taste and warm in property, and metal can control wind, thus it has the power of bow and arrow. Therefore, it can mainly eliminate strange pathogenic factors like ghosts. Tianma (tall gastrodiatuber) pertains to earth as it is sweet in taste and mild in property, and earth can predominate dampness, thus it is at the center of the five circuits. Therefore, it can be used to resolve worm toxin and vicious qi. The shape of Tianma (tall gastrodiatuber) is like that of Yukui [芋魁, dasheen tuber, Tuber Colocasiae Esculentae]. It has twelve pieces of circling halimasch in accordance with the twelve ancient constellations. The outside twelve pieces of halimasch correspond with six qi dominating the heaven. Tianma (tall gastrodiatuber) obtains major qi and essence, just like Polaris at the center, so its effect is the same as that of five kinds of Zhi [芝, fragrant herb], and is much better than that of five kinds of Shen［参, sage herb］. Thus, it is a top-grade herb taken by those pursuing immortality. Therefore, long-term taking of it will replenish qi and energy, nourish yin and fortify the body.

Li Shizhen（李时珍）said, "Among the top-grade tonifying medicinal, Tianma（tall gastrodiatuber）is the best. However, people only use it to treat the disease caused by wind. What a pity！"

22. 干地黄

干地黄　气味甘寒,无毒。主伤中,逐血痹,填骨髓,长肌肉,作汤,除寒热积聚,除痹,疗折跌绝筋。久服轻身不老。生者尤良。

地黄《本经》名地髓。《尔雅》名芐,又名芑。始出咸阳川泽黄土地者佳,今处处有之,近似怀庆者为上。根色通黄,干则微黑,古时种子,今时种根,以根节多者,寸断而莳植之。制干地黄法,以细小者捣烂取汁,拌肥大者,晒干。

地黄色黄,味甘性寒,禀太阴中土之专精,兼少阴寒水之气化。主治伤中者,味甘质润,补中焦之精汁也。血痹,犹脉痹。逐血痹者,横纹似络脉,通周身之经络也。得少阴寒水之精,故填骨髓,得太阴中土之精,故长肌肉。地黄性唯下行,故字从芐。藉汤饮,则上行外达,故曰作汤除寒热集聚。除集聚,上行也。除寒热,外达也。又曰除痹,言不但逐血痹,更除皮肉筋骨之痹也,除皮肉筋骨之痹,则折跌绝筋,亦可疗矣。久服则精血充足,故轻身不老。生者尤良,谓生时多津汁而尤良,惜不能久贮远市也。后人蒸熟合丸,始有生地、熟地之分。熟地黄功力与生地黄相等,性稍减,补肾相宜,所以然者,蒸熟,则甘中之苦味尽除,故寒性稍减,蒸熟则黑,故补肾相宜。

愚按:地黄入土最深,性唯下行,作汤则助其上达。日华子有天黄、地黄、人黄之分,谬矣。

22. Gandihuang［干地黄, dried rehmannia, Radix Rehmanniae］

It is sweet in taste, cold and non-toxic in property, and it is mainly used to treat internal damage, expel blood impediment, enrich marrow and promote the growth of the muscles. When it is made into decoction, it can eliminate the accumulation of cold and heat, expel impediment and treat the fracture of the bones and sinews due to falling. Long-term taking of it will keep healthy and prevent aging. The effect of Shengdihuang〔生地黄, raw rehmannia, Rehmanniae Radix Exsiccata seu Recens〕is better.

Dihuang〔地黄, rehmannia, Radix Rehmanniae〕is mentioned as Disui (地髓) in *Shen Nong Ben Cao Jing*〔《神农本草经》, *Shennong's Classic of Materia Medica*〕and Hu（苄）or Qi（芑）in *Er Ya*〔《尔雅》, *On Elegance*〕. Those firstly recorded to be growing in the river and lake as well as the yellow soil of Xianyang（咸阳）were of good quality, and now it grows everywhere. Those growing near Huaiqing（怀庆）are of better quality. Its roots are thoroughly yellow and turn light black when they are dried. People planted seeds in ancient times while people plant roots nowadays. Cut roots with many nodes into smaller parts and plant them. The way to make Gandihuang（dried rehmannia）is to pound the small one to extract juice, mix the juice with the big one, dry the big one in the sun.

Dihuang（rehmannia）, sweet in taste, cold in property and yellow in color, receives the essence of center earth from greater yin and qi transformation of cold water from lesser yin. It can mainly treat internal damage, because it can tonify the essence-juice of the middle energizer with its sweet taste and moist property. Blood impediment is like meridian impediment. It can expel blood impediment, because it has transverse creases similar to collaterals that can connect the meridians of the whole body. It obtains the essence of cold water from lesser yin, so it can enrich marrow. It receives the essence of center earth from greater yin, so it can promote the growth of the muscles. It tends to go downward, so its Chinese name has the character "苄"（Hu）. When it is made into decoction, it can go upward and reach outside, so it can then eliminate the accumulation of cold and heat. To eliminate accumulation needs to go upward, and to eliminate cold and heat needs to reach outside. It can also eliminate impediment. That is to say, it can not only expel blood impediment, but also can eliminate the impediment in the skin, muscles, sinews and bones, thus it can further treat the fracture of the bones and sinews due to falling. Long-term taking of it will have sufficient essence and blood, so it can keep healthy and prevent aging. The effect of Shengdihuang（raw rehmannia）is better, because the raw one is full of juice. However, it is a pity that it cannot be stored for a long time to be sold in distant markets. People later on steamed Shengdihuang (raw rehmannia) to make pills. Till then it began to be divided into Shengdihuang (raw rehmannia) and Shudihuang [熟地黄, cooked rehmannia, Rehmanniae Radix Praeparata]. Shudihuang (cooked rehmannia) has the same effects as those of Shengdihuang (raw rehmannia), but it is slightly lighter in property, thus it is suitable to be used to tonify the kidney. The reason is that the bitterness in the sweet taste can be eliminated thoroughly when it is steamed, so its cold property can be slightly reduced. It turns black after it is steamed, so it is suitable to tonify the kidney.

Note by Zhang Zhicong (张志聪): Dihuang (rehmannia) is a medicinal herb which goes into the deepest earth and tends to go downward. However, it can go upward in property when it is made into decoction. It is divided into Tianhuang (天黄), Dihuang (地黄) and Renhuang (人黄) in *Ri Hua Ben Cao* [《日华本草》, *Rihuazi's Materia Medica*], which is a false statement.

23. 麦门冬

麦门冬 气味甘平,无毒。主心腹结气,伤中,伤饱,胃络脉绝,羸瘦短气。久服轻身不老,不饥。

麦门冬。始出函谷、川谷,叶如细韭,凌冬不死,根色黄白,中心贯通,延蔓相引,古时野生,宛如麦粒,故名麦冬,今江浙皆莳植矣。一本横生,根颗联络,有十二枚者,有十四五枚者。所以然者,手足三阳、三阴之络共有十二,加任之尾翳,督之长强,共十四,又加脾之大络,共十五,此物性之自然而合于人身者也,唯圣人能体察之,故用麦冬以通络脉,并无去心二字,后人不详经义,不穷物理,相沿去心久矣,今表正之。

麦门冬气味甘平,质性滋润,凌冬青翠,盖禀少阴冬水之精,上与阳明胃土相合。主治心腹结气者,麦冬一本横生,能通胃气于四旁,则上心下腹之结气皆散除矣。伤中者,经脉不和,中气内虚也。伤饱者,饮食不节,胃气壅滞也。麦门禀少阴癸水之气,上合阳明戊土,故治伤中、伤饱。胃之大络,内通于脉,胃络脉绝者,胃络不通于脉也。麦冬颗分心贯,横生土中,连而不断,故治胃络脉绝。胃虚则羸瘦,肾虚则短气,麦冬助胃补肾,故治羸瘦、短气。久服则形体强健,故身轻,精神充足,故不老不饥。

23. Maimendong [麦门冬, ophiopogon, Ophiopogonis Radix]

It is sweet in taste, mild and non-toxic in property, and it is mainly used to disperse the qi stagnation of the heart and abdomen, resolve internal damage and dyspepsia, relieve the exhaustion of the collateral vessels of the stomach and treat emaciation and shortness of breath. Long-term taking of it will keep healthy, prevent aging and tolerate hunger.

Maimendong (ophiopogon) was firstly recorded to be growing in Hangu (函谷) and Chuangu (川谷). Its leaves are as thin as Jiucai [韭菜, Chinese leek, Allii Tuberosi Folium] and do not wither even in winter. Its roots are white-yellow in color and hollow in shape, twining with each other like vines. In ancient times, it grew in wild like the grain, so it is called Maidong (麦冬). Now it is planted in Jiangsu (江苏) and Zhejiang (浙江). There are root tubers on its root which grows sideways. One root may have twelve, fourteen or fifteen root tubers. The reason is that each hand or foot has three yang collaterals or three yin collaterals, which altogether have twelve collaterals. There will be fourteen when adding Weiyi [尾翳, Tail Screen] of conception vessel and Changqiang [长强, Long Strong] of governor vessel and fifteen when further adding the great collateral of the spleen. So the above description manifests that natural principles are in accordance with the human body, which can only be understood by sages. Therefore, Maimendong (ophiopogon) is used to free the collateral vessels without mentioning the need of removing its inner heart. Without knowing true meanings of the classics and laws of things, People later on just followed the old traditions to remove its inner heart. Now this is corrected here.

Maimendong (ophiopogon) is sweet in taste and mild and moist in property. It keeps green even in winter, because it receives the essence of winter water from lesser yin and it is in accordance with yang brightness and stomach earth in the upper. It can mainly disperse the qi stagnation of the heart and abdomen, because its roots grow sideways and thus can make the stomach transport nutrients to other organs. Therefore, the qi stagnation of the upper heart and lower abdomen can be dispersed. Internal damage is the disharmony of the meridians and the insufficiency of center qi. Dyspepsia is caused by improper diet and stagnant stomach qi. Maimendong (ophiopogon) receives the qi of Guishui (癸水) from lesser yin and it is in accordance with Wutu (戊土) from yang brightness in the upper. Therefore, it can be used to resolve internal damage and dyspepsia. The great collateral of the stomach connects with the meridians internally, and the exhaustion of the collateral vessels of the stomach means that the stomach collateral cannot connect with the meridians. Its roots grow separately but their inner hearts connect one after another inherently, thus although the roots grow sideways, they actually connect with each other. So it can be used to relieve the exhaustion of the collaterals of the stomach meridian. Stomach deficiency causes emaciation while kidney deficiency causes shortness of breath. Maimendong (ophiopogon) can tonify the stomach and aid the kidney, so it can be used to treat emaciation and shortness of breath. Long-term taking of it will fortify the body, so it can keep healthy. With sufficient essence and energy, it can prevent aging and tolerate hunger.

24. 天门冬

天门冬 气味苦平,无毒。主诸暴风湿偏痹,强骨髓,杀三虫,去伏尸。久服轻身益气,延年不饥。

天门冬,一名天棘,又名颠棘。始出奉高山谷,此山最高,上奉于天,故名曰天、曰颠。藤引蔓延,茎稍有刺,故名曰棘。其根白色或黄紫色,柔润多汁,长二三寸,一科一二十枚,与百部相类。

天门冬,《本经》言:气味苦平。《别录》言:甘寒。新出土时,其味微苦,曝干则微甘也。性寒无毒,体质多脂,始生高山,盖禀寒水之气,而上通于天,故有天冬之名。主治诸暴风湿偏痹者,言风湿之邪,暴中于身,而成半身不遂之偏痹,天冬禀水天之气,环转运行,故可治也。强骨髓者,得寒水之精也。杀三虫、去伏尸者,水阴之气,上通于天也,水气通天,则天气下降,故土中之三虫,泉下之伏尸,皆杀去也。太阳为诸阳主气,故久服轻身益气,天气通贯于地中,故延年不饥。

伏尸者,传尸鬼疰,泉下尸鬼,阴而为病也。天门冬能启水中之生阳,上通于天,故去伏尸。凡治传尸之药,皆从阴达阳,由下升上。

天、麦门冬,皆禀少阴水精之气。麦门冬禀水精而上通于阳明。天门冬禀水精而上通于太阳。夫冬主闭藏,门主开转,咸名门冬者,咸能开转闭藏而上达也。后人有天门冬补中有泻,麦门冬泻中有补之说,不知从何处引来,良可嗤也。

24. Tianmendong [天门冬, asparagus, Radix Asparagi]

It is bitter in taste, mild and non-toxic in property, and it is mainly used to treat the hemiplegia caused by sudden wind-dampness, strengthen the bones and marrow, kill three kinds of worms and eliminate Fushi (伏尸, a serious disease caused by overstrain). Long-term taking of it will keep healthy, replenish qi, prolong life and tolerate hunger.

It is also called Tianji (天棘) or Dianji (颠棘). Firstly recorded to be growing in the valley of Fenggao Mountain (奉高山) which is the highest mountain and can connect the heaven, so its name has the characters "天" (Tian) or "颠" (Dian). Its main stem grows upward, and its vines grow sideways. Its stem has a few thorns, so it is called Ji [棘, thorn]. Its roots, white or yellowish-purple in color, soft and juicy, are two or three Cun long. One root of Tianmendong (asparagus) has ten or twenty root tubers, which is similar to Baibu [百部, stemona, Stemonae Radix].

According to *Shen Nong Ben Cao Jing* [《神农本草经》, *Shennong's Classic of Materia Medica*], Tianmendong (asparagus) is bitter in taste and mild in property. According to *Ming Yi Bie Lu* [《名医别录》, *Miscellaneous Records of Famous Physicians*], it is sweet in taste and cold in property. It is slightly bitter in taste when newly dug out while it is slightly sweet in taste after it is dried in the sun. It is cold and non-toxic in property as well as rich in fat. Firstly recorded to be growing in the high mountain, it receives the qi of cold water and moves upward to connect with the heaven, so it is also called Tiandong (天冬). It can mainly treat the hemiplegia caused by sudden wind-dampness. The pathogen of wind-dampness suddenly attacks the body, resulting in hemiplegia. It receives the qi of water and heaven and circulates in the body, so it can treat the hemiplegia caused by sudden wind-dampness. It can strengthen the bones and marrow, because it receives the essence of cold water. It can kill three kinds of worms and eliminate Fushi〔伏尸, a serious disease caused by overstrain〕, because the qi of water yin moves upward to connect the heaven. Water qi connects the heaven, then heaven qi descends, so three kinds of worms in earth and Fushi in the nether world can be eliminated. Greater yang is the major qi of all yang, so long-term taking of it will keep healthy and replenish qi. Heaven qi connects with earth center, so it can prolong life and tolerate hunger.

Fushi〔伏尸, serious diseases caused by overstrain〕, also known as Chuanshi〔传尸, infectious consumptive diseases〕or Guizhu〔鬼疰, multiple infixation abscess〕, is caused by the haunting of ghosts in the nether world. Tianmendong (asparagus) can activate the kidney-yang in water and make it move upward to connect the heaven, so it can eliminate Fushi〔伏尸, serious diseases caused by overstrain〕. Any medicinal that can be used to treat Chuanshi〔传尸, infectious consumptive diseases〕reaches yang from yin and goes upward from downward.

Both Tianmendong (asparagus) and Maimendong〔麦门冬, phiopogon, Ophiopogonis Radix〕receive the qi of water essence from lesser yin. Maimendong (phiopogon) receives water essence and moves upward to connect with yang brightness. Tianmendong (asparagus) receives water essence and moves upward to connect with greater yang. Dong〔冬, winter〕governs closure and storage, and Men〔门, door〕governs opening and turning. All things which are called Mendong (门冬) mean that they can all open, turn, close, store and move upward. People later on had a statement saying that Tianmendong (asparagus) can mainly tonify, but can have the reducing effect as well, and Maimendong (phiopogon) can mainly reduce, but can have the tonifying effect as well. The origin of the above statement cannot be traced, so it can be sneered.

25. 葳 蕤

葳蕤　气味甘平,无毒。主中风暴热,不能动摇,跌筋结肉,诸不足。久服去面黑䵟,好颜色,润泽,轻身不老。

《本经》名女萎。《吴氏本草》名葳蕤。《别录》名玉竹。《拾遗》名青黏。始出太山山谷及丘陵，今处处有之。女萎者，性阴柔而质滋润，如女之委顺相随也。葳蕤者，女子娇柔之意。玉竹者，根色如玉，茎节如竹也。青黏，茎叶青翠，根汁稠粘也。春生苗，茎直有节，其叶如竹，两两相对，其根横生如黄精，色白微黄，性柔多脂，最难干。

按：葳蕤叶密者，似乎对生，而实不相对。或云：其叶对生者，即是黄精矣。今浙中采药人拣根之细长者为玉竹，根之园而大者为黄精，其实只是一种年未久者，故根细而长。年久者，其根大而园。余求真黄精，种数十年不能得。

葳蕤气味甘平，质多津液，禀太阴湿土之精，以资中焦之汁。中风暴热者，风邪中人，身热如曝也。不能动摇者，热盛于身，津液内竭，不濡灌于肌腠也。跌筋者，筋不柔和，则踒蹶而如跌也。结肉者，肉无膏泽，则涩滞而如结也。诸不足者，申明中风暴热，不能动摇，跌筋结肉，是诸不足之证也。久服则津液充满，故去面上之黑皯，好颜色而肌肤润泽，且轻身不老。

愚按：葳蕤润泽滑腻，禀性阴柔，故《本经》主治中风暴热，古方主治风温灼热，所治皆主风热之病。近医谓葳蕤有人参之功，无分寒热燥湿，一概投之，以为补剂，不知阴病内寒此为大忌，盖缘不考经书，咸为耳食所误。

25. Weirui［葳蕤，stem of October clematis，Caulis Clematidis Apiifoliae］

It is sweet in taste，mild and non-toxic in property，and it is mainly used to treat the wind stroke with sudden heat，inability to move，the convulsion of the sinews and the tension of the muscles as well as syndromes of various deficiency. Long-term taking of it can remove chloasma，luster complexion，moisten the skin，keep healthy and prevent aging.

It is mentioned as Nüwei（女萎）in *Sheng Nong Ben Cao Jing*［《神农本草经》，*Shennong's Classic of Materia Medica*］，Weirui（葳蕤）in *Wu Shi Ben Cao*［《吴氏本草》，*Wu Pu's Studies of Materia Medica*］，Yuzhu（玉竹）in *Ming Yi Bie Lu*［《名医别录》，*Miscellaneous Records of Famous Physicians*］and Qingnian（青黏）in *Ben Cao Shi Yi*［《本草拾遗》，*Supplement to Materia Medica*］. Firstly recorded to be growing in the valleys and hills of Taishan Mountain（太山），now it grows everywhere. Nüwei（女萎）means being tender and moist in property, which is like a tender girl accompanying her lover. Weirui (葳蕤) means the charm and gentleness of a girl. Yuzhu (玉竹) means that the color of its roots is as green as the jade, and its stems and joints are like those of bamboos. Qingnian (青黏) means that its stems and leaves are green in color, and the juice of its roots is sticky. It sprouts in spring. Its stems are straight with nodes. Its leaves are like those of bamboos, which grow on opposite sides. Its root, growing sideways like Huangjing [黄精, yellow essence, Polygonati Rhizoma], is white and light yellow in color, tender in property, rich in fat and very difficult to become dry.

Note by Gao Shishi (高世栻): The flourish leaves of Weirui (stem of October clematis) seem to grow on opposite sides, but in fact they do not. It is also stated that those with leaves growing opposite sides are actually Huangjing (yellow essence). Nowadays, herbalists in Zhezhong (浙中) regard those with long and thin roots as Yuzhu (玉竹) and those with round and big roots as Huangjing (yellow essence). Yuzhu (玉竹) and Huangjing (yellow essence) are in fact one kind of herbs. Those with long and thin roots are young ones, and those with round and big roots are old ones. I have searched for genuine Huangjing (yellow essence) and tried to plant it for decades, but ending in vain.

Weirui (stem of October clematis), sweet in taste, mild in property and rich in juice, can nourish the juice of the middle energizer by receiving the essence of wet earth from greater yin. The wind stroke with sudden heat means that wind pathogen attacks people, and their bodies are as hot as being exposed to the sun. Inability to move means that the body is filled with heat, and fluids inside are exhausted, so the interstices of the muscles cannot be moistened. The convulsion of the sinews means that the sinews are not soft, which leads to limp and the spasm of the legs. The tension of the muscles means that muscles have no fat, which leads to the tension-like stagnation of the muscles. The syndromes of various deficiency are manifested as the wind stroke with sudden heat, inability to move as well as the convulsion of the sinews and the tension of the muscles. Long-term taking of it can make the body full of fluids, thus can remove chloasma, luster complexion, moisten the skin, keep healthy and prevent aging.

Note by Zhang Zhicong（张志聪）: Weirui（stem of October clematis）is moist, slippery and tender in property, so *Shen Nong Ben Cao Jing* [《神农本草经》, *Shennong's Classic of Materia Medica*] says that it can mainly treat the wind stroke with sudden heat. In ancient formulas it was mainly used to treat the diseases caused by wind warmth and scorching heat. The diseases mentioned above are all mainly wind-heat diseases. Doctors recently state that Weirui（stem of October clematis）has the same action as that of Renshen [人参, ginseng, Ginseng Radix]. Without differentiating the nature of diseases as cold, hot, dry or damp, they just use it as tonic formula. They do not know that it is a taboo to use Weirui（stem of October clematis）for internal cold of yin diseases. This is because they do not study the classics and are therefore misled by erroneous hearsay.

26. 牛 膝

牛膝 气味苦酸平,无毒。主寒湿痿痹、四肢拘挛、膝痛不可屈伸,逐血气伤热火烂,堕胎。久服轻身耐老。

牛膝《本经》名百倍。始出河内川谷及临朐,今江淮闽粤关中皆有,然不及怀庆川中者佳。春生苗,枝节两两相对,故又名对节草,其根一本直下,长二三尺,以肥阔粗大者为上。

《本经》谓:百倍气味苦酸,概根苗而言也。今时所用,乃根下之茎,味甘臭酸,其性微寒。《易》曰:乾为马,坤为牛,牛之力在膝,取名牛膝者,禀太阴湿土之气化,而能资养筋骨也。主治寒湿痿痹,言或因于寒,或因于湿,而成痿痹之证也。痿痹则四肢拘挛,四肢拘挛,则膝痛不可屈伸。牛膝禀湿土柔和之化,而资养筋骨,故能治之。血气伤热火烂,言血气为热所伤,则为火烂之证。牛膝味甘性寒,故可逐也。根下之茎,形如大筋,性唯下泄,故堕胎。久服则筋骨强健,故轻身耐老。

26. Niuxi [牛膝, root of twotooth achyranthes, Radix Achyranthis Bidentatae]

It is bitter and sour in taste, mild and non-toxic in property, and it is mainly used to treat the flaccidity impediment due to cold and dampness, the spasm of the four limbs, the inability of the knees to extend and bend due to pain, resolve the fire canker caused by blood qi being hurt by heat and induce abortion. Long-term taking of it will keep healthy and prevent aging.

Niuxi (root of twotooth achyranthes) is mentioned as Baibei (百倍) in *Sheng Nong Ben Cao Jing* [《神农本草经》, *Shennong's Classic of Materia Medica*]. Firstly recorded to be growing in the valleys of Heinei (河内) and Linqu (临朐), now it grows everywhere in Jianghuai (江淮), Minyue (闽粤) and Guanzhog (关中), which is not as good as that growing in Huaiqing (怀庆) and Chuangzhong (川中) in terms of quality. In spring it sprouts. Its branches and nodes grow on opposite sides, so it is also called Duijiecao [对节草, herb with nodes on opposite sides]. Its root, growing straight downward, is two or three Chi deep. The root which is fat, wide, thick and big is of better quality.

Sheng Nong Ben Cao Jing [《神农本草经》, *Shennong's Classic of Materia Medica*] says that Baibei (百倍) is bitter and sour in taste in terms of its root and seedlings. Nowadays, the rhizome is used as medicinal, which is sweet in taste, sour in smell and slightly cold in property. *Yi Jing* [《易经》, *The Book of Changes*] says that the horse pertains to the heaven, the cattle pertains to the earth, and the strength of the cattle originates from its knees. It is called Niuxi [牛膝, cattle's knees] because it receives the qi transformation of wet earth from greater yin to foster the sinews and bones. It can mainly treat the flaccidity impediment due to cold and dampness. It is said that flaccidity impediment is caused by cold or dampness. The flaccidity impediment will cause the spasm of the four limbs, which further causes the inability of the knees to extend and bend due to pain. It receives the softness transformation of wet earth to foster the sinews and bones, so it can treat the diseases mentioned above. Blood qi is hurt by heat, resulting in fire cranker. Niuxi (root of twotooth achyranthes) is sweet in taste and cold in property, so it can treat the diseases mentioned above. The rhizome is like the large sinew, which tends to go downward and discharge, so it can induce abortion. Long-term taking of it will strengthen the sinews and bones, so it can keep healthy and prevent aging.

27. 杜 仲

杜仲 气味辛平,无毒。主腰膝痛,补中,益精气,坚筋骨,强志,除阴下痒湿,小便余沥。久服轻身耐老。

杜仲木皮,状如厚朴,折之有白绵相连,故一名木绵。杜字从土,仲者中也,此木始出豫州山谷,得中土之精,《本经》所以名杜仲也。李时珍曰:昔有杜仲,服此得道,因以名之谬矣。在唐宋本草或有之矣,《神农本经》未必然也。

杜仲皮色黑而味辛平,禀阳明、少阴金水之精气。腰膝痛者,腰乃肾府,少阴主之。膝属大筋,阳明主之。杜仲禀少阴、阳明之气,故腰膝之痛可治也。补中者,补阳明之中土也。益精气者,益少阴肾精之气也。坚筋骨者,坚阳明所属之筋,少阴所主之骨也。强志者,所以补肾也。阳明燥气下行,故除阴下痒湿,小便余沥。久服则金水相生,精气充足,故轻身耐老。

愚按:桑皮、桑叶有丝,蚕食桑而结茧,其色洁白,其质坚牢,禀金气也。藕与莲梗有丝,生于水中,得水精也。杜仲色黑味辛而多丝,故兼禀金水之气化。

27. Duzhong [杜仲, eucommia bark, Cortex Eucommiae]

It is pungent in taste, mild and non-toxic in property, and it is mainly used to relieve the pain in the waist and spine, tonify the middle, replenish essential qi, strengthen the sinews and bones, strengthen memory, eliminate genital itching and dampness and treat dribbling urination. Long-term taking of it will keep healthy and prevent aging.

The shape of its bark is like that of Houpu [厚朴, magnolia bark, Cortex Magnoliae Officinalis], and there is gutta percha, looking like white silk, between the broken parts, so it is also called Mumian (木绵). "杜" (Du) has the character "土" (Tu), and "仲" (Zhong) means middle. Firstly recorded to be growing in the mountain valleys of Yuzhou (豫州), it obtains the essence of center earth. Therefore, in *Sheng Nong Ben Cao Jing* [《神农本草经》, *Shennong's Classic of Materia Medica*] it is mentioned as Duzhong (杜仲). Li Shizhen (李时珍) said, "There was a person called Duzhong (杜仲) who became an immortal after taking it, so it was called Duzhong（杜仲）." What he said was not true. The origin of its name may be recorded in the works on materia medica in the Tang or Song Dynasty, and the origin was not necessarily recorded in *Sheng Nong Ben Cao Jing*［《神农本草经》, *Shennong's Classic of Materia Medica*］.

Duzhong（eucommia bark）is pungent in taste and mild in property with black bark. It receives the essential qi of metal and water from yang brightness and lesser yin. It can relieve the pain in the waist and spine, because the waist is the house of the kidney and is governed by lesser yin, and the knee pertains to the large sinew and is governed by yang brightness. It receives the qi of lesser yin and yang brightness, so it can relieve the pain in the waist and spine. To tonify the middle is to tonify the center earth of yang brightness. To replenish essential qi is to replenish the qi of kidney essence from lesser yin. To strengthen the sinews and bones is to strengthen the sinews pertaining to yang brightness and the bones pertaining to lesser yin. To strengthen memory is to tonify the kidney. The dry qi of yang brightness moves downward, so it can eliminate the genital itching and dampness and treat dribbling urination. Long-term taking of it will result in mutual generation of metal and water and produce sufficient essential qi, thus it will keep healthy and prevent aging.

Note by Zhang Zhicong（张志聪）: There is mucus in Sangpi［桑皮, mulberry bark, Mori Cortex］and Sangye［桑叶, mulberry leaf Mori Folium］. Silkworms eat them to spin cocoons which are pure white in color and firm in texture, because they receive metal qi. There are fibers in Ou［藕, lotus root, Nelumbinis Rhizoma］and Liangeng［莲梗, lotus stalk, Nelumbinis Petiolus seu Pedicellus］, because they grow in water and receive water essence. Duzhong（eucommia bark）, black in color and pungent in taste, has a lot of gutta percha, so it receives the qi transformation of both water and metal.

28. 枸　杞

枸杞　味苦寒，无毒。主五内邪气、热中、消渴、周痹风湿。久服坚筋骨，轻身不老，耐寒暑。

枸杞始出常山平泽及丘陵阪岸,今处处有之,以陕西甘州者为胜。春生,苗叶如石榴,叶软嫩可食,七月开小紫花,随结实,圆红如樱桃,凌冬不落。李时珍曰:枸杞二树名,此木棘如枸刺,茎若杞条,故兼而名之。《本经》气味主治概根苗花实而言,初未分别,后人以实为枸杞子,根名地骨皮,主治稍不同矣。

枸杞根苗苦寒,花实紫赤,至严冬霜雪之中,其实红润可爱,是禀少阴水阴之气,兼少阴君火之化者也。主治五内邪气,热中、消渴。谓五藏正气不足,邪气内生,而为热中、消渴之病。枸杞得少阴水阴之气,故可治也。主治周痹风湿者,兼得少阴君火之化也。岐伯曰:周痹者,在于血脉之中,随脉以上,随脉以下,不能左右,各当其所。枸杞能助君火之神,出于血脉之中,故去周痹而除风湿。久服坚筋骨,轻身不老,耐寒暑。亦得少阴水火之气,而精神充足,阴阳交会也。

28. Gouqi〔枸杞, barbary wolfberry fruit, Fructus Lycii〕

It is bitter in taste, cold and non-toxic in property, and it is mainly used to expel the pathogenic qi in the five zang-organs, treat heat strike, resolve consumptive thirst, cure generalized impediment and wind-dampness. Long-term taking of it will strengthen the sinews and bones, keep healthy, prevent aging and tolerate severe cold and heat.

Firstly recorded to be growing in the lakes, hills and scarps of Changshan Mountain (常山), now it grows everywhere, and those growing in Ganzhou (甘州) of Shaanxi (陕西) Province are of much better quality. In spring it grows seedlings and leaves which are like those of Shiliu〔石榴, pomegranate, Granati Fructus〕. Its leaves are soft, tender and edible. It blossoms in the seventh lunar month with little purple flowers. Then it will bear round fruits which are as red as cherries and will not fall even in winter. Li Shizhen (李时珍) said, "Gou (枸) is the name of one plant, and Qi (杞) is the name of another plant. The thorns of Gouqi (barbary wolfberry fruit) are like Gouci〔枸刺, cition, Citrus Medica L.〕, and its stems are like Qitiao〔杞条, osier, Salix Integra〕. Thus, it got its name, Gouqi (barbary wolfberry fruit), from Gouci (cition) and Qitiao (osier)." *Shen Nong Ben Cao Jing*〔《神农本草经》, *Shennong's Classic of Materia Medica*〕describes its taste, property and actions, which are mainly about its root, seedlings, flowers and fruits without telling the differences. People later on called its fruits Gouqizi〔枸杞子, lycium, Lycii Fructus〕and its root Digupi〔地骨皮, lycium bark, Lycii Cortex〕, which are slightly different in their actions.

Its root and seedlings are bitter in taste and cold in property, and its flowers are firm in property and purple-red in color. It bears red and lovely fruits in snow and frost. It receives the qi of water yin from lesser yin and the transformation of sovereign fire from lesser yin. It can mainly expel the pathogenic qi in the five zang-organs, treat heat strike and resolve consumptive thirst. The insufficient healthy qi in the five-zang organs will cause pathogenic qi arising internally, which further leads to heat strike and consumptive thirst. It receives the qi of water yin from lesser yin, so it can treat the disease mentioned above. The it can also mainly cure generalized impediment and wind-dampness, because it receives the transformation of sovereign fire from lesser yin. Qibo（歧伯）said, "Generalized impediment is caused by the invasion of pathogenic factors into the blood vessels and moves upward and downward along the channels. But it corresponds to each other the left side and the right side. So the pain occurs in the affected regions respectively." Gouqi（barbary wolfberry fruit）can assist the spirit of sovereign fire to reach the blood vessels, so it can cure generalized impediment and wind dampness. Long-term taking of it will strengthen the sinews and bones, keep healthy, prevent aging and tolerate severe cold and heat, because it also receives the qi of water and fire from lesser yin, which can produce sufficient essence and lead to the interaction of yin and yang.

29. 枸杞苗 附

枸杞苗 附　气味苦寒,主除烦,益志,补五劳七伤,壮心气,去皮肤、骨节间风,消热毒,散疮肿。《日华本草》附

29. Gouqimiao〔枸杞苗, lycium leaf, Lycii Folium〕*supplement*

It is bitter in taste and cold in property, and it is mainly used to relieve vexation, strengthen memory, tonify five kinds of overstrains and seven kinds of damages, strengthen heart qi, eliminate the wind pathogen in the skin and joints, disperse heat toxin and dissipate swollen sore. Supplemented in *Ri Hua Ben Cao* [《日华本草》, *Rihuazi's Materia Medica*].

30. 地骨皮 附

地骨皮 附　气味苦寒。主去骨热、消渴。

30. Digupi [地骨皮, Chinese wolfberry root-bark, Cortex Lycii] *supplement*

It is bitter in taste and cold in property, and it is mainly used to eliminate bone-steaming syndrome and treat consumptive thirst.

31. 枸杞子 附

枸杞子 附　气味甘寒。主坚筋骨,耐老,除风,去虚劳,补精气。《食疗本草》附。

31. Gouqizi [枸杞子, barbary wolfberry fruit, Fructus Lycii] *supplement*

It is sweet in taste and cold in property, and it is mainly used to strengthen the sinews and bones, prevent aging, expel wind pathogen, resolve consumptive diseases and replenish essential qi. Supplemented in *Shi Liao Ben Cao* [《食疗本草》, *Materia Medica for Dietotherapy*].

32. 女贞实

女贞实　气味苦平,无毒。主补中,安五脏,养精神,除百病。久服肥健,轻身不老。

女贞木始出武陵山谷,今处处有之。叶似冬青,凌冬不落。五月开细青白花,结实,九月熟,紫黑色,放虫造成白蜡者,女贞也。无蜡者,冬青也。

三阳为男,三阴为女,女贞禀三阴之气,岁寒操守,因以为名。味苦性寒,得少阴肾水之气也。凌冬不凋,得少阴君火之气也。作蜡坚白,得太阴肺金之气也。结实而园,得太阴脾土之气也。四季常青,得厥阴肝木之气也。女贞属三阴而禀五脏五行之气,故主补中,安五脏也。水之精为精,火之精为神,禀少阴水火之气,故养精神。人身百病,不外五行,女贞备五脏五行之气,故除百病。久服则水火相济,五脏安和,故肥健,轻身不老。

32. Nüzhenshi〔女贞实, glossy privet fruit, Fructus Ligustri Lucidi〕

It is bitter in taste, mild and non-toxic in property, and it is mainly used to tonify the middle, harmonize the five zang-organs, nourish essence and spirit, and eliminate all diseases. Long-term taking of it will fortify the body, keep healthy and prevent aging.

Firstly recorded to be growing in the mountains and valleys of Wuling (武陵), now it grows everywhere. Its leaves are like those of Dongqing〔冬青, Chinese ilex, Ilicis Chinensis〕and do not wither even in winter. It blossoms in the fifth lunar month with little green-white flowers and then bears fruits which will turn purple-black when getting ripe in the ninth lunar month. If there is secretion of the male Bailachong〔白蜡虫, white wax insect, Ericerus pela (Chavannes) Guerin〕, which can be further processed into Chongbaila〔虫白蜡, insect wax, Cera Chinensis Cera〕on the leaves, it is Nüzhenshi (glossy privet fruit), otherwise it is Dongqing (Chinese ilex).

Three yang represents the man and three yin represents the woman. Nüzhenshi (glossy privet fruit) receives the qi of three yin, and its leaves do not wither even in winter. That is why it gets such a name. It is bitter in taste and cold in property, because it receives the qi of kidney water from lesser yin. Its leaves do not wither even in winter, because it receives the qi of sovereign fire from lesser yin. Chongbaila (insect wax), made of secretion of the male Bailachong (white wax insect) on the leaves, and it is strong in property and white in color, because it receives the qi of lung metal from greater yin. It bears round fruits, because it receives the qi of spleen earth from greater yin. It is evergreen, because it receives the qi of liver wood from reverting yin. It pertains to three yin and receives the qi of five elements from the five zang-organs, so it can mainly tonify the middle and harmonize the five zang-organs. The essence of water is called essence, and the essence of fire is called spirit. Nüzhenshi (glossy privet fruit) receives the qi of water and fire from lesser yin, so it can nourish essence and spirit. All diseases are related to five elements. Nüzhenshi (glossy privet fruit) has the qi of five elements from the five zang-organs, so it can eliminate all diseases. Long-term taking of it will make fire and water aid each other and harmonize the five zang-organs, so it can fortify the body, keep healthy and prevent aging.

33. 五加皮

五加皮　气味辛温,无毒。主治心腹疝气、腹痛,益气,疗躄、小儿五岁不能行,疽疮阴蚀。

五加木始出汉中冤句,今江淮、湖南州郡皆有。春生苗,叶青茎赤似藤蒌,高三五尺,上有黑刺,一枝五叶交加,每叶上生一刺,三四月开白花,根若荆根,皮黄色,肉白色。

五加皮色备五行,花叶五出,乃五车星之精也,为修养家长生不老之药。主治心腹疝气,乃心病而为少腹有形之疝也。黄帝问曰:诊得心脉而急,此为何病? 病形何如? 岐伯曰:病名心疝,少腹当有形者是也,腹痛,乃脾病而致腹痛也。益气,乃肺病气虚,五加皮能益其气也。疗躄,乃肝病筋虚,五加皮能强筋疗躄也。小儿五岁不能行,乃肾病骨虚,五加皮补肾坚骨,故治小儿五岁不能行。治疽疮者,诸疮痛痒,皆属心火。五加皮助精水上滋,而能济其火也。治阴蚀者,虫乃阴类,阳虚则生,五加皮能益君火,而下济其阴也。夫五加皮、女贞实,咸禀五运之气化,女贞皆言养正,五加皆言治病,须知养正则病自除,治病则正自养。

按:《东华真人煮石经》云:何以得长久,何不食金盐,何以得长寿,何不食玉豉。玉豉,地榆也。金盐,五加也。取名金盐、玉豉者,盐乃水味,豉乃水谷,得先天水精,以养五脏之意。昔人有言曰:宁得一把五加,不用金玉满车。宁得一斤地榆,不用明月宝珠。又,鲁定公母服五加酒,以致不死,尸解而去。张子声、杨建始、王叔牙、于世彦等,皆服此酒,而房室不绝,得寿三百岁。亦可为散,以代茶汤。又曰:五加者,五车星之精也,水应五湖,人应五德,位应五方,物应五车,故青精入茎,则有东方之液。白气入节,则有西方之津。赤气入华,则有南方之光。玄精入根,则有北方之饴。黄烟入皮,则有戊已之灵。五神镇生,相转育成,饵之者真仙,服之者反婴。是五加乃服食养生之上品,而《本经》不言久服延年,或简脱也。

33. Wujiapi〔五加皮, slenderstyle acanthopanax bark, Cortex Acanthopanacis Radicis〕

It is pungent in taste, warm and non-toxic in property, and it is mainly used to treat the hernia in the heart and abdomen, relieve abdominal pain, replenish qi, cure atrophy-flaccidity, treat the children's difficulty in walking even when they are five years old, resolve carbuncles, sores and genital erosion.

Firstly recorded to be growing in Hanzhong (汉中) and Yuanju (冤句), now it grows everywhere in Jianghuai (江淮) and Hunan (湖南). It sprouts in spring. Like vines, its leaves are green. Its stalk is red in color. It is three to five Chi high with black thorns. There are five intertwining leaves on one branch, and there is one thorn on one leaf. It blossoms with white flowers in the third and fourth lunar months. Like Jinggen〔荆根, negundo vitex root, Viticis Negundinis Radix〕, its root has a yellow bark and white flesh.

It has five colors which correspond with five elements. Its flower has five petals, and one leaf is composed of five small leaves. It receives the essence of Wuche (five coaches) Star. Therefore, it is the elixir of life for people who cultivate immortality. It can mainly treat the hernia in the heart and abdomen, which is caused by heart disease involving the lower abdomen. Huangdi (黄帝) asked, "What disease does rapid heart pulse indicate? And what are its symptoms and signs?" Qibo (歧伯) answered, "The disease is called heart hernia involving the lower abdomen." The abdominal pain is caused by spleen diseases. Qi deficiency is caused by lung diseases, and Wujiapi (slenderstyle acanthopanax bark) can replenish qi. Atrophy-flaccidity results from sinew deficiency caused by liver diseases, and Wujiapi (slenderstyle acanthopanax bark) can strengthen the sinews and thus treat atrophy-flaccidity. Children's difficulty in walking even when they are five years old results from bone deficiency caused by kidney diseases, and

Wujiapi（slenderstyle acanthopanax bark）can tonify the kidney and strengthen the bones, so it can treat the above disease. Carbuncles, sores, pain and itching all pertain to heart fire. Wujiapi（slenderstyle acanthopanax bark）can assist essential water to nourish upward so as to aid the fire. The genital erosion is aching and itching like being bitten by worms, and worms pertain to yin which generates when yang is deficient. Wujiapi（slenderstyle acanthopanax bark）can benefit sovereign fire and move downward to aid yin. Both Wujiapi（slenderstyle acanthopanax bark）and Nüzhenshi［女贞实, glossy privet fruit, Fructus Ligustri Lucidi］receive the qi transformation of five circuits. It is commonly believed that Nüzhenshi（glossy privet fruit）can invigorate healthy qi, and Wujiapi（slenderstyle acanthopanax bark）can treat diseases. It should be known that invigorating healthy qi will lead to the curing of diseases, and treating diseases will lead to the invigorating of healthy qi.

Note by Zhang Zhicong（张志聪）: *Dong Hua Zhen Ren Zhu Shi Jing*［《东华真人煮石经》, *Immortal Donghua's Canon of Boiling Stone*］says, "How do people live a long life? Eat Jinyan（金盐）. How do people prolong life? Eat Yuchi（玉豉）." Yuchi（玉豉）is Diyu［地榆, garden burnetroot, Radix Sanguisorbae］, and Jinyan（金盐）is Wujiapi（slenderstyle acanthopanax bark）. The reason why they get such names is that Yan［盐, salt］has the taste of water, and Chi［豉, fermented soybean］means grain and water. Both of them receive the water essence of earlier heaven to nourish the five zang-organs. Ancient people said that they would rather have a handful of Wujiapi（slenderstyle acanthopanax bark）than a cartful of gold and jade, and would rather have one Jin of Diyu（garden burnet root）than the bright moon and valuable pearls. The mother of Duke Ding of Lu State in the Spring and Autumn Period left her human body in the secular world and flew up to the heaven to be an immortal by drinking liquor made from Wujiapi（slenderstyle acanthopanax bark）. Zhang Zisheng（张子声）, Yang Jianshi（杨建始）, Wang Shuya（王叔牙）, Yu Shiyan（于世彦）, etc. all drank the liquor, which made them able to have excessive sexual activities and have a lifespan of 300 years. It can also be made into powder to replace tea for drinking. It is also said to be the essence of Wuche（five coaches）Star. Water corresponds with five lakes, human beings with five virtues, positions with five directions and things with five Che（coaches）. So green essence enters the stalk, which will have the liquid of the east. White qi enters the node, which will have fluids of the west. Red qi enters the flower, which will have light of the south. Black essence enters the root, which will have maltose of the north. Yellow qi enters the bark, which will have center（Wu and Ji）sprit. The interchange and transformation of spirit qi of the five positions produces Wujiapi（slenderstyle acanthopanax bark）. Taking it can become immortal and rejuvenated. It is a top-grade medicinal for health preservation. There is no record that long-term taking of it will prolong life in *Shen Nong Ben Cao Jing*［《神农本草经》, *Shennong's Classic of Materia Medica*］, probably because such record was lost in handing down the book.

34. 肉苁蓉

肉苁蓉 气味甘,微温,无毒。主五劳七伤,补中,除茎中寒热痛,养五脏,强阴,益精气,多子,妇人症瘕。久服轻身。

肉苁蓉《吴氏本草》名松容,又名黑司命。始出河西山谷及代州雁门,今以陇西者为胜,北国者次之,乃野马之精入于土中而生。陇西者形扁色黄,柔润多花,其味甘。北国者形短少花,生时似肉,三四月掘根,长尺余,绳穿阴干,八月始好。皮有松子鳞甲,故名松容。马属午畜,以少阴为正化,子水为对化,故名黑司命。朱丹溪曰:肉苁蓉罕得,多以金莲根用盐制而伪充,或以草苁蓉代之,用者宜审。苏恭曰:草苁蓉功用稍劣。

马为火畜,精属水阴,苁蓉感马精而生,其形似肉,气味甘温,盖禀少阴水火之气,而归于太阴坤土之药也。土性柔和,故有苁蓉之名。五劳者,志劳、思劳、烦劳、忧劳、恚劳也。七伤者,喜、怒、忧、悲、思、恐、惊,七情所伤也。水火阴阳之气,会归中土,则五劳七伤可治矣。得太阴坤土之精,故补中。得少阴水火之气,故除茎中寒热痛。阴阳水火之气,归于太阴坤土之中,故养五脏。强阴者,火气盛也。益精者,水气盛也。多子者,水火阴阳皆盛也。妇人症瘕,乃血精留聚于郛郭之中,土气盛,则症瘕自消。而久服轻身。

34. Roucongrong［肉苁蓉, desertliving cistanche, Herba Cistanches］

It is sweet in taste, slightly warm and non-toxic in property, and it is mainly used to treat five kinds of overstrains and seven kinds of damages, tonify the middle, resolve cold and heat as well as the pain in the penis, nourish the five zang-organs, strengthen yin, replenish essence and qi, increase fertility and disperse female abdominal mass. Long-term taking of it will keep healthy.

It is mentioned as Songrong (松容) or Heisiming (黑司命) in *Wu Shi Ben Cao* [《吴氏本草》, *Wu Pu's Studies of Materia Medica*]. Firstly recorded to be growing in the valleys of Hexi (河西) and in Yanmen (雁门) of Daizhou (代州), now those growing in Longxi (陇西) are of better quality, and those growing in Beiguo (北国) are next to them. It grows out of the essence of wild horse seeping into the earth. Flat in shape, yellow in color, sweet in taste, those growing in Longxi (陇西) are soft with a lot of flowers. Short in shape, those growing in Beiguo (北国) grow fewer flowers and are like flesh when they are raw. Its root dug out in the third and fourth lunar months is about one Chi long. Rope its roots and dry them in the shade till the eighth lunar month. Its bark has imbricate fleshy scales, so it is called Songrong (松容). Horses, pertaining to Wu [午, the seventh of the twelve Earthly Branches], use lesser yin as normal transformation and Zi [子, the first of the twelve Earthly Branches] water as opposite transformation, so it is called Heisiming (黑司命). Zhu Danxi (朱丹溪) said, "Roucongrong (desertliving cistanche) is very rare, so people mostly use the salted root of Diyong Jinlian [地涌金莲, musella, Musellae Flos] to fake it or Caocongrong [草苁蓉, boschniakia, Boschniakiae Herba] to replace it. So we should carefully examine it when using it." Sugong (苏恭) said, "Caocongrong (boschniakia) is of slightly inferior effect."

The horse is an animal pertaining to fire, and its essence pertains to water yin. Roucongrong (desertliving cistanche), growing out of horse essence, is flesh-like in shape, sweet in taste and warm in property, because it is a medicinal which pertains to Kun earth from greater yin by receiving the qi of water and fire from lesser yin. Earth is soft in property, so it is called Congrong (苁蓉). Five kinds of overstrains are the overstrains caused by memory, thought, vexation, anxiety and anger. Seven kinds of damages are the damages caused by seven affects which are joy, anger, anxiety, sorrow, thought, fear, and fright. The qi of water, fire, yin and yang all pertain to center earth, and then five kinds of overstrains and seven kinds of damages can be treated. It receives the essence of Kun earth from greater yin, so it can be used to tonify the middle. It receives the qi of water and fire from lesser yin, so it can be used to resolve cold and heat as well as the pain in the penis. The qi of water, fire, yin and yang all pertain to Kun earth from greater yin, so it can be used to nourish the five zang-organs. Strengthening yin will need exuberant fire qi. Replenishing essence will need exuberant water qi. Increasing fertility will need to be exuberant in water, fire, yin and yang. Female abdominal mass is caused by the retention of blood and essence in the uterus. It will be treated when earth qi is exuberant. So long-term taking of it will keep healthy.

35. 巴戟天

巴戟天 气味辛甘,微温,无毒。主大风邪气,阴痿不起,强筋骨,安五脏,补中,增志,益气。

巴戟天一名不凋草,始出巴郡及下邳山谷,今江淮河东州郡亦有,然不及川蜀者佳。叶似茗,经冬不凋,根如连珠,白紫色,以连珠多,肉厚者为胜。

巴戟生于巴蜀,气味辛甘,禀太阴金土之气化。其性微温,经冬不凋,又禀太阳标阳之气化。主治大风邪气者,得太阴之金气,金能制风也。治阴痿不起,强筋骨者,得太阳之标阳,阳能益阴也。安五脏,补中者,得太阴之土气,土气盛,则安五脏而补中。增志者,肾藏志而属水,太阳天气,下连于水也。益气者,肺主气而属金,太阴天气,外合于肺也。

35. Bajitian [巴戟天, morinda root, Radix Morindae Officinalis]

It is pungent and sweet in taste, slightly warm and non-toxic in property, and it is mainly used to treat the leprosy caused by pathogenic qi, resolve impotence, strengthen the sinews and bones, harmonize the five zang-organs, tonify the middle, increase intelligence and replenish qi.

It is also called Budiaocao [不凋草, non-withered grass]. Firstly recorded to be growing in the mountain valleys of Bajun (巴郡) and Xiapi (下邳), now it also grows in Jianghuai (江淮) and Hedong (河东), but it is not of better quality than that growing in Chuanshu (川蜀). Its leaves are like those of tea and do not wither even in winter. Its root, white-purple in color, is like a chain of pearls. Those with more chains of pearls and thick flesh are of better quality.

Growing in Bashu（巴蜀）, pungent and sweet in taste, it receives the qi transformation of metal and earth from lesser yin. Slightly warm in property, it does not wither even in winter and also receives the qi transformation of branch yang from greater yang. It can mainly treat the leprosy caused by pathogenic qi, because it receives metal qi from lesser yin, and metal can control wind. It can resolve impotence and strengthen the sinews and bones, because it receives branch yang from greater yang, and yang can benefit yin. It can also harmonize the five zang-organs and tonify the middle, because it receives the earth qi from lesser yin, and if the earth qi is exuberant, then the five zang-organs will be harmonized, and the middle will be tonified. It can increase intelligence, because intelligence is stored in the kidney which pertains to water, and the heaven qi from greater yang connects water downward. It can replenish qi, because the lung, pertaining to metal, governs qi, and the heaven qi from lesser yin corresponds with the lung externally.

36. 五味子

五味子 气味酸温,无毒。主益气,咳逆上气,劳伤羸瘦,补不足,强阴,益男子精。

五味子《别录》名玄及,始出齐山山谷及代郡,今河东陕西州郡尤多,杭越间亦有,故有南北之分。南产者,色红核圆。北产者,色红兼黑,核形似猪肾。凡用以北产者为佳。蔓生,茎赤色,花黄,白子,生青熟紫,亦具五色,实具五味,皮肉甘酸,核中辛苦,都有咸味,味虽有五,酸味居多。名玄及者,谓禀水精而及于木也。都有咸味,则禀水精。酸味居多,则及于木。盖五行之气,本于先天之气,而生后天之木也。

五味子色味咸五,乃禀五运之精,气味酸温,得东方生长之气,故主益气。肺主呼吸,发原于肾,上下相交,咳逆上气,则肺肾不交。五味子能启肾脏之水精,上交于肺,故治咳逆上气。本于先天之水,化生后天之木,则五脏相生,精气充足,故治劳伤羸瘦,补不足。核形象肾,入口生津,故主强阴。女子不足于血,男子不足于精,故益男子精。

36. Wuweizi〔五味子, Chinese magnoliavine fruit, Fructus Schisandrae Chinensis〕

It is sour in taste, warm and non-toxic in property, and it is mainly used to replenish qi, treat cough with dyspnea, descend adverse-rising qi, resolve overstrain with emaciation, tonify insufficiency, strengthen yin and replenish the male semen.

Wuweizi (Chinese magnoliavine fruit) is mentioned as Xuanji (玄及) in *Ming Yi Bie Lu* 〔《名医别录》, *Miscellaneous Records of Famous Physicians*〕. Firstly recorded to be growing in the valleys of Qishan Mountain (齐山) and Daijun (代郡), now it grows in a large amount in Hedong (河东) and Shaanxi (陕西) Province and also in Hangyue (杭越). So those growing in the south are different from those growing in the north. Those growing in the south are red in color with round pits while those growing in the north are red-black in color with pig-kidney-like pits. For medicinal use, those growing in the north are of better quality. It is a kind of trailing plant and has red stalks, yellow flowers and white seeds. It is green when unripe and purple when ripe. Altogether it can be in five colors and have five tastes. Its skin and flesh are sour-sweet in taste, and the inside of the pit is pungent and bitter in taste. All of them can be salty in taste. Although it has five tastes, it is mainly sour in taste. It is also called Xuanji (玄及), because it receives water essence and can grow into wood. All its parts are salty in taste, because it receives water essence. It is mainly sour in taste, manifesting that it can grow into wood. This is because the qi of five elements originates from earlier heaven qi and generates later heaven wood.

It is in five colors and has five tastes, because it receives the essence of five circuits. It is sour in taste and warm in property, because it obtains the growing qi of the east. Therefore, it can mainly replenish qi. The lung governs the breath, which originates from the kidney. The lung in the upper part and the kidney in the lower part interact with each other. The cough with dyspnea and adverse-rising qi manifests that the lung and the kidney do not interact with each other. It can activate the water essence of the kidney to make the kidney interact upward with the lung, so it can be used to treat cough with dyspnea and descend adverse-rising qi. It originates from earlier heaven water and transforms into later heaven wood. Thus, the five zang-organs will promote each other, and essential qi will be sufficient. So it can be used to resolve overstrain with emaciation and tonify insufficiency. Its pit is kidney-like in shape and engenders fluid in the mouth. So it can mainly strengthen yin. Insufficiency of the female lies in the blood while insufficiency of the male lies in the semen. So it can replenish male semen.

37．蛇床子

蛇床子 气味苦辛,无毒。主男子阴痿湿痒,妇人阴中肿痛,除痹气,利关节,癫痫,恶疮。久服轻身,好颜色。辛,旧作平,今改正。

蛇床子《本经》名蛇粟,又名蛇米。《尔雅》名虺床,以虺蛇喜卧于下,嗜食其子,故有此名。始出临淄川谷及田野湿地,今所在皆有。三月生苗,高二三尺,叶青碎作丛似蒿,每枝上有花头百余,同结一窠,四五月开花白色,子如黍粒,黄褐色。

蛇床子气味苦辛,其性温热,得少阴君火之气。主治男子阴痿湿痒,妇人阴中肿痛,禀火气而下济其阴寒也。除痹气,利关节,禀火气而外通其经脉也。心气虚而寒邪盛,则癫痫。心气虚而热邪盛,则生恶疮。蛇床味苦性温,能助心气,故治癫痫恶疮。久服则火土相生,故轻身。心气充盛,故好颜色。

蛇,阴类也。蛇床子性温热,蛇虺喜卧于中,嗜食其子,犹山鹿之嗜水龟,潜龙之嗜飞燕,盖取彼之所有,以资己之所无,故阴痿虚寒,所宜用也。

李时珍曰:蛇床子,《神农》列之上品,不独助男子,且有益妇人,乃世人舍此而求补药于远域,且近时但用为疮药,惜哉。

37. Shechuangzi〔蛇床子, common chidium fruit, Fructus Cnidii〕

It is bitter in taste, pungent and non-toxic in property, and it is mainly used to treat impotence, resolve man's itching due to dampness, treat swelling and the pain of the vulva, eliminate impediment, dredge the joints, and treat epilepsy and malign sores. Long-term taking of it will keep healthy and luster complexion. It was mild rather than pungent in property in the past. Now this is corrected.

In *Shen Nong Ben Cao Jing* [《神农本草经》, *Shennong's Classic of Materia Medica*], it is mentioned as Shesu (蛇粟) or Shemi (蛇米). In the book *Er Ya* [《尔雅》, *On Elegance*], it is mentioned as Huichuang (虺床), because Hui (虺) snake (poisonous snake) likes lying in it and eating its seeds. Firstly recorded to be growing in the valleys, fields and wetlands of Linzi (临淄), now it grows everywhere. It grows seedlings in the third lunar month, which will be two to three Chi high. It has fine green leaves, forming clumps like those of Qinghao [青蒿, sweet wormwood, Artemisiae Annuae Herba]. Every branch has hundreds of flower heads sharing one base. It blossoms with white flowers in the fourth and fifth lunar month, and its seeds are like Shumi [黍米, broomcorn millet, Panici Miliacei Semen] with yellowish-brown color.

Shechuangzi (common chidium fruit), bitter in taste, pungent, warm and hot in property, obtains the qi of sovereign fire from lesser yin. It can mainly treat impotence, resolve man's itching due to dampness, and treat swelling and the pain of the vulva, because it can go downward to aid yin cold by receiving fire qi. It can eliminate impediment and dredge the joints, because it can go outside to dredge the meridians by receiving fire qi. Insufficient heart qi and intense cold pathogen will cause epilepsy while insufficient heart qi and intense hot pathogen will cause malign sores. Shechuangzi (common chnidium fruit) is bitter in taste and warm in property and can assist heart qi, so it can treat epilepsy and malign sores. Long-term taking of it will lead to the mutual generation of fire and earth, so it can keep healthy. Sufficient and exuberant heart qi will luster complexion.

The snake pertains to the category of yin. Shechuangzi (common chnidium fruit) is warm and hot in property. Hui snakes (poisonous snakes) like lying in Shechuangzi (common chnidium fruit) and eating its seeds, which is like that deer are fond of eating turtles and dragons are fond of eating flying swallows. All these show that they take what they do not have from others to improve themselves, so Shechuangzi (common chnidium fruit) is suitable for impotence and deficiency cold.

Li Shizhen (李时珍) said, "In *Shen Nong Ben Cao Jing* [《神农本草经》, *Shennong's Classic of Materia Medica*], it is classified as top grade. It not only assists men, but benefits women. However, people ask for tonic formula in remote areas instead of using it, and use it only as medicinal for sores nowadays. What a pity!"

38. 覆盆子

覆盆子 气味酸平,无毒。主安五脏,益精气,长阴,令人坚,强志倍力,有子。久服轻身不老。

《别录》名覆盆。《本经》名蓬蘽。始出荆山平泽及冤句,今处处有之。藤蔓繁衍,茎有倒刺,就蒂结实,生则青黄,熟则紫黯,微有黑色,状如熟葚,至冬苗叶不凋。马志曰:蓬蘽乃覆盆之苗,覆盆乃蓬蘽之子,李时珍曰:蓬蘽、覆盆一类二种,覆盆早熟,蓬蘽晚熟。然近时只知有覆盆,不知有蓬蘽矣。愚以覆盆、蓬蘽功用相同,故合而为一。

《本经》名蓬蘽,以其藤蔓繁衍,苗叶不凋,结子则蓬蓬而蘽蘽也。《别录》名覆盆,以其形圆而扁,如釜如盆,就蒂结实,倒垂向下,一如盆之下覆也。气味酸平,藤蔓繁衍,具春生夏长之气,覆下如盆。得秋时之金气,冬叶不凋。得冬令之水精,结实形圆。具中央之土气,体备四时,质合五行,故主安五脏。肾受五脏之精而藏之,故益精气而长阴。肾气充足,则令人坚,强志倍力,有子。是覆盆虽安五脏,补肾居多,所以然者,水天上下之气,交相轮应也。天气下覆,水气上升,故久服轻身不老。

38. Fupengzi〔覆盆子, palmleaf raspberry fruit, Fructus Rubi〕

It is sour in taste, mild and non-toxic in property, and it is mainly used to harmonize the five zang-organs, replenish essential qi, enlarge and harden the penis, strengthen memory, replenish energy and enable people to conceive babies. Long-term taking of it will keep healthy and prevent aging.

It is also mentioned as Fupen (覆盆) in *Ming Yi Bie Lu*〔《名医别录》, *Miscellaneous Records of Famous Physicians*〕and Penglei (蓬蘽) in *Shen Nong Ben Cao Jing*〔《神农本草经》, *Shennong's Classic of Materia Medica*〕. Firstly recorded to be growing in the lakes and fields of Jingshan (荆山) and Yuanju (冤句), now it grows everywhere. It has luxuriant vines, and its stalk has barbed thorns. Its fruit grows from the base, which is green-yellow in color when unripe and dark purple with slight blackness in color when ripe. The shape of its fruit is similar to that of the ripe Sangshenzi［桑葚子, mulberry, Mori Fructus］. Its seedlings and leaves do not wither even in winter. Mazhi（马志）said, "Its seedling is called Penglei（蓬蘽）, and its fruit is called Fupen（覆盆）."Li Shizhen（李时珍）said, "Penglei（蓬蘽）and Fupen（覆盆）are two species pertaining to the same family. Fupen（覆盆）is early-maturing and Penglei（蓬蘽）is late-maturing."But nowadays, only Fupen（覆盆）is commonly known while Penglei（蓬蘽）is seldom known. I think that Fupen（覆盆）and Penglei（蓬蘽）have the same effect, so I merge them into one.

It is mentioned as Penglei（蓬蘽）in *Shen Nong Ben Cao Jing*［《神农本草经》, *Shennong's Classic of Materia Medica*］, because it has luxuriant vines, evergreen seedlings and leaves and clusters of fruits. It is mentioned as Fupen（覆盆）in *Ming Yi Bie Lu*［《名医别录》, *Miscellaneous Records of Famous Physicians*］, because its fruit is round and flat in shape, just like a pan or a basin. Its fruit grows from the base and droops like an overturned basin. Sour in taste and mild in property, it has the qi of spring resuscitation and summer growth with luxuriant vines. Its fruit is like an overturned basin. It obtains the metal qi of autumn, which allows it to have evergreen leaves. It obtains the water essence of winter, which allows it to bear round fruits. With earth qi of the center, it is in accordance with the four seasons and five elements, so it can mainly harmonize the five zang-organs. The kidney stores the essence of the five zang-organs which can in turn nourish the kidney, so it is used to replenish essential qi and enlarge the penis. With sufficient kidney qi, the penis will be hardened, memory will be strengthened, energy will be replenished and people will be able to conceive babies. So although it is used to harmonize the five zang-organs, it is mainly used to tonify the kidney. The reason is that the upward qi and downward qi of water and heaven are interrelated and interact on each other. Heaven qi goes downward while water qi goes upward, so long-term taking of it will keep healthy and prevent aging.

39. 菟丝子

菟丝子　气味辛甘平,无毒。主续绝伤,补不足,益气力,肥健人。《别录》

云：久服明目、轻身延年。

　　菟丝子《尔雅》名玉女。《诗》名女萝。始出朝鲜川泽田野，盖禀水阴之气，从东方而生，今处处有之。夏生苗，如丝遍地，不能自起，得他草梗则缠绕而上，其根即绝于地，寄生空中，无叶有花，香气袭人，结实如秕豆而细，色黄。法当温水淘去沙泥，酒浸一宿，曝干捣用。又法，酒浸四五日，蒸曝四五次，研作饼，焙干用。

　　凡草木子实，得水湿清凉之气后能发芽。菟丝子得沸汤火热之气，而有丝芽吐出，盖禀性纯阴，得热气而发也。气味辛甘，得手足太阴天地之气化，寄生空中，丝茎缭绕，故主续绝伤。续绝伤，故能补不足。补不足，故能益气力。益气力，故能肥健人。兔乃明月之精，故久服明目。阴精所奉其人寿，故轻身延年。

39. Tusizi［菟丝子, dodder seed, Semen Cuscutae］

It is pungent and sweet in taste, mild and non-toxic in property, and it is mainly used to treat the fracture of bones and sinews, tonify insufficiency, replenish qi and energy, and fortify the body. *Ming Yi Bie Lu*［《名医别录》, *Miscellaneous Records of Famous Physicians*］says that long-term taking of it will improve vision, keep healthy and prolong life.

It is mentioned as Yunü（玉女）in *Er Ya*［《尔雅》, *On Elegance*］and Nüluo（女萝）in *Shi Jing*［《诗经》, *The Book of Songs*］. Firstly recorded to be growing in the rivers, lakes and fields of Chaoxian（朝鲜）, because it receives the qi of water yin, which makes it originate from the east. Now it grows everywhere. In summer, it sprouts, with its seedlings covering the ground like silk and unable to go upright naturally. When the seedlings are close to other plants, they will twine around them. Then its root will be out of the soil and grow in the air. Without leaves, it has fragrant flowers. Its fruit, yellow in color, is like a blighted bean, but thinner. For medicinal use, wash its dirt out with warm water, soak it in liquor overnight, dry it in the sun and pound it. Or soak it in liquor for four or five days, steam and dry it in the sun four or five times and grind it to make a cake before baking.

The seeds or fruit of any plant will sprout after obtaining the cool qi of wet water. However, it cannot sprout unless it obtains the hot qi of boiling water because it is pure yin in property. Therefore, it can only sprout after it obtains hot qi. Pungent and sweet in taste, it receives the qi transformation of hand greater yin lung channel (heaven) and foot greater yin spleen channel (earth). Growing in the air, its thin stalks twine, so it can mainly treat the fracture of the bones and sinews, which further leads to the tonification of insufficiency. Tonifying insufficiency can lead to the replenishing of qi and energy, which further leads to the fortifying of the body. The rabbit grows out of the essence of the bright moon, so long-term taking of it can improve vision. Those who are nourished by yin essence will live a long life, so it can keep healthy and prolong life.

40. 沙 参

沙参　气味苦,微寒,无毒。主血结惊气,除寒热,补中,益肺气。《别录》云:久服利人。

　　沙参一名白参,以其根色名也。又名羊乳。俚人呼为羊婆奶,以其根茎折之皆有白汁也。始出河内川谷及冤句、般阳,今淄齐、潞随、江淮、荆湖州郡,及处处山原有之。喜生近水沙地中。

　　沙参生于近水之沙地,其性全寒,苦中带甘,故曰微寒,色白多汁,禀金水之精气。血结惊气者,荣气内虚,故血结而惊气也。寒热者,卫气外虚,故肌表不和而寒热也。补中者,补中焦之精汁。补中则血结惊气可治矣。益肺者,益肺气于皮毛,益肺则寒热可除矣。所以然者,禀水精而补中,禀金精而益肺也。久服则血气调而荣卫和,故利人。

　　愚按:《本经》人参味甘,沙参味苦,性皆微寒。后人改人参微温,沙参味甘,不知人参味甘,甘中稍苦,故曰微寒。沙参全寒,苦中带甘,故曰微寒。先圣立言自有深意,后人不思体会而审察之,擅改圣经,误人最甚。

40. Shashen [沙参, root of coastal glehnia, Radix Glehniae]

It is bitter in taste, slightly cold and non-toxic in property, and it is mainly used to resolve the blood stasis with fright and convulsion, eliminate cold and heat, tonify the middle and replenish lung qi. According to *Ming Yi Bie Lu* [《名医别录》, *Miscellaneous Records of Famous Physicians*], long-term taking of it will be beneficial to people's health.

It is also called Baishen（白参）due to the white color of its roots. It is also called Yangru（羊乳）, and the people of Li（俚）nationality called it Yangponai（羊婆奶）, because there will be white juice when its root or stalk is broken. Firstly recorded to be growing in the valleys of Henei（河内）and in Yuanju（冤句）and Banyang（般阳）, now it grows in Ziqi（淄齐）, Lusui（潞随）, Jianghuai（江淮）and Jinghu（荆湖）as well as everywhere in the mountain and on the plain. It tends to grow in the sandy area near water.

Growing in the sandy area near water, it is totally cold in property and bitter with sweetness in taste. So it can be said to be slightly cold in property. It is juicy and white in color and receives the essential qi of metal and water. The blood stasis with fright and convulsion is caused by the insufficiency of nutrient qi. Cold and heat is caused by the insufficiency of defensive qi and the resulting disharmony of fleshy exterior. To tonify the middle is to tonify the essential juice of the middle energizer. Tonifying the middle can treat the blood stasis with fright and convulsion. To tonify the lung is to replenish lung qi by acting on the skin and hair. Tonifying lung can eliminate cold and heat. The reason is that receiving water essence will tonify the middle, and receiving metal essence will tonify the lung. Long-term taking of it can lead to the harmony of blood and qi which will further lead to the harmony of nutrient qi and defensive qi. So it will be beneficial to people's health.

Note by Zhang Zhicong（张志聪）: According to *Shen Nong Ben Cao Jing* [《神农本草经》, *Shennong's Classic of Materia Medica*], Renshen [人参, ginseng, Ginseng Radix] is sweet in taste while Shashen（root of coastal glehnia）is bitter in taste, but both of them are slightly cold is property. However, people later on changed the property of Renshen（ginseng）into slightly warm and the taste of Shashen（root of coastal glehnia）into sweet. Neither did they know that Renshen（ginseng）is said to be slightly cold in property because it is sweet with slightly bitterness in taste. Nor did they know that Shashen（root of coastal glehnia）is also said to be slightly cold in property because although totally cold in property, it is bitter with sweetness in taste. There is a deep meaning in what the ancestor sages wrote. People later on did not understand and study it carefully, but just revised the classic works related to materia medica arbitrarily, which has caused the most misleading and harmful consequence.

41. 泽 泻

泽泻 气味甘寒,无毒。主风寒湿痹,乳难,养五脏,益气力,肥健,消水。久服耳目聪明,不饥延年,轻身,面生光,能行水上。

泽泻《本经》名水泻,主泻水上行故名。始出汝南池泽,今近道皆有,唯汉中者为佳。生浅水中,独茎直上,根圆如芋,有毛。

泽泻,水草也。气味甘寒,能启水阴之气上滋中土。主治风寒湿痹者,启在下之水津,从中土而灌溉于肌腠皮肤也。乳者,中焦之汁,水津滋于中土,故治乳难。五脏受水谷之精,泽泻泻泽于中土,故养五脏。肾者作强之官,水精上资,故益气力。从中土而灌溉于肌腠,故肥健。水气上而后下,故消水。久服耳目聪明者,水济其火也。不饥延年者,水滋其土也。轻身面生光者,水泽外注也。能行水上者,言此耳目聪明,不饥延年,轻身,面生光,以其能行在下之水,而使之上也。

41. Zexie〔泽泻, oriental waterplantain rhizome, Rhizoma Alismatis〕

It is sweet in taste, cold and non-toxic in property, and it is mainly used to treat the impediment due to wind, cold and the dampness and the difficulty in lactation, nourish the five zang-organs, replenish qi and energy, fortify the body and relieve edema. Long-term taking of it can improve hearing and vision, tolerate hunger, prolong life, keep healthy, luster complexion and make people feel weightless just like walking over the river.

In *Shen Nong Ben Cao Jing*〔《神农本草经》, *Shennong's Classic of Materia Medica*〕it is mentioned as Shuixie (水泻), because it is mainly used to drain water so as to make it flow upward. Firstly recorded to be growing in the lakes and pools of Runan (汝南), now it grows everywhere nearby, and those growing in Hanzhong (汉中) are of good quality. Growing in shallow water, its stalks grow straight upward. Its hairy root is round in shape like Yutou〔芋头, taro, Colocasiae Tuber〕.

In fact, it is a kind of water weed. Sweet in taste and cold in property, it can activate the qi of water yin to move upward to nourish center earth. It can mainly treat the impediment due to wind, cold and dampness, because it can activate the water fluid of the lower part to nourish the interstices of the muscles and the skin from center earth. Milk is the juice of the middle energizer. Water fluid is nourished by center earth, so it can be used to treat the difficulty in lactation. The five-zang organs are nourished by the essence of water and grain. Zexie (oriental waterplantain rhizome) drains water into center earth, so it can be used to nourish the five zang-organs. The kidney is the organ similar to an official with great power, which is nourished by upward water essence, so it can be used to replenish qi and energy. The interstices of the muscles are nourished by center earth, so it can be used to fortify the body. Water qi moves upward and then downward, so it can be used to relieve edema. Long-term taking of it can improve hearing and vision, because water can aid fire. It can be used to tolerate hunger and prolong life, because water can nourish earth. It can be used to keep healthy and luster complexion, because water can nourish the external. It can be used to make people feel weightless just like walking over a river, because it can be used to improve hearing and vision, tolerate hunger, prolong life, keep healthy and luster complexion, which means it can make the water in the lower part move upward.

42. 菖 蒲

菖蒲 气味辛温,无毒。主风寒湿痹,咳逆上气,开心孔,补五脏,通九窍,明耳目,出音声,主耳聋痈疮,温肠胃,止小便利。久服轻身、不忘、不迷惑,延年,益心智,高志,不老。

菖蒲处处有之,种类不一。其生流水中,根茎络石,略无少土,稍有泥滓即易凋萎,此种入药为良。李时珍曰:菖蒲凡五种,生于水石之间,根细节密者,名石菖蒲,可入药。余皆不堪。此草新旧相代,四时常青,《罗浮山记》言:山中菖蒲一寸二十节。抱朴子言:服食以一寸九节、紫花者尤善。苏东坡曰:凡草生石上者,必须微土,以附其根,唯石菖蒲濯去泥土,渍以清水置盆中,可数十年不枯。

太阳之气,生于水中,上与肺金相合而主表,与君火相合而主神。菖蒲生于水石之中,气味辛温,乃禀太阳寒水之气,而上合于心肺之药也。主治风寒湿痹,咳逆上气者,太阳之气,上与肺气相合而出于肌表也。开心孔者,太阳之气,上与心气相合而运其神机也。五脏在内,九窍在外,肝开窍于二目,心开窍于二耳,肺开窍于二鼻,脾开窍于口,肾开窍于前后二阴。菖蒲禀寒水之精,能濡五脏之窍,故内补五脏,外通九窍,明耳目,出音声,是通耳目口鼻之上窍也。又曰:主耳聋、痈疮者,言耳不能听而为耳痈、耳疮之证。菖蒲并能治之。温肠胃,止小便利,是通前后二阴之下窍也。菖蒲气味辛温,性唯上行,故温肠胃而止小便之过利。久服则阳气盛,故轻身。心气盛,故不忘,寒水之精,太阳之阳,标本相合,故不迷惑而延年。益心智者,菖蒲益心,心灵则智生,高志不老者,水精充足,则肾志高强,其人能寿而不老。

42. Changpu〔菖蒲, acorus, Acorus Calamus〕

It is pungent in taste, warm and non-toxic in property, and it is mainly used to treat the impediment due to wind, cold and dampness as well as cough with dyspnea, descend adverse-rising qi, open heart orifice, tonify the five zang-organs, relieve the nine orifices and improve hearing, vision and voice. It is also mainly used to treat deafness as well as welling-abscesses and the sores of the ears, warm the intestines and stomach, and resolve frequent urination. Long-term taking of it can keep healthy, prevent amnesia, avoid confusion, prolong life, improve mentality, strengthen memory and prevent aging.

Growing everywhere, it has a variety of kinds. It grows in running water. Seldom is there earth on its root and stalks which twine around the rock, otherwise it will wither. Those growing like this are good to be used as medicinal. Li Shizhen (李时珍) said, "There are five kinds of Changpu (acorus). Those growing on rocks in water with thin roots and dense nodes are called Shichangpu〔石菖蒲, acorus, Acori Tatarinowii Rhizoma〕, which can be used as medicinal, and the other four kinds cannot." It is continuously replaced by the new one, so it is evergreen all the year round. *Luo Fu Shan Ji*〔《罗浮山记》, *Essays Written in Luofu Mountain*〕says, "Changpu (acorus) growing in the mountain is one Cun long with twenty nodes." Baopuzi (抱朴子)

said, "It is the best to eat the one which is one Cun long with nine nodes and purple flowers." Su Dongpo（苏东坡）said, "Any plant growing on the rock should have some earth for its root to grow, but only earth on Shichangpu（石菖蒲）can be washed off, and it will not wither for decades if it is put in a basin full of water."

The qi of greater yang, originating from water, is in accordance with lung metal upward to govern branch and is in accordance with sovereign fire to govern spirit. Growing in water and on the rock, Changpu (acorus) is pungent in taste and warm in property. Receiving the qi of cold water from greater yang, it is a medicinal in accordance with the heart and lung upward. It is mainly used to treat the impediment due to wind, cold and dampness as well as cough with dyspnea and descend adverse-rising qi, because the qi of greater yang can be in accordance with lung qi upward to move out to reach the fleshy exterior. It is used to open heart orifice, because the qi of greater yang can be in accordance with heart qi upward to invigorate vital activity. The five zang-organs are inside while the nine orifices are outside. The liver opens the two orifices at the eyes, the heart opens the two orifices at the ears, the lung opens the two orifices at the nostrils, the spleen opens the orifice at the mouth, and the kidney opens the two orifices at anterior yin (genital orifice) and posterior yin (the anus). Changpu (acorus) receives the essence of cold water to moisten the orifices of the five-zang organs. So it can be used to tonify the five zang-organs inside and relieve the nine orifices outside. To improve hearing, vision and voice is to dredge the upper orifices of the ears, eyes, mouth and nostrils. It can also mainly treat deafness as well as welling-abscesses and the sores of the ears. Deafness can cause welling-abscesses and the sores of the ears. All the diseases mentioned above can be treated by Changpu (acorus). To warm the intestines and stomach and resolve frequent urination are to dredge the lower orifices of anterior yin (genital orifice) and posterior yin (the anus). Changpu (acorus) is pungent in taste and warm in property. It tends to go upward, so it can be used to warm the intestines and stomach and resolve frequent urination. Long-term taking of it can make yang qi exuberant thus to keep healthy. Exuberant heart qi will prevent amnesia. The combination of the essence of cold water and yang of greater yang is the combination of branches and roots. So it can be used to avoid confusion and prolong life. It can be used to improve mentality, because it is beneficial to mind, and a keen mind leads to the increase of intelligence. It can be used to strengthen memory and prevent aging, because sufficient water essence can strengthen kidney will, which will help people live a long life and prevent aging.

43. 远 志

远志 气味苦温,无毒。主咳逆伤中,补不足,除邪气,利九窍,益智慧,耳目聪明,不忘,强志倍力。久服轻身不老。

远志始出太山及冤句川谷,今河洛陕西州郡皆有之。苗名小草,三月开红花,四月采根晒干,用者去心取皮。李时珍曰:服之主益智强志,故有远志之称。

远志气味苦温,根荄骨硬,禀少阴心肾之气化。苦温者,心也。骨硬者,肾也。心肾不交,则咳逆伤中。远志主交通心肾,故治咳逆伤中。补不足者,补心肾之不足。除邪气者,除心肾之邪气。利九窍者,水精上濡空窍于阳,下行二便于阴也。神志相通,则益智慧。智慧益,则耳目聪明。心气盛,则不忘。肾气足,则强志倍力。若久服,则轻身不老。抱朴子云:陵阳子仲服远志二十年,有子三十七人,开书所视,记而不忘,此轻身不老之一征也。

43. Yuanzhi〔远志, milkwort root, Radix Polygalae〕

It is bitter in taste, warm and non-toxic in property, and it is mainly used to treat cough with dyspnea and internal damage, tonify insufficiency, eliminate pathogenic qi, disinhibit the nine orifices, enhance wisdom, improve hearing and vision, prevent amnesia, strengthen memory and replenish energy. Long-term taking of it will keep healthy and prevent aging.

Firstly recorded to be growing in the river valleys of Taishan Mountain (太山) and those of Yuanju (冤句), now it grows everywhere in Heluo (河洛) and Shaanxi (陕西) Province. Its seedlings are called Xiaocao (小草). It blossoms with red flowers in the third lunar month. Collect its roots in the fourth lunar month and dry them in the sun. Peel the dried ones and remove their inner hearts for medicinal use. Li Shizhen（李时珍）said, "Taking it can mainly enhance wisdom and strengthen memory, so it is called Yuanzhi（远志）."

It is bitter in taste and warmin property, and its root is as hard as bones. It receives the qi transformation of the heart and kidney from lesser yin. Being bitter in taste and warmin property is related to the heart. Its root being as hard as bones is related to the kidney. If the heart and kidney do not interact with each other, it will cause cough with dyspnea and internal damage. It can mainly connect the heart and kidney, so it can be used to treat cough with dyspnea and internal damage. To tonify insufficiency is to tonify the insufficiency of the heart and kidney. To eliminate pathogenic qi is to eliminate the pathogenic qi of the heart and kidney. The process of disinhibiting the nine orifices is that water essence goes upward to moisten the upper yang orifices and downward to disinhibit urination and purge defecation in the two lower yin orifices. If spirit and memory are connected, wisdom will be enhanced. If wisdom is enhanced, hearing and vision will be improved. If heart qi is exuberant, amnesia will be prevented. If kidney qi is sufficient, memory will be strengthened and energy will be replenished. Long-term taking of it will keep healthy and prevent aging. Bao Puzi（抱朴子）said, "Zi Zhong（子仲）of Lingyang（陵阳）has taken Yuanzhi（milkwort root）for twenty years, so he can have thirty-seven sons. He can memorize anything he reads. It is an example of Yuanzhi's（milkwort root）action to keep healthy and prevent aging."

44. 细 辛

细辛 气味辛温,无毒。主咳逆上气,头痛脑动,百节拘挛,风湿痹痛,死肌。久服明目,利九窍,轻身长年。

细辛始出华阴山谷,今处处有之。一茎直上,端生一叶,其茎极细,其味极辛,其叶如葵,其色赤黑。辽冀产者,名北细辛,可以入药。南方产者,名杜衡,其茎稍粗,辛味稍减,一茎有五七叶,俗名马蹄香,不堪入药。

细辛气味辛温,一茎直上,其色赤黑,禀少阴泉下之水阴,而上交于太阳之药也。少阴为水脏,太阳为水府。水气相通,行于皮毛,皮毛之气,内合于肺。

若循行失职,则病咳逆上气,而细辛能治之。太阳之脉,起于目内眦,从巅络脑,若循行失职,则病头痛脑动。而细辛亦能治之。太阳之气主皮毛,少阴之气主骨髓,少阴之气不合太阳,则百节拘挛。节,骨节也。百节拘挛,致有风湿相侵之痹痛。风湿相侵,伤其肌腠,故曰死肌。而细辛皆能治之。久服则水精之气,濡于空窍,故明目,利九窍。九窍利,则轻身而长年。

愚按:细辛乃《本经》上品药也,味辛臭香,无毒。主明目利窍。宋元祐陈承谓:细辛单用末,不可过一钱,多则气闭不通而死。近医多以此语忌用,嗟嗟。凡药所以治病者也,有是病,服是药,岂辛香之药而反闭气乎?岂上品无毒而不可多服乎?方书之言,俱如此类,学者不善详察而遵信之,伊黄之门,终身不能入矣。

44. Xixin〔细辛, manchurian wildginger, Herba Asari〕

It is pungent in taste, warm and non-toxic in property, and it is mainly used to treat cough with dyspnea, descend adverse-rising qi, resolve headache, head shaking, the spasm of the joints, impediment and the pain caused by wind and dampness, and the numbness of the muscles. Long-term taking of it will improve vision, disinhibit the nine orifices, keep healthy and prolong life.

Firstly recorded to be growing in the mountain valleys of Huayin（华阴）, now it grows everywhere. It has a stalk growing straight, on top of which grows one leaf. The stalk is very thin. It is very pungent in taste. Its leaves, red-black in color, are just like those of Xiangrikui〔向日葵, sunflower, Helianthus annuus L.〕. Those growing in Liaoji（辽冀）are called Beixixin（北细辛）, which can be used as medicinal. Those growing in the south are called Duheng（杜衡）, which has slightly thicker stalks and slightly less pungent taste. There are five or seven leaves on one stalk. The leaves are popularly called Matixiang（马蹄香）, which cannot be used as medicinal.

Xixin（manchurian wildginger）, pungent in taste and warm in property, has a stalk growing straight which is red-black in color. It is a medicinal which receives the water yin from lesser yin underground and connects greater yang upward. Lesser yin is the water viscus while the greater yang is the water house. Water and qi connect with each other and move on the skin and hair. The qi of the skin and hair is in accordance with the lung inside. The failure of the smooth flowing in the above process will lead to cough with dyspnea and adverse-rising qi, which can be treated by Xixin (manchurian wildginger). The greater yang meridian starts from Muneizi [目内眦, Inner Canthus] and connects the brain through the vertex. The failure of the smooth flowing in the above process will lead to headache and head shaking, which can also be treated by Xixin (manchurian wildginger). The qi of greater yang governs the skin and hair while the qi of lesser yin governs the marrow. The qi of lesser yin is not in accordance with greater yang, resulting in the spasm of the joints. The joints are the ones of the bones. The spasm of the joints will lead to impediment and the pain caused by the invasion of wind and dampness. The invasion of wind and dampness will hurt the interstices of the muscles, resulting in the numbness of the muscles, all of which can be treated by Xixin (manchurian wildginger). Long-term taking of it will impel the qi of water essence to moisten the orifices thus to improve vision and disinhibit the nine orifices. The disinhibiting of the nine orifices will keep healthy and prolong life.

Note by Zhang Zhicong (张志聪): Xixin (manchurian wildginger), the top-grade medicinal in *Shen Nong Ben Cao Jing* [《神农本草经》, *Shennong's Classic of Materia Medica*], is pungent in taste, fragrant in smell and non-toxic in property. It can mainly improve vision and dredge the orifices. Chen Cheng (陈承) of the Yuanyou Reign of the Song Dynasty said, "Xixin (manchurian wildginger) should only be used in the form of powder for medicinal use, and the dose should be no more than one Qian. Otherwise, it will lead to qi block which can further cause death." Nowadays, doctors avoid using it due to what he said. What a pity! The reason the medicinal can be used to treat diseases is that what a patient suffers from is diseases while what a patient takes is medicinal. How can a medicinal which is pungent in taste and fragrant in smell lead to qi block? Why can people not take the non-toxic top-grade medicinal much? The statements in the books of formula are all like this. The scholars who do not study and examine these statements carefully but just take them completely and blindly will not become true practitioners of TCM in their whole life.

45. 柴 胡

柴胡 气味苦平,无毒。主心腹肠胃中结气,饮食积聚,寒热邪气,推陈致新。久服轻身明目益精。

　　柴胡一名地薰,叶名芸蒿,始出宏农川谷及冤句,今长安及河内近道皆有。二月生苗甚香,七月开黄花,根淡赤色,苗之香气直上云间,有鹤飞翔于上,过往闻者,皆神气清爽。柴胡有硬软二种,硬者名大柴胡,软者名小柴胡。小柴胡生于银州者为胜,故又有银柴胡之名。今市肆中另觅草根白色而大,不知何种,名银柴胡,此伪充也,不可用。古茈从草,今柴从木,其义相通。

　　柴胡春生白蒻,香美可食,香从地出,直上云霄。其根苦平,禀太阴坤土之气,而达于太阳之药也。主治心腹肠胃中结气者。心为阳中之太阳而居上,腹为至阴之太阴而居下,肠胃居心腹之中,柴胡从坤土而治肠胃之结气,则心腹之正气自和矣。治饮食积聚,土气调和也。治寒热邪气,从阴出阳也。从阴出阳,故推陈堃而致新谷。土地调和,故久服轻身。阴气上出于阳,故明目。阳气下交于阴,故益精。

　　愚按:柴胡乃从太阴地土、阳明中土而外达于太阳之药也。故仲祖《卒病论》言:伤寒中风,不从表解,太阳之气逆于中土,不能枢转外出,则用小柴胡汤达太阳之气于肌表,是柴胡并非少阳主药,后人有病在太阳,而用柴胡,则引邪入于少阳之说,此庸愚无稽之言,后人宗之,鄙陋甚矣。

45. Chaihu〔柴胡, **Chinese thorowax root**, **Radix Bupleuri**〕

　　It is bitter in taste, mild and non-toxic in property, and it is mainly used to treat the qi stagnation in the heart, abdomen, stomach and intestines, eliminate the accumulation of undigested food, remove pathogenic cold qi and heat qi and get rid of the stale to bring forth the fresh. Long-term taking of it will keep healthy, improve vision and replenish essence.

　　It is also called Dixun（地薰）. Its leaves are called Yunhao（芸蒿）. Firstly recorded to be growing in the valleys of Hongnong（宏农）and in Yuanju（冤句）, now it grows everywhere nearby Chan'an（长安）and Henei

（河内）. It grows seedlings in the second lunar month, smelling quite fragrant. It blossoms with yellow flowers in the seventh lunar month. Its root is light purple in color. The fragrance of its seedlings goes upward to the sky where cranes fly by. People all feel refreshed when smelling it. There are two kinds of Chaihu（Chinese thorowax root）. One is hard which is called Dachaihu［大柴胡, major bupleurum, Materia Medica Dachaihu］, and the other one is soft which is called Xiaochaihu［小柴胡, minor bupleurum, Bupleurum tenue］. Xiaochaihu（minor bupleurum）growing in Yinzhou（银州）is of better quality, so it is also called Yinchaihu（银柴胡）. Nowadays, some unknown white and big roots are sold to fake Yinchaihu（银柴胡）in the market, which cannot be used as medicinal. The ancient character "茈"（Chai）has part of the character "草"（Cao）while the character "柴"（Chai）now has the character "木"（Mu）. In fact, they have the same meaning.

Chaihu（Chinese thorowax root）grows white seedlings in spring which are edible, tasting sweet and delicious. Its fragrance comes out of the underground and goes upward to the sky. Its root, bitter in taste and mild in property, is a medicinal which can reach greater yang by receiving the qi of Kun earth from greater yin. It can mainly treat the qi stagnation in the heart, abdomen, stomach and intestines, because the heart is the greater yang of yang and stays in the upper part, the abdomen is the beginning of the yin of consummate yin and stays in the lower part, and the intestines and stomach stay between the heart and the abdomen. Chaihu（Chinese thorowax root）can treat the qi stagnation in the intestines and stomach through Kun earth, thus the healthy qi in the heart and abdomen will be harmonized naturally. It can eliminate the accumulation of undigested food, because earth qi is harmonized with it. It can remove pathogenic cold qi and heat qi because it can pass pathogenic qi from greater yin to greater yang. When the above process is finished, it can thus get rid of the stale to bring forth the fresh. The earth spleen is harmonized, so long-term taking of it will keep healthy. Yin qi comes upward from yang, so it can improve vision. Yang qi goes downward to connect yin, so it can replenish essence.

Note by Zhang Zhicong（张志聪）: Chaihu（Chinese thorowax root）is a medicinal which goes out to reach greater yang from the spleen earth of greater yin and the central earth of yang brightness. According to *Shang Han Zu Bing Lun* [《伤寒卒病论》, *Treatise on Cold Damage and Sudden Diseases*] written by Zhang Zhongjing (张仲景), cold damage and wind strike should not be treated from branch, and if the qi of greater yang is not in accordance with center earth and cannot perform the pivot function and go outside, Xiaochaihu Tang [小柴胡汤, Minor Bupleurum Decoction] can be used to send the qi of greater yang to the fleshy exterior. This is because Chaihu (Chinese thorowax root) is not the main medicinal for the disease in lesser yang. Patients later on suffered from the disease in greater yang and were treated with it, which would then lead to a statement that pathogen was conducted to lesser yang. This was quite absurd, but was held in esteem by people later on. How shallow and ignorant they were!

46. 升　麻

升麻　气味甘苦平,微寒,无毒。主解百毒,杀百精老物殃鬼,辟瘟疫、瘴气、邪气,蛊毒入口皆吐出,中恶腹痛,时气毒疠,头痛寒热,风肿诸毒,喉痛口疮。久服不夭,轻身长年。

升麻今蜀汉、陕西、淮南州郡皆有,以川蜀产者为胜。一名周麻。春苗夏花,叶似麻叶,其根如蒿根,其色紫黑,多须。

升麻气味甘苦平,甘者土也,苦者火也。主从中土而达太阳之气。太阳标阳本寒,故微寒。盖太阳禀寒水之气而行于肤表,如天气之下连于水也。太阳在上,则天日当空,光明清湛。清湛,故主解百毒。光明,故杀百精老物殃鬼。太阳之气,行于肤表,故辟瘟疫、瘴气、邪气。太阳之气,行于地中,故蛊毒入口皆吐出。治蛊毒,则中恶腹痛自除。辟瘟疫瘴气邪气,则时气毒疠,头痛寒热自散。寒水之气,滋于外而济于上,故治风肿诸毒,喉痛口疮。久服则阴精上滋,故不夭。阳气盛,故轻身,阴阳充足,则长年矣。

愚按:柴胡、升麻,皆达太阳之气,从中土以上升,柴胡从中土而达太阳之标阳,升麻兼启太阳之寒水,细辛更启寒水之气于泉下,而内合少阴,三者大义相同,功用少别。具升转周遍之功,故又名周麻。防风、秦艽、乌药、防己、木通、升麻,皆纹如车辐,而升麻更觉空通。

46. Shengma〔升麻, largetrifoliolious bugbane rhizome, Rhizoma Cimicifuga〕

It is sweet and bitter in taste, mild, slightly cold and non-toxic in property, and it is mainly used to resolve various toxins, kill various ghost-like pathogens causing various diseases, repel pestilence, miasmic qi and pathogenic qi, help people vomit the pathogenic worm toxin in the mouth, and eliminate the attack of noxious factor, abdominal pain, seasonal epidemic, toxic pestilence, headache, diseases caused by pathogenic cold and heat, the rubella caused by various toxins, sore throat and mouth sores. Long-term taking of it will help people live longer, keep healthy and prolong life.

It grows in Shuhan (蜀汉), Shaanxi (陕西) and Huainan (淮南). Those growing in Chuanshu (川蜀) are of better quality. It is also called Zhouma (周麻). It sprouts in spring and blossoms in summer. Its leaves are like Maye〔麻叶, hemp leaf, Cannabis Folium〕, and its roots are like Qinghaogen〔青蒿根, sweet wormwood root, Artemisiae Annuae Radix〕, which is purple-black in color with many branching roots.

It is sweet and bitter in taste and mild in property. Sweetness pertains to earth, and bitterness pertains to fire. It can move qi from center earth to greater yang. The branch yang of greater yang is cold in property. So Shengma (largetrifoliolious bugbane rhizome) is slightly cold in property. It is because that greater yang receives the qi of cold water to flow on the fleshy exterior like heaven qi going downward to connect water. The greater yang is sufficient, which is like the sun being in the sky, and then it will make people have a bright and clear mind, which is like the sky being bright and clear. Being clear will resolve various toxins, and being bright will kill various ghost-like pathogens causing various diseases. The qi of greater yang flows on the fleshy exterior, so it can repel pestilence, miasmic qi and pathogenic qi. The qi of greater yang moves in the inner part of earth, so it can help people vomit the pathogenic worm toxin in the mouth. The worm toxin is resolved, and then the attack of noxious factor and abdominal pain will be eliminated naturally. Pestilence, miasmic qi and pathogenic qi are repelled, then seasonal epidemic, toxic pestilence, headache and diseases caused by pathogenic cold and heat can be treated naturally. The qi of cold water can nourish the exterior and aid the upper part, so it can be used to treat the rubella caused by various toxins, sore throat and mouth sores. Long-term taking of it will impel yin essence to nourish upward, so it will help people live longer. Yang qi is exuberant, and then it will keep healthy. Yin qi and yang qi are sufficient, and then it will prolong life.

Note by Zhang Zhicong（张志聪）: Both Chaihu［柴胡, Chinesethorowax root, Radix Bupleuri］and Shengma（largetrifoliolious bugbane rhizome）can go upward from center earth to reach the qi of greater yang. Chaihu（Chinese thorowax root）goes from center earth to reach the branch yang of greater yang. Besides that, Shengma（largetrifoliolious bugbane rhizome）can also activate the qi of cold water of greater yang, and Xixin［细辛, manchurian wildginger, Herba Asari］can also activate the qi of cold water underground to be in accordance with lesser yin inside. All the three almost have the same effect, but with slight differences. Shengma（largetrifoliolious bugbane rhizome）has the effect of impelling qi to rise and flow in the whole body, so it is also called Zhouma（周麻）. Fangfeng［防风, divaricate saposhnikovia root, Radix Saposhnikoviae］, Qinjiao［秦艽, largeleaf gentian root, Radix Gentianae Macrophyllae］, Wuyao［乌药, combined spicebush fruit, Radix Linderae］, Fangji［防己, fourstamen stephania root, Radix Stephaniae Tetrandrae］, Mutong［木通, trifoliate akebia, Akebiae Trifoliatae Caulis］and Shengma（largetrifoliolious bugbane rhizome）all have lines which are like spokes. However, those of Shengma（largetrifoliolious bugbane rhizome）are looser and hollower.

47. 桂

桂 气味辛温, 无毒。主上气咳逆, 结气, 喉痹, 吐吸, 利关节, 补中益气。久服通神, 轻身不老。

《本经》有牡桂、菌桂之别, 今但以桂摄之。桂木臭香, 性温, 其味辛甘。始出桂阳山谷及合浦、交趾、广州、象州、湘州诸处。色紫黯, 味辛甘者为真。若皮色黄白, 味不辛甘, 香不触鼻, 名为柳桂, 又名西桂。今药肆中此桂居多。真广者,百无一二。西桂只供发散,不能助心主之神,壮木火之气,用者不可不择。上体枝干质薄,则为牡桂。牡,阳也。枝干治阳本乎上者,亲上也。下体根荄质浓,则为菌桂。菌,根也。根荄治阴本乎下者,亲下也。仲祖《伤寒论》有桂枝加桂汤,是牡桂、菌桂并用也。又云:桂枝去皮,去皮者,只取稍尖嫩枝,外皮内骨皆去之不用。是枝与干又各有别也,今以枝为桂枝,干为桂皮,为官桂,即《本经》之牡桂也。根为肉桂,去粗皮为桂心,即《本经》之菌桂也。生发之机在于干枝,故录《本经》牡桂主治,但题以桂而总摄焉。

桂木凌冬不凋,气味辛温,其色紫赤,水中所生之木火也。上气咳逆者,肺肾不交,则上气而为咳逆之证。桂启水中之生阳,上交于肺,则上气平而咳逆除矣。结气喉痹者,三焦之气,不行于肌腠,则结气而为喉痹之证。桂秉少阳之木气,通利三焦,则结气通而喉痹可治矣。吐吸者,吸不归根,即吐出也。桂能引下气与上气相接,则吸入之气,直至丹田而后出,故治吐吸也。关节者,两肘两腋、两髀两腘,皆机关之室。周身三百六十五节,皆神气之所游行。桂助君火之气,使心主之神,而出入于机关,游行于骨节,故利关节也。补中益气者,补中焦而益上下之气也。久服则阳气盛而光明,故通神。三焦通会元真于肌腠,故轻身不老。

47. Gui [桂, cinnamon bark, Cortex Cinnamomum Cassia]

It is pungent in taste, warm and non-toxic in property, and it is mainly used to treat the cough with dyspnea due to adverse-rising qi, the throat impediment due to stagnation of qi, and the breath with the mouth due to the severe impediment of the throat, dredge the joints, tonify the middle and replenish qi. Long-term taking of it will invigorate the spirit and mind, keep healthy and prevent aging.

There are two different herbs recorded in *Shen Nong Ben Cao Jing* [《神农本草经》, *Shennong's Classic of Materia Medica*], which are called Mugui (牡桂) and Jungui (菌桂), but they are both represented by Gui (桂) there. The tree of Gui (桂) is fragrant in smell, warm in property and pungent and sweet in taste. It was firstly recorded to be growing in the valleys of Guiyang (桂阳) and in Hepu (合浦), Jiaozhi (交趾), Guangzhou (广州), Xiangzhou (象州) and Xiangzhou (湘州). It is dark purple in color. The genuine one is pungent and sweet in taste. If the bark is yellow-white in color and the herb is not pungent and sweet in taste with very slight fragrance, the herb is called Liugui（柳桂）or Xigui（西桂）, which is sold in a larger amount in today's drug stores. Hardly can the genuine one growing in Guangzhou（广州）be found. Xigui（西桂）can only be used to dissipate and cannot assist the spirit governed by the heart and strengthen the qi of wood and fire. Users should make a careful choice concerning the use of Xigui（西桂）. The one whose bark of the upper twig is thin in texture, and it is called Mugui （牡桂）. Mu（牡）means yang. Twigs of Mugui（牡桂）in accordance with yang grow on the upper part of the tree, so it can enter the upper part of human body and treat the diseases developing there. The one whose bark of the lower root is thick in texture is called Jungui（菌桂）. Jun（菌）means root. The root of Jungui（菌桂）in accordance with yin grows in the lower part of the tree, so it can enter the lower part of human body and treat the diseases developing there. There is Guizhi Jiagui Tang［桂枝加桂汤, Cinnamon Twig Decoction with Extra Cinnamon］in *Shang Han Lun*［《伤寒论》, *Treatise on Cold Damage Diseases*］written by Zhang Zhongjing（张仲景）, which used both Mugui（牡桂）and Jungui（菌桂）. It is also stated to remove the bark from the twig of Gui（桂）, only use slightly pointed tender twigs and discard the bark and other parts. The twig and the bark are used in a different way. The twigs are called Guizhi［桂枝, cinnamon twig, Cinnamomi Ramulus］, and the bark of the trunk is called Guipi［桂皮, thin cinnamon bark, Cinnamomi Cortex Tenuis］. Both of them are called Guangui［官桂, quilled cinnamon, Cinnamomi Cortex Tubiformis］, which is also Mugui（牡桂）mentioned in *Shen Nong Ben Cao Jing*［《神农本草经》, *Shennong's Classic of Materia Medica*］. The root is called Rougui［肉桂, cinnamon bark, Cinnamomi Cortex］, and it is also called Guixin［桂心, shaved cinnamon bark, Cinnamomi Cortex Rasus］when its bark is removed. Both Rougui（cinnamon bark）and Guixin （shaved cinnamon bark）are also Jungui（菌桂）mentioned in *Shen Nong Ben Cao Jing*［《神农本草经》, *Shennong's Classic of Materia Medica*］. The key to its growth and development lies in its twigs and bark, so the actions recorded under Gui（桂）in *Shen Nong Ben Cao Jing*［《神农本草经》, *Shennong's Classic of Materia Medica*] are actually those of Mugui（牡桂）, but it is represented by Gui（桂）there.

Gui（cinnamon bark）does not wither even in winter. Pungent in taste, warm in property, and purple-red in color, it is wood and fire originating from water. The cough with dyspnea due to adverse-rising qi results from that the lung and the kidney do not interact with each other. It can activate the kidney-yang in water to connect the lung upward, so adverse-rising qi can be calmed, and the cough with dyspnea can be treated. The throat impediment due to the stagnation of qi results from that the qi of the triple energizer does not flow on the interstices of the muscles. It can dredge the triple energizer by receiving the wood qi of lesser yang, then the stagnation of qi can be disinhibited, and the throat impediment can therefore be treated. The breath with the mouth due to the severe impediment of the throat results from that inhaled qi is exhaled before reaching the kidney. It can guide the lower qi to connect with upper qi. Then inhaled qi can reach the cinnabar field before exhalaton, so it can treat the breath with the mouth due to the severe impediment of the throat. The joints, including two elbows, two axillae, two thighs and two popliteal fossae, are all the pivots of limbs. There are three hundred and sixty-five joints in the whole body where spirit and qi can move in and out. Gui（cinnamon bark）can assist the qi of sovereign fire to make the spirit governed by the heart go in and out of pivots and move in and out of the joints, so it can dredge the joints. To tonify the middle and replenish qi is to tonify the middle energizer and replenish the upward and downward qi. Long-term taking of it will make yang qi exuberant and sufficient, so it can be used to invigorate the spirit and mind. The triple energizer can send primordial qi to the interstices of the muscles, so it can also be used to keep healthy and prevent aging.

48. 羌 活

羌活　气味苦甘辛,无毒。主风寒所击,金疮止痛,奔豚、痫痓,女人疝瘕。久服轻身耐老。甘辛旧本作甘平,误,今改正。

　　羌活始出雍州川谷及陇西南安,今以蜀汉、西羌所出者为佳。《本经》只言独活,不言羌活,说者谓其生苗,一茎直上,有风不动,无风自摇,故名独活。后人以独活而出于西羌者,名羌活。出于中国,处处有者,名独活。羌活色紫赤,节密轻虚。羌活之中复分优劣,西蜀产者,性优。江淮近道产者,性劣。独活出土黄白,晒干褐黑,紧实无节,其气香烈,其味辛腥。

羌活初出土时,苦中有甘,曝干则气味苦辛,故《本经》言气味苦甘辛,其色黄紫,气甚芳香,生于西蜀,禀手足太阴金土之气化。风寒所击,如客在门而扣击之,从皮毛而入肌腠也。羌活禀太阴肺金之气,则御皮毛之风寒。禀太阴脾土之气,则御肌腠之风寒,故主治风寒所击。金疮止痛,禀土气而长肌肉也。奔豚乃水气上奔,土能御水逆,金能益子虚,故治奔豚。痫痓、风痫,风痓也。金能制风,故治痫痓。肝木为病,疝气,瘕聚。金能平木,故治女子疝瘕。久服则土金相生,故轻身耐老。

48. Qianghuo〔羌活, incised notopterygium rhizome and root, Rhizoma et Radix Notopterygii〕

It is bitter and sweet in taste, pungent and non-toxic in property, and it is mainly used to treat wind-cold attack, relieve the pain caused by incised wound, resolve running piglet, epilepsy and convulsion and hernia and movable abdominal mass in woman. Long-term taking of it will keep healthy and prevent aging. It was recorded in the past as being sweet in taste and mild in property instead of being sweet in taste and pungent in property, which was a false statement. Now this is corrected.

Firstly recorded to be growing in the valleys of Yongzhou (雍州) and in Nan'an (南安) of Longxi (陇西), now those growing in Shuhan (蜀汉) and Xiqiang (西羌) are of good quality. In *Shen Nong Ben Cao Jing*〔《神农本草经》, *Shennong's Classic of Materia Medica*〕it is only called Duhuo (独活) instead of Qianghuo (incised notopterygium rhizome and root). The reason why it is called Duhuo (独活) is that it sprouts and has a stalk growing straight which never moves when there is a wind, but spontaneously moves when there is no wind. People later on called those originating from Xiqiang (西羌) Qianghuo (incised notopterygium rhizome and root). Those growing everywhere in the central plains are called Duhuo (独活). Purple-red in color, Qianghuo (incised notopterygium rhizome and root) has dense nodes but it is light and loose in quality. It can be further divided into two kinds of either good or bad quality. Those growing in Xishu（西蜀）are of good quality while those growing in areas near Jianghuai（江淮）are of bad quality. Duhuo（独活）is yellow-white in color when it is just dug out while brown-black in color when it is dried in the sun. Without nodes, it will be firm with strong and fragrant smell and pungent and stinky taste.

Qianghuo（incised notopterygium rhizome and root）is bitter with sweetness in taste when it is just dug out and will be bitter in taste and pungent in property when it is dried in the sun. That is the reason why in *Shen Nong Ben Cao Jing* [《神农本草经》, *Shennong's Classic of Materia Medica*] it is mentioned to be bitter and sweet in taste and pungent in property. It is yellow-purple in color and extremely fragrant in smell. Growing in Xishu（西蜀）, it receives the qi transformation of metal and earth from hand greater yin and foot greater yin. Wind-cold attack is like a guest knocking at a door, which can enter the interstices of the muscles from the skin and hair. Qianghuo（incised notopterygium rhizome and root）receives the qi of lung metal from greater yin, so it can be used to protect the skin and hair from wind cold. It also receives the qi of spleen earth from greater yin, so it can be used to protect the interstices of muscles from wind cold. Therefore, it can be used to treat wind-cold attack. It can be used to relieve the pain caused by incised wound, because it can promote the growth of the muscles by receiving earth qi. Running piglet is caused by water qi going upward. Earth can restrict water counterflow, and metal can benefit vacuous children, so Qianghuo（incised notopterygium rhizome and root）can be used to resolve running piglet. Epilepsy and convulsion and wind epilepsy are wind convulsion. Metal can control wind, so it can be used to resolve epilepsy and convulsion. Liver wood is ill, and then there will be hernia-conglomeration. Metal can calm wood, so it can be used to treat the hernia and movable abdominal mass in women. Long-term taking of it will lead to the mutual generation of earth and metal, so it can keep healthy and prevent aging.

49. 防 风

防风 气味甘温,无毒。主大风头眩痛,恶风风邪,目盲无所见,风行周身,骨节疼痛烦满。久服轻身。

防风始出沙苑川泽及邯郸、琅琊、上蔡,皆属中州之地。春初发嫩芽,红紫色,三月茎叶俱青,五月开细白花,六月结实黑色,九月、十月采根,色黄空通。

防风茎、叶、花、实,兼备五色,其味甘,其质黄,其臭香,禀土运之专精,治周身之风证。盖土气厚,则风可屏,故名防风。风淫于头,则大风头眩痛。申明大风者,乃恶风之风邪,眩痛不已,必至目盲无所见,而防风能治之。又,风邪行于周身,甚至骨节疼痛,而防风亦能治之,久服则土气盛,故轻身。

元人王好古曰:病头痛、肢节痛、一身尽痛,非羌活不能除,乃却乱反正之主君药也。李东垣曰:防风治一身尽痛,随所引而至,乃卒伍卑贱之职也。

愚按:《神农》以上品为君,羌活、防风皆列上品,俱散风治病,何以贵贱迥别若是。后人发明药性,多有如此谬妄之论,虽曰无关治法,学者遵而信之,陋习何由得洗乎。

49. Fangfeng [防风, divaricate saposhnikovia root, Radix Saposhnikoviae]

It is sweet in taste, warm and non-toxic in property, and it is mainly used to treat the diseases caused by severe pathogenic wind, the headache with vertigo, the aversion to wind, the damage due to wind pathogen, poor vision, invasion of wind in the whole body, the pain in the bones and joints, and vexation and fullness. Long-term taking of it will keep healthy.

It was firstly recorded to be growing in the rivers and lakes of Shayuan (沙苑) as well as in Handan (邯郸), Langya (琅琊) and Shangcai (上蔡), which all belong to central plains. At the beginning of spring, it begins to grow red-purple seedlings. In the third lunar month both its stalks and leaves are green in color. In the fifth lunar month it blossoms with fine white flowers. In the sixth lunar month it bears black fruits. In the ninth or tenth lunar month its root can be collected, which is yellow in color and hollow in shape.

Its stalks, leaves, flowers and fruits have five colors. Sweet in taste, yellow in color and fragrant in smell, it receives the essence of earth motion and can be used to treat the diseases caused by pathogenic wind in the whole body. Abundant earth qi can be used to prevent wind, so it is called Fangfeng［防风, which means wind prevention］. Wind invades the head, resulting in diseases caused by severe pathogenic wind and the headache with vertigo. The clear explanation of severe pathogenic wind is malign wind pathogen which leads to endless dizziness and headache, which is certain to cause poor vision and can be treated by Fangfeng（divaricate saposhnikovia root）. The invasion of wind in the whole body and even the pain in the bones and joints can also be treated by Fangfeng（divaricate saposhnikovia root）. Long-term taking of it will lead to exuberant earth qi, so it can be used to keep healthy.

Wang Haogu（王好古）of the Yuan Dynasty said, "The headache, pain in the joints and pain in the whole body can only be relieved by Qianghuo［羌活, pubescent angelica, Radix Angelicae Pubescentis］, which is a kind of sovereign medicinal to relieve pain and regain health." Li Dongyuan（李东垣）said, "The pain in the whole body can be treated by Fangfeng（divaricate saposhnikovia root）, which can be used at any time with meridian conductor. Its role in treating diseases is the same as that of a soldier at the lowest level."

Note by Zhang Zhicong（张志聪）: *Shen Nong Ben Cao Jing*［《神农本草经》, *Shennong's Classic of Materia Medica*］regards the top-grade medicinals as sovereign medicinals. Both Qianghuo（羌活）and Fangfeng（防风）are listed as top-grade medicinal. Both of them can be used to dissipate wind and treat diseases. Why do people classify medicinals as the noble or the mean? People later on labeled properties to various medicinals, but some of the properties do not make sense. Although this is irrelevant to therapy as well as therapeutic rules, some scholars still accept and take it. How will the corrupt customs be eliminated?

50. 紫 苏

紫苏 气味辛微温，无毒。主下气杀谷，除饮食，辟口臭，去邪毒，辟恶气。久服通神明，轻身耐老。《纲目》误列中品，今改入上品。

紫苏《本经》名水苏，始生九真池泽，今处处有之，好生水旁，因名水苏，其叶面青背紫，昼则森挺，暮则下垂。气甚辛香，开花成穗，红紫色，穗中有细子，其色黄赤，入土易生。后人于壤土莳植，面背皆紫者，名家紫苏。野生瘠土者,背紫面青。《别录》另列紫苏,其实一种,但家野之不同耳。又一种面背皆青,气辛臭香者,为荠苧。一种面背皆白者,名白苏,俱不堪入药。

紫苏气味辛温,臭香色紫,其叶昼挺暮垂,禀太阳天日晦明之气。天气下降,故主下气。下气则能杀谷,杀谷则能除饮食。除,消除也。味辛臭香,故辟口臭。辟口臭,则能去邪毒。去邪毒,则能辟恶气。久服则天日光明,故通神明。天气下降,则地气上升,故轻身耐老。

愚按:紫苏配杏子,主利小便,消水肿,解肌表,定喘逆,与麻黄同功而不走泄正气,故《本经》言:久服通神明,轻身耐老。列于上品。

50. Zisu〔紫苏, perilla, Perillae Folium〕

It is pungent in taste, slightly warm and non-toxic in property, and it is mainly used to descend qi, promote digestion, remove the retention of food, eliminate fetid mouth odor, remove pathogenic toxin and repel malign qi. Long-term taking of it will invigorate spirit and mentality, keep healthy and prevent aging. It was a mistake to classify it as the medium-grade herb in *Ben Cao Gang Mu*〔《本草纲目》, *Compendium of Materia Medica*〕, and now it is corrected to be in the top grade.

It is mentioned as Shuisu（水苏）in *Shen Nong Ben Cao Jing*〔《神农本草经》, *Shennong's Classic of Materia Medica*〕. Firstly recorded to be growing in the lakes and pools of Jiuzhen（九真）, now it grows everywhere. It tends to be growing by the water, so it is called Shuisu（水苏）. The leaves, with blue surfaces and purple backs, are upright in the day and nutant in the evening. It is extremely pungent and fragrant in smell. It grows red-purple flowers in flower clusters, and the flower clusters have fine yellow-red seeds which can easily grow in the soil. Those cultivated in the loam by people later on with purple surfaces and backs are called Jiazisu（家紫苏）. Those growing in the infertile soil in the wild have purple backs and green surfaces. The wild one is listed as another medicinal in *Ming Yi Bie Lu*〔《名医别录》, *Miscellaneous Records of Famous Physicians*〕. But in fact, they pertain to the same species, just with the difference of being cultivated or growing in the wild. Another one which is pungent in taste and fragrant in smell with black surface and back is called Jining

[荠苧, Chinese mosla, Mosla chinensis]. Another one which has the white surface and back is called Baisu [白苏, white perilla, Perilla frutescens (L.) Britt.]. Both of them cannot be used as medicinal.

Pungent in taste, slightly warm in property, fragrant in smell, and purple in color, it has leaves which are upright in the day and nutant in the evening. It receives the dark and bright qi from greater yang. Heaven qi goes downward, so it can mainly descend qi, which can promote digestion. When digestion is promoted, the retention of food can be removed. Here "remove" means "eliminate". It is pungent in taste and fragrant in smell, so it can be used to eliminate fetid mouth odor, which is effective in removing pathogenic toxin. When pathogenic toxin is removed, malign qi will be repelled. Long-term taking of it will lead to sufficient healthy qi, so it can be used to invigorate spirit and mentality. Heaven qi descends, and earth qi will then ascend, so it can keep healthy and prevent aging.

Note by Zhang Zhicong (张志聪): The combination of Zisu (perilla) and Xingzi [杏子, apricot, Armeniacae Fructus] is quite effective in disinhibiting urination, relieving swelling, resolving the fleshy exterior and curing asthma, which performs the same action as Mahuang [麻黄, ephedra, Herba Ephedrae] without discharging healthy qi. So *Shen Nong Ben Cao Jing* [《神农本草经》, *Shennong's Classic of Materia Medica*] says that long-term taking of it will invigorate spirit and mentality, keep healthy and prevent aging. It is therefore classified as the top grade.

51. 苏　子 附

苏子 附　气味辛温，无毒。主下气，除寒，温中。《别录》附。

51. Suzi [苏子, **perilla fruit**, **Perillae Fructus**] *supplement*

It is pungent in taste, slightly warm and non-toxic in property, and it is mainly used to descend qi, eliminate cold and warm the middle. Supplemented in *Ming Yi Bie Lu* [《名医别录》, *Miscellaneous Records of Famous Physicians*].

52. 苏 枝 附

苏枝 附 气味辛平,无毒。主宽中行气,消饮食,化痰涎,治噎膈反胃,止心腹痛,通十二经关窍脉络。《新增》附。

苏枝是茎上傍枝,非老梗也。

52. Suzhi〔苏枝, perilla twig, Perillae Ramulus〕 *supplement*

It is pungent in taste, mild and non-toxic in property, and it is mainly used to smooth the middle, move qi, promote digestion, resolve phlegm and fluid retention, treat dysphagia and stomach reflux, relieve the pain in the heart, and abdomen, and dredge the twelve meridians and meridians and the collateral vessels of the joints and orifices. Supplemented in *Xin Zeng*〔《新增》, *New Supplement to Materia Medica*〕.

Suzhi (perilla twig) is the side branch growing on the stem instead of the stem itself.

53. 橘 皮

橘皮 气味苦辛温,无毒。主治胸中瘕热逆气,利水谷。久服去臭,下气,通神。

橘生江南及山南山谷,今江浙荆襄湖岭皆有。枝多坚刺,叶色青翠,经冬不凋,结实青圆,秋冬始熟,或黄或赤,其臭辛香,肉味酸甜,皮兼辛苦。

橘实形圆色黄,臭香肉甘,脾之果也。其皮气味苦辛,性主温散,筋膜似络脉,皮形若肌肉,宗眼如毛孔,乃从脾脉之大络而外出于肌肉毛孔之药也。胸中瘕热逆气者,谓胃上郛郭之间,浊气留聚,则假气成形,而为瘕热逆气之病。橘皮能达胃络之气,出于肌腠,故胸中之瘕热逆气可治也。利水谷者,水谷入胃,藉脾气之散精,橘皮能达脾络之气,上通于胃,故水谷可利也。久服去臭者,去中焦腐秽之臭气,而整肃脾胃也。下气通神者,下肺主之气,通心主之神,橘皮气味辛苦,辛入肺,而苦入心也。

愚按:上古诸方,只曰橘皮个用不切,并无去白之说。李东垣不参经义,不礼物性,承《雷敩炮制》谓:留白则理脾健胃,去白则消痰止嗽。后人习以为法,每用橘红治虚劳咳嗽。夫咳嗽非只肺病，有肝气上逆而咳嗽者，有胃气壅滞而咳嗽者，有肾气奔迫而咳嗽者，有心火上炎而咳嗽者，有皮毛闭拒而咳嗽者，有脾肺不和而咳嗽者。《经》云：五脏六腑皆令人咳，非独肺也。橘皮里有筋膜，外黄内白，其味先甘后辛，其性从络脉而外达于肌肉、毛孔，以之治咳，有从内达外之义。若去其白，其味但辛，只行皮毛，风寒咳嗽似乎相宜，虚劳不足，益辛散矣。后人袭方书糟粕，不穷物性本原，无怪以讹传讹，而莫之止。须知雷敩乃宋人，非黄帝时雷公也。业医者当以上古方制为准绳，如《金匮要略》用橘皮汤治干呕哕，义可知矣。日华子谓：橘瓤上筋膜，治口渴吐酒，煎汤饮甚效。以其能行胸中之饮而行于皮肤也。夫橘皮从内达外，凡汗多里虚，阳气外浮者，宜禁用之。

53. Jupi〔橘皮, tangerine peel, Citri Reticulatae Pericarpium〕

It is bitter and pungent in taste, warm and non-toxic in property, and it is mainly used to disperse the accumulation of heat and descend the adverse-rising qi in the chest, and promote the digestion of food. Long-term taking of it will remove halitosis, descend qi and invigorate spirit.

Firstly recorded to be growing in Jiangnan（江南）and in the valleys of Shannan（山南）, now it grows everywhere in the mountains and lakes of Jiangzhe（江浙）and Jingxiang（荆襄）. The branches usually have hard thorns. The leaves are green and do not wither even in winter. Its fruits are green in color and round in shape, which will turn yellow or red when they start to ripen in autumn and winter with pungent and fragrant smell. The flesh is sweet and sour in taste, and the peel is pungent and bitter in taste.

Its fruit, round in shape, yellow in color, fragrant in smell and sweet in taste, can fortify the spleen. Its peel is bitter in taste and pungent in property with the main action of warming and dissipating. Juluo〔橘络, tangerine pith, Citri Reticulatae Fructus Fasciculus Vascularis〕looks like the collateral vessel, the peel resembles the muscle and its sacs are like the pores. It is a medicinal which goes out from the great collateral of the spleen meridian to reach the muscles and pores. The accumulation of heat and adverse-rising qi in the chest is caused by the turbid qi in the chest, which leads to the formation of conglomeration qi. Jupi (tangerine peel) can move the qi of the stomach collateral out to reach the interstices of the muscles, so it can be used to treat the accumulation of heat and descend the adverse-rising qi in the chest. It is used to promote the digestion of food, because Jupi (tangerine peel) can move the qi of the spleen collateral to go upward to connect the stomach when food enters the stomach with the help of the spleen's function of distributing essence. So it can be used to promote the digestion of food. Long-term taking of it will remove halitosis, because it can remove the rotten and dirty qi in the middle energizer and purify the spleen and stomach. To descend qi and invigorate spirit are to descend the qi governed by the lung and invigorate the spirit governed by the heart. Jupi (tangerine peel) is bitter in taste and pungent in property, and pungency enters the lung while bitterness enters the heart.

Note by Zhang Zhicong (张志聪): It was just mentioned in ancient formulas that Jupi (tangerine peel) can be used as a whole without being cut into parts. Removing Jubai [橘白, white tangerine peel, Citri Reticulatae Periocarpium Album] was never mentioned. Li Dongyuan (李东垣) did not grasp the true meaning of the classics or understand the nature of medicinal, but blindly followed what was recorded in *Lei Xiao Pao Zhi* [《雷敩炮制》, *Lei Xiao's Study on Processing of Medicinals*]. He said that it can regulate the spleen and strengthen the stomach by keeping Jubai (white tangerine peel) while it can disperse phlegm and stop cough by removing Jubai (white tangerine peel). People later on learned from him and usually used Juhong [橘红, red tangerine peel, Citri Reticulatae Pericarpium Rubrum] to treat consumptive diseases and cough. However, cough is not caused by the diseases related to the lung alone. It can be caused by adverse-rising liver qi, the congestion of stomach qi, running piglet, The up-flaming of heart fire, the closure of the skin and hair, or disharmony between the spleen and the lung. *Huang Di Nei Jing* [《黄帝内经》, *Huangdi's Internal Classic*] says that instead of the lung alone, the five zang-organs and the six fu-organscan all lead to cough. Yellow outside and white inside, and having Juluo (tangerine pith) inside, Jupi (tangerine peel) is at first sweet and then pungent in taste, and it has the function of going outside to reach the muscles and pores from the collateral vessels. Treating cough with it has the meaning of reaching the outside from the inside. Without Jubai (white tangerine peel), it is only pungent in taste and can only move on the skin and hair, which seems to be suitable for treating wind-cold cough, but will actually cause more serious consumptive diseases because pungency will disperse gradually. People later on just followed the worst parts of books of formula without deep understanding of the nature and origin of medicinal. It is no wonder that errors have been handed down continuously. It must be kept in mind that Lei Xiao（雷敩）lived in the Song Dynasty of the Southern Dynasties and he was not Leigong（雷公）of the Huangdi（黄帝）times. True practitioners of TCM should take ancient formulas as criterion. For example, *Jin Gui Yao Lüe* [《金匮要略》, *Synopsis of the Golden Chamber*] uses Jupi Tang [橘皮汤, Tangerine Peel Decoction] to treat retching, whose reason can be understood. *Ri Hua Ben Cao* [《日华本草》, *Rihuazi's Materia Medica*] says that Juluo (tangerine pith) can be used to treat thirst and vomiting after drinking, which is quite effective when it is decocted because it can promote the alcohol in the stomach to discharge from the skin. Jupi (tangerine peel) has the effect of reaching the outside from the inside, so it is prohibited for those with profuse sweating, interior deficiency and yang qi floating outward.

54. 青橘皮 附

青橘皮 附 气味苦辛温,无毒。主治气滞,下食,破积结及膈气。《图经本草》附。

54. Qingjupi [青橘皮, unripe tangerine peel, Citri Reticulatae Pericarpium Viride] *supplement*

It is bitter and in taste, pungent, mild and non-toxic in property, and it is mainly used to treat qi stagnation, stimulate the digestion of retained food, eliminate the accumulation lump due to retained food and free diaphragm qi. Supplemented in *Tu Jing Ben Cao* [《图经本草》,*Illustrated Classic of Materia Medica*].

55. 橘 核 附

橘核 附 气味苦平,无毒。主治肾疰腰痛,膀胱气痛,肾冷。《日华本草》附。

55. Juhe〔橘核，tangerine pip，Citri Reticulatae Semen〕*supplement*

It is bitter in taste，mild and non-toxic in property，and it is mainly used to treat kidney infixation，lumbar pain，the pain due to the invasion of pathogenic qi in the bladder and kidney cold. Supplemented in *Ri Hua Ben Cao*〔《日华本草》，*Rihuazi's Materia Medica*〕.

56. 橘　叶　附

橘叶 附　气味苦平，无毒。主导胸膈逆气，入厥阴。行肝气，消肿散毒。乳痈胁痛，用之行经。《本草衍义补遗》附。

56. Juye〔橘叶，tangerine leaf，Citri Reticulatae Folium〕*supplement*

It is bitter in taste，mild and non-toxic in property，and it is used to conduct the adverse-rising qi in the chest and the diaphragm into reverting yin，move liver qi，disperse swelling，resolve toxin，treat acute mastitis，rib-side pain and regulate menstruation. Supplemented in *Ben Cao Yan Yi Bu Yi*〔《本草衍义补遗》，*Supplement to the Amplification on Materia Medica*〕.

57. 辛　夷

辛夷　气味辛温，无毒。主治五脏身体寒热，风头脑痛，面黚。久服下气，轻身，明目，增年耐老。

辛夷始出汉中、魏兴、梁州川谷，今近道处处有之。人家园亭亦多种植。树高丈余，花先叶后，叶苞有茸毛。花开白色者，名玉兰，谓花色如玉，花香如兰也。红紫色者，名木笔，谓花苞尖长，俨然如笔也。入药红白皆用，取含苞未开者收之。

辛夷味辛臭香，苞毛花白，禀阳明土金之气化也。阳明者土也，五脏之所归也。故主治五脏不和而为身体之寒热。阳明者金也，金能制风，故主治风淫头脑之痛。阳明之气有余，则面生光，故治面黚。黚，黑色也。《经》云：阳明者，胃脉也，其气下行，故久服下气，土气和平，故轻身。金水相生，故明目。下气轻身明目,则增年耐老。

57. Xinyi〔辛夷, immature flower of biond magnolia, Flos Magnoliae〕

It is pungent in taste, warm and non-toxic in property, and it is mainly used to treat the cold-heat disease in the body caused by the disharmony of the five-zang organs, the headache caused by wind excess in the head and black facial spots. Long-term taking of it will descend qi, keep healthy, improve vision, prolong life and prevent aging.

Firstly recorded to be growing in the river valleys of Hanzhong (汉中), Weixing (魏兴) and Liangzhou (梁州), now it grows everywhere in nearby places. It is also planted in household gardens. It is more than one Zhang high. Its leaves with hairy bracts come out later than flowers. Those with white flowers are called Yulan (玉兰), which means that the color of the flower is the same as jade and the flower smells like orchid. Those with red-purple flowers are called Mubi (木笔), for the bud is long and pointed, and looks like a Chinese brush. Both Yulan (玉兰) and Mubi (木笔) can be collected and used as medicinal when they are in bud.

Pungent in taste and fragrant in smell, it has hairy buds and white flowers and receives the qi transformation of earth and metal from yang brightness. Yang brightness pertains to earth from which the qi of the five-zang organs comes. So it can mainly treat the cold-heat disease in the body caused by the disharmony of the five-zang organs. Yang brightness also pertains to metal, and metal can control wind. So it can also mainly treat the headache caused by the wind excess in the head. The abundant qi of yang brightness will lead to lustering complexion. So it can be used to treat Miangan〔面鼾, black facial spots〕. Gan (鼾) means being black. *Huang Di Nei Jing*〔《黄帝内经》, *Huangdi's Internal Classic*〕says that yang brightness is related to the meridian of the stomach, and the qi of yang brightness will go downward. So long-term taking of it will descend qi. Then earth qi can be harmonized, and health can be kept. The mutual generation of metal and water will lead to the improvement of vision. Descending qi, keeping healthy and improving vision will prolong life and prevent aging.

58. 木 香

木香 气味辛温，无毒。主治邪气，辟毒疫温鬼，强志，主淋露。久服不梦寤魇寐。

木香始出永昌山谷，今皆从外国舶上来，昔人谓之青木香，后人呼马兜铃根为青木香，改呼此为广木香以别之。《三洞珠囊》云：五香者，木香也。一株五根，一茎五枝，一枝五叶，叶间五节，故名五香。根条左旋，采得二十九日方硬，形如枯骨，烧之能上彻九天，以味苦粘牙者为真，一种番白芷伪充木香，皮带黑而臭腥，不可不辨。

木香其臭香，其数五，气味辛温，上彻九天，禀手足太阴天地之气化，主交感天地之气，上下相通。治邪气者，地气四散也。辟毒疫温鬼者，天气光明也。强志者，天一生水，水生则肾志强。主淋露者，地气上腾，气腾则淋露降。天地交感，则阳阳和，开合利，故久服不梦寤魇寐。梦寤者，寤中之梦。魇寐者，寐中之魇也。

58. Muxiang［木香, common aucklandia root, Radix Aucklandiae］

It is pungent in taste, warm and non-toxic in property, and it is mainly used to eliminate pathogenic qi, prevent the invasion of toxin and pestilence, strengthen memory, and treat severe heat disease and the diseases caused by rain, fog and dew. Long-term taking of it will avoid sudden waking up due to fright and nightmare.

Firstly recorded to be growing in the mountain valleys of Yongchang（永昌）, now it is all imported from abroad. It used to be called Qingmuxiang（青木香）and was renamed Guangmuxiang（广木香）in order to avoid confusion, because people later on also called the root of Madouling［马兜铃, aristolochia fruit, Aristolochiae Fructus］Qingmuxiang（青木香）. *San Dong Zhu Nang* ［《三洞珠囊》, *Essence of Books on Taoism*］says that Wuxiang（五香）is Muxiang（common aucklandia root）, because each herb has five roots, each stem has five branches, each branch has five leaves and each leaf has five transverse leaf veins. Its root grows left and will not be strong until it is dug out for twenty-nine days, which is like a dry bone. Its fragrance can go upward to the sky when the root is burnt. The genuine ones are sticky and bitter in taste. Fanbaizhi [番白芷, Dahurian angelica, Angelicae Dahuricae Radix] is used to fake Muxiang (common aucklandia root). However, Fan Baizhi (Dahurian angelica) smells stinky with blackish peel. Thus, we should carefully examine Muxiang (common aucklandia root) when using it.

It is fragrant in smell and it is related to the number five. It is pungent in taste and mild in property, and its fragrance can go upward to the sky. It receives the qi transformation of heaven and earth from hand greater yin and foot greater yin. It is mainly used to interact heaven qi with earth qi, which leads to the heaven qi and the earth qi aiding each other. It is used to eliminate pathogenic qi, because earth qi spreads in all directions. It is used to prevent the invasion of toxin and pestilence and treat severe heat disease, because heaven qi is bright. It is used to strengthen memory because Heaven One (天一) generates water, which will strengthen kidney will. It is used to treat the disease caused by rain, fog and dew because earth qi goes upward, which will lead to forming of rain, fog and dew. The interaction of heaven qi and earth qi will make yin and yang harmonized and make opening and closing smooth, so long-term taking of it will avoid sudden waking up due to fright and nightmare. The sudden waking up due to fright means having bad dreams in half asleep, and nightmare means having bad dream when sleeping.

59. 续　断

续断　气味苦微温,无毒。主治伤寒,补不足,金疮痈疡,折跌,续筋骨,妇人乳难。久服益气力。

续断始出常山山谷,今所在山谷皆有,而以川蜀者为胜。三月生苗,四月开花红白色,或紫色,似益母草花,根色赤黄,晒干则黑。

续断气味苦温,根色赤黄,晒干微黑,折有烟尘,禀少阴阳明火土之气化,而治经脉三因之证。主治伤寒者,经脉虚而寒邪侵入,为外因之证也,补不足者,调养经脉之不足,为里虚内因之证也。金疮者,金伤成疮,为不内外因之证也。经脉受邪,为痈为疡,亦外因也。折跌而筋骨欲续,亦不内外因也。妇人经脉不足而乳难,亦里虚内因也。续断禀火土之气,而治经脉三因之证者如此。久服则火气盛,故益气。土气盛,故益力也。

59. Xuduan〔续断, root of Himalayan teasel, Radix Dipsaci〕

It is bitter in taste, slightly warm and non-toxic in property, and it is mainly used to treat cold damage, tonify insufficiency, resolve incised wounds, abscesses and ulcers, cure traumatic injury, invigorate the sinews and bones, and treat the difficulty in lactation. Long-term taking of it will replenish qi and energy.

Firstly recorded to be growing in the valleys of Changshan Mountain（常山）, now it grows in all valleys, and those growing in Chuanshu（川蜀）are of better quality. It has seedlings in the third lunar month and blossoms red-white or purple flowers in the fourth lunar month. The flowers look like those of Yimucao〔益母草, leonurus, Leonuri Herba〕. The root is red-yellow in color, but turns black after dried in the sun.

It is bitter in taste and slightly warm in property. Its root is red-yellow in color, but turns slightly black when it is dried in the sun. There is smoke dust when the root is broken. It receives the qi transformation of fire and earth from lesser yin and yang brightness to treat the diseases in the meridians of three types of cause. It can mainly treat the cold damage, which is caused by deficient meridians followed by the attack of cold pathogen, and it is a kind of disease of external cause. To tonify insufficiency is to regulate and nourish the insufficiency of the meridians, which is a kind of disease of interior deficiency and internal cause. The incised wound is the sore caused by metal injury, which is a kind of disease of non-internal and non-external cause. The meridians attacked by pathogen will lead to abscesses and ulcers, which is also a kind of disease of external cause. The traumatic injury whose treatment needs to invigorate the sinews and bones is also a kind of disease of non-internal and non-external cause. The difficulty in lactation caused by insufficiency in the meridians is also a kind of disease of interior deficiency and internal cause. That is the reason why Xuduan（root of Himalayan teasel）can treat the diseases in the meridians of the three types of cause by receiving the qi of fire and earth. Long-term taking of it leads to the exuberance of fire qi, so it will replenish qi. The exuberance of earth qi is good for replenishing energy.

60. 蒺 藜

蒺藜 气味苦温,无毒。主治恶血,破瘕症积聚,喉痹,乳难。久服长肌肉,明目,轻身。

蒺藜始出冯翊平泽或道旁,今西北地多有。春时布地,蔓生细叶,入夏做碎小黄花,秋深结实,状如菱米,三角四刺,其色黄白,实内有仁,此刺蒺藜也。《尔雅》名茨。《诗》言:墙有茨者是也。又,同州沙苑一种,生于牧马草地上,亦蔓生布地,茎间密布细刺,七月开花黄紫色,九月结实作荚,长寸许,内子如脂麻,绿色,状如羊肾,味甘微腥,今人谓之沙苑蒺藜,即白蒺藜也。今市肆中以茨蒺藜为白蒺藜,白蒺藜为沙苑蒺藜,古今名称互异,从俗可也。

蒺藜子坚劲有刺,禀阳明之金气,气味苦温,则属于火。《经》云:两火合并,故为阳明,是阳明禀火气而属金也。金能平木,故主治肝木所瘀之恶血,破肠胃郛郭之症瘕积聚,阴阳交结之喉痹,阳明胃土之乳难,皆以其禀锐利之质而攻伐之力也。久服则阳明土气盛,故长肌肉。金水相生,故明目。长肌肉,故轻身。

其沙苑蒺藜一种,生于沙地,形如羊肾,主补肾益精,治腰痛虚损,小便遗沥。所以然者,味甘带腥,禀阳明土金之气,土生金而金生水也。

60. Jili〔蒺藜，puncturevine caltrop fruit，Fructus Tribuli〕

It is bitter in taste, warm and non-toxic in property, and it is mainly used to resolve blood stasis, disperse the accumulation of abdominal mass, and treat throat impediment and difficult lactation. Long-term taking of it will promote the growth of the muscles, improve vision and keep healthy.

Firstly recorded to be growing in the pools or at the roadsides of Fengyi (冯翊), it now commonly grows in the northwest. In spring, it grows all over the land with spires rambling; in summer, small yellow flowers blossom; in late autumn, it bears water-caltrop-shaped fruits. The fruits are covered by thorns with three protrusions, and they are yellow and white in color with seeds inside. It is called Cijili (刺蒺藜). It is mentioned as puncture vine (茨) in *Er Ya*〔《尔雅》, *On Elegance*〕. *Shi Jing*〔《诗经》, *The Book of Songs*〕says that it is all right to have some puncture vines on the wall. There is another type of it growing in Shayuan（沙苑）of Tongzhou（同州）. It grows all over the grassland where horses graze, and fine thorns densely cover its stem. The yellow and purple flowers blossom in the seventh lunar month and the fruits in the ninth lunar month. Its fruit is about one Cun in length, with sesame-sized seeds inside, green in color, goat's-kidney-like in shape, and sweet in taste with slightly stinky smelling. Today, it is called Shayuan Jili（沙苑蒺藜）or Baijili（白蒺藜）. In shops nowadays, Cijili（刺蒺藜）is often regarded as Baijili（白蒺藜）, and Baijili（白蒺藜）is often regarded as Shayuan Jili（沙苑蒺藜）. This is because the herbal names are different from the ancient times to the present, so it is all right to follow the local customs.

Jilizi〔蒺藜子, fruit of puncturevine caltrap, Fructus Tribuli〕is hard and thorny. Receiving the metal qi from yang brightness, it is bitter in taste and mild in property and pertains to fire. *Huang Di Nei Jing*〔《黄帝内经》, *Huangdi's Internal Classic*〕says that the combination of double fire is yang brightness which receives fire qi and pertains to metal. Metal can restrain wood, so Jilizi（fruit of puncturevine caltrap）can be used to resolve the blood stasis of liver wood, break abdominal mass and accumulation-gathering surrounding the stomach and intestines, and treat the pharyngitis due to yin-yang connection and the difficult lactation due to stomach earth from yang brightness, this is all because it is sharp in nature and has an effect of violent attack. Long-term taking of it can boost the earth qi from yang brightness, so as to promote the growth of the muscles. The mutual generation between metal and water improves vision. The growth of the muscles helps keep healthy.

One type of Shayuan Jili（沙苑蒺藜）grows in sand, looking like goat's kidney. It is mainly used to tonify the kidney and boost essence, treat lumbago, deficiency and detriment, and dribbling urination. The reason lies in that it is sweet and slightly stinky smelling in taste and receives earth qi and the metal qi from yang brightness. Earth generates metal and metal generates water.

61. 桑根白皮

桑根白皮　气味甘寒,无毒。主治伤中,五劳六极,羸瘦崩中,绝脉,补虚,益气。

　　《纲目》误书中品,夫桑上之寄生得列上品,岂桑反在中品也,今改入上品。桑处处有之,而江浙独盛。二月发叶,深秋黄陨,四月椹熟,其色赤黑,味甘性温。

　　桑名白桑,落叶后望之,枝干皆白,根皮作纸,洁白而绵,蚕食桑精,吐丝如银,盖得阳明金精之气。阳明属金而兼土,故味甘。阳明主燥而金气微寒,故气寒,主治伤中,续经脉也。五劳,志劳、思劳、烦劳、忧劳、恚劳也。六极,气极、血极、筋极、骨极、肌极、精极也。羸瘦者,肌肉消减。崩中者,血液下注。脉绝者,脉络不通。桑皮禀阳明土金之气,刈而复茂,生长之气最盛,故补续之功如此。

61. Sanggen Baipi〔桑根白皮, bark of white mulberry, Cortex Mori〕

It is sweet in taste, cold and non-toxic in property, and it is mainly used to treat the damage of the middle, five kinds of strain and six extremes, weakness and emaciation, metrorrhagia and no pulsation, tonify deficiency and replenish qi.

　　It is mistakenly classified as the medium grade in *Ben Cao Gang Mu*〔《本草纲目》, *Compendium of Materia Medica*〕. Since Sangshang Jisheng〔桑上寄生, Mistletoe, Taxilli Herba〕is classified as the top grade, how should the mulberry be classified as the medium grade? So it is corrected into top grade in this book. It abounds exceptionally in Jiangsu（江苏）and Zhejiang（浙江）although it grows everywhere. Its leaves come out in the second lunar month and turn yellow and fall in late autumn. The mulberry fruit turns ripe in the fourth lunar month, which is reddish-black in color, sweet in taste and warm in property.

The mulberry is also known as white mulberry（白桑）because its branches and trunks appear white after its leaves fall. Its root bark can be used to make white and soft paper. Silkworms eating the essence of mulberry produces silver-like silk as it receives the metal qi from yang brightness. Yang brightness pertains to metal and earth, so the mulberry is sweet in taste. Yang brightness governs dryness while metal is slightly cold, so its qi is cold and can be used to treat the damage of the middle and continue the vessels and collaterals. Five kinds of strain include the strain of mind, thought, vexation, anxiety and anger. Six extremes include the extreme disorder of qi, blood, sinews, bones, muscles and essence. Weakness and emaciation is featured with the decrease of the muscles. Metrorrhagia is manifested by profuse vaginal bleeding, and the expiry of vessels is manifested by the obstruction of vessels and collaterals. The mulberry bark receives the qi of metal and earth from yang brightness and can restore to flourish very soon even after its being chopped down, so it has the greatest qi of growth, making it effective in improving deficiency and continuing qi.

62. 桑 叶

桑叶　气味苦寒,主除寒热,出汗。

　　按:《夷坚志》云:严州山寺有一游僧,形体赢瘦,饮食甚少,每夜就枕,遍身汗出,迨旦衣皆湿透,如此二十年无药能疗,期待尽耳。监寺僧曰:吾有药绝验,为汝治之,三日宿疾顿愈,其方单用桑叶一味,乘露采摘,焙干碾末,每用二钱,空腹温米饮调服。或值桑落时,干者亦堪用,但力不如新采者,桑叶是止盗汗之药,非发汗药。《本经》盖谓桑叶主治能除寒热,并除出汗也,恐人误读作发汗解故表而明之。

62. Sangye [桑叶, mulberry leaf, Mori Folium]

It is bitter in taste and cold in property, and it is mainly used to treat cold and heat and stop sweating.

　　Note by Gao Shishi (高世栻): *Yi Jian Zhi* [《夷坚志》, *Record of Yijian*] says that in a mountain temple of Yanzhou (严州) lived a wandering monk who was weak and emaciated with very little diet. For every night in sleep, he was sweating all over so that the clothes were soaked by dawn. It lasted for twenty years and no medicinal was found to treat him. He even stopped holding any expectations. The monk in charge of the temple told him: "I have an effective medicine which can cure you in three days. The formula contains only a single herb—Sangye (mulberry leaf), which must be picked in morning dew, dried and ground into powder. Take two Qian each time with warm rice soup on an empty stomach. The fallen dry leaves can be used, but they are not as effective as the fresh ones. " Sangye (mulberry leaf) is a medicinal for stopping night sweat, rather than inducing sweat. *Shen Nong Ben Cao Jing* [《神农本草经》, *Shennong's Classic of Materia Medica*] says that Sangye (mulberry leaf) is mainly used to treat cold and heat and stop sweating. To avoid the original words being misinterpreted as inducing sweat, hereby it is specified.

63. 桑　枝 附

桑枝 附　气味苦平,主治遍体风痒干燥,水气,脚气,风气,四肢拘挛,上气,眼运,肺气咳嗽,消食,利小便。久服轻身,聪明耳目,令人光泽。《图经本草》附。

63. Sangzhi [桑枝, mulberry twig, Ramulus Mori] *supplement*

It is bitter in taste and mild in property, and it is mainly used to treat the pruritus and dryness all over the body, edema, leg qi, wind qi, the spasm of four limbs, the abnormal rising of qi and dizziness. It is also effective in treating the cough due to the damage of lung qi, dispersing food accumulation and disinhibiting urination. Long-term taking of it can keep healthy, improve hearing and vision and luster the skin. Supplemented in *Tu Jing Ben Cao* [《图经本草》, *Illustrated Classic of Materia Medica*].

64. 桑　椹

桑椹 止消渴《唐本草》,利五脏,关节痛,安魂,镇神,令人聪明,变白不老。《本草拾遗》附。

64. Sangshen [桑椹, mulberry fruit, Fructus Mori] *supplement*

It can be used to treat consumptive thirst [*Tang Ben Cao*,《唐本草》, *Tang Materia Medica*], promote the functions of the five zang-organs, relieve the pain of joints, tranquilize the ethereal soul and set mind, make people brighter, and slow aging even with gray hair. Supplemented in *Ben Cao Shi Yi* [《本草拾遗》, *Supplement to Materia Medica*].

65. 桑 花 ^附

桑花 ^附　气味苦暖,无毒。主治健脾,涩肠,止鼻洪,吐血,肠风,崩中,带下。《日华本草》附。

桑花生桑枝上白藓也,如地钱花样,刀刮取炒用,非是桑椹花。

65. Sanghua［桑花, mulberry flower, Flos Mori］*supplement*

It is bitter in taste, warm and non-toxic in property, and it is mainly used to invigorate the spleen, astringe the intestines, stop nosebleed, treat hematemesis, bloody defecation, metrorrhagia and leukorrhea. Supplemented in *Ri Hua Ben Cao*［《日华本草》, *Rihuazi's Materia Medica*］.

Sanghua (mulberry flower) here refers to the dittany growing on Sangzhi［桑枝, mulberry twig, Ramulus Mori］rather than the mulberry flower. It looks like the liverwort flower. Scrape it with a knife and stir-fry it to make it medicinal.

66. 桑上寄生

桑上寄生　气味苦平,无毒。主腰痛,小儿背强痈肿,充肌肤,坚发齿,长须眉,安胎。

桑寄生始出弘农川谷及近海州邑海外之境,其地暖而不蚕。桑无剪伐之苦,气厚力充,故枝节间有小木生焉,是为桑上寄生,寄生之叶如橘而厚软。寄生之茎,如槐而肥脆。四月开黄白花,五月结黄赤实,大如小豆,有汁稠粘,断茎视之色深黄者良。寄生木枫槲榉柳水杨等树上皆有之。须桑上生者可用。世俗多以寄生他树者伪充,不知气性不同,用之非徒无益,而反有害。一种黄寄生,形如石斛,一种如柴,不黄色者,皆伪也。

寄生感桑气而寄生枝节间,生长无时,不假土力,夺天地造化之神功。主治腰痛者,腰乃肾之外候,男子以藏精,女子以系胞。寄生得桑精之气,虚系而生,故治腰痛。小儿肾形未足,似无腰痛之证,应有背强痈肿之疾。寄生治腰痛,则小儿背强痈肿,亦能治之。充肌肤,精气外达也。坚发齿,精气内足也。精气外达而充肌肤,则须眉亦长。精气内足而坚发齿,则胎亦安。盖肌肤者,皮肉之余。齿者,骨之余。发与须眉者,血之余。胎者,身之余。以余气寄生之物,而治余气之病,同类相感如此。

66. Sangshang Jisheng〔桑上寄生, Chinese taxillus herb, Herba Taxilli〕

It is bitter in taste, mild and non-toxic in property, and it is mainly used to treat lumbago, infantile back rigidity and carbuncle, enrich the muscles, strengthen the hair and teeth, promote beards and eyebrows and prevent abortion.

　　Sangshang Jisheng (Chinese taxillus herb) was firstly recorded to be growing in the river valleys of Hongnong (弘农) and the offshore areas near Haizhou (海州) County. Mulberry trees in these areas do not have to suffer from chopping down because it is warm and not suitable to raise silkworms here. So the trees are growing in full vigor, and small twigs parasitically grow out between branches and knots, which are Sangshang Jisheng (Chinese taxillus herb). Its leaves are thick and soft like tangerines and its stalks are thick and crisp like those of pagoda trees. Yellow and white flowers blossom in the fourth lunar month, and yellow-red fruits grow in the fifth lunar month. The fruits are in size of a bean with sticky juice. Sangshang Jisheng (Chinese taxillus herb) is of good quality if the transection of the interior of stalks appears dark yellow in color. Jisheng〔寄生, mistletoe, Taxilli Herba〕can be found on various trees and timbers such as maple, Mongolian oak, zelkova schneideriana, willow, bigcatkin willow, etc. Only those growing on mulberry trees can be used as medicinal. People often take Jisheng (mistletoe) growing on other trees as fake Sangshang Jisheng (Chinese taxillus herb). They don't realize that the two are different in taste and property, and the fake ones are not beneficial but harmful. There is a type of Jisheng (mistletoe) with the color of yellow, like Shihu〔石斛, dendrobium, Herba Dendrobii〕, and another type looks like firewood, without the color of yellow, both of which are fake.

Sangshang Jisheng (Chinese taxillus herb) receives the qi of mulberry and grows parasitically out of branches and knots. It can grow any time with no need of soil fertility as it receives the essence of heaven and earth. It is mainly used to treat lumbago because the waist is the external manifestation of the kidney, where men's semen is stored and women's uterus is nourished. Sangshang Jisheng (Chinese taxillus herb) obtains the essence qi of mulberry, grows parasitically on mulberry trees, so it can treat lumbago. For infants, their kidneys have not developed into full shape, so it seems they do not have lumbago, but they have back rigidity and carbuncle. Since Sangshang Jisheng (Chinese taxillus herb) can treat lumbago, it can also treat the infantile back rigidity and carbuncle. If the muscles are enriched, essence qi has reached outward; if the hair and teeth are strengthened, essence qi has been sufficient internally; if beards and eyebrows are promoted, essence qi has gone outward and the muscles have been enriched; if the fetus is quiet, essence qi has reached outward and the teeth have been strengthened. This is because the muscles are a part of skin and flesh; teeth are a part of bones; hair, beards and eyebrows are part of blood, and the fetus is a part of mother's body. Sangshang Jisheng (Chinese taxillus herb), an extra parasitic twig of the mulberry tree, can be used to treat the diseases of extension parts of the body. It draws an analogy between the two.

67. 桑寄生实

桑寄生实 气味甘平,无毒。主明目,轻身,通神。

67. Sangjisheng Shi〔桑寄生实, Chinese taxillus herb fruit, Materia Medica Sangjisheng Shi〕

It is sweet in taste, mild and non-toxic in property, and it is mainly used to improve vision, keep healthy and invigorate the spirit and mentality.

68. 柏子仁

柏子仁 气味甘平,无毒。主治惊悸,益气,除风湿,安五脏。久服令人润泽美色,耳目聪明,不饥不老,轻身延年。

柏木处处有之，其实先以大山者为良，今以陕州、宜州、乾州为胜。柏有数种，叶扁而侧生者，名侧柏叶，可以入药。其实皆圆柏所生，若侧柏之实，尤为佳妙，但不可多得尔，仁色黄白，其气芬香，最多脂液。万木皆向阳，柏独西顾，故字从白，白者西方也。《埤雅》云：柏之指西，犹针之指南也。寇宗奭曰：予官陕西登高望柏，千万株皆一一西指。

柏叶经冬不凋，禀太阳之水气也。仁黄臭香，禀太阴之土气也。水精上资，故治心肾不交之惊悸。土气内充，故益气，除风湿。夫治惊悸，益气，除风湿，则五脏皆和，故安五脏也。仁多脂液，久服则令人润泽而美色，且耳目聪明。五脏安和，津液濡灌，故不饥不老，轻身延年。

68. Baiziren [柏子仁, Chinese arborvitae kernel, Semen Platycladi]

It is sweet in taste, mild and non-toxic in property, and it is mainly used to treat fright and palpitation, replenish qi, eliminate wind dampness and pacify the five zang-organs. Long-term taking of it can luster and beautify the complexion, improve hearing and vision, make people feel no hunger, slow aging, keep healthy and prolong life.

The arborvitae grows everywhere. Its fruit originally growing in mountains is of good quality. Today, those growing in Shanzhou (陕州), Yizhou (宜州) and Qianzhou (乾州) are better. There are several kinds of arborvitaes, one of which used as medicinal is called Cebaiye [侧柏叶, Chinese arborvitae twig and leaf, Cacumen Platycladi] with flatten and lateral leaves. The fruits of the oriental arborvitae are exceptionally good and rare because most fruits are actually from the sabina chinensis. Its kernel is yellow-white in color with fragrance and abundant juice. All trees grow facing the sun while only the arborvitae grows westward. So its name is "Bai" [柏, cypress], the same pronunciation as Bai [白, white] which refers to the west. *Pi Ya* [《埤雅》, *Piya*] says that the arborvitae's pointing to the west is like the compass's pointing to the south. Kou Zongshi (寇宗奭), the famous pharmacologist of the Song Dynasty, once said, "When I worked as an officer in Shaanxi, I once climbed a mountain to overlook the arborvitaes, and thousands of them all pointed to the west."

The arborvitae leaves do not wither and fall even in winter as it receives the water qi from greater yang. Its yellow kernels smell fragrant as it receives the earth qi from greater yin. Water essence goes upward, so it can treat fright and palpitation due to the non-interaction between the heart and the kidney. Earth qi is sufficient inside the body, so it can replenish qi, eliminate wind dampness, and harmonize the five zang-organs, making them pacified. Since its kernel is abundant with juice, long-term taking of it can luster and beautify the complexion and improve hearing and vision. When the five zang-organs are harmonized and pacified, the body fluid is sufficient to perform the effect of moistening and nourishing, so taking it can make people feel no hunger, keep healthy and prolong life.

69. 侧柏叶 附

侧柏叶 附 气味苦,微温,无毒。主治吐血、衄血、痢血、崩中赤白,轻身益气,令人耐寒暑。去湿痹,生肌。《别录》附。

凡草木耐岁寒,冬不落叶者,阴中有阳也。冬令主太阳寒水,而水府属太阳,水脏属少阴,柏叶禀寒水之气,而太阳为标,禀少阴之气而君火为本,故气味苦,微温。主治吐血、衄血、痢血、崩中赤白者,得水阴之气而资养其血液也。轻身益气,令人耐寒暑,去湿痹,生肌者,得太阳之标,少阴之本,而补益其阳气也。柏子仁气味甘平,故禀太阳寒水而兼得太阴之土气。侧柏叶气味苦微温,故禀太阳寒水而兼得少阴之君火。叶实之所以不同者如此。

69. Cebaiye [侧柏叶, Chinese arborvitae twig and leaf, Cacumen Platycladi] supplement

It is bitter in taste, slightly warm and non-toxic in property, and it is mainly used to treat hematemesis, epistaxis, blood dysentery and mixed red and white metrorrhagia. It can replenish qi and keep healthy, make people tolerate cold and summer-heat, eliminate dampness impediment and regenerate the muscles. Supplemented in *Ming Yi Bie Lu* [《名医别录》, *Miscellaneous Records of Famous Physicians*].

There is yang within yin for all cold-resistant grass and trees whose leaves do not wither and fall in winter. Winter governs cold water from greater yang; the bladder pertains to greater yang and the kidney pertains to lesser yin. Arborvitae twigs and leaves receives qi from cold water with greater yang as branch, and it receives the qi of lesser yin with the sovereign fire as root. So it is bitter in taste and slightly warm in property. It can treat hematemesis, epistaxis, blood dysentery, mixed red and white metrorrhagia as it obtains the qi of water yin and can nourish blood. It can replenish qi and keep healthy, make people tolerate cold and summer-heat, eliminate dampness impediment and regenerate muscles, as it obtains the branch of greater yang and the root of lesser yin to replenish yang qi. Baiziren〔柏子仁, Chinese Arborvitae Kernel, Semen Platycladi〕is sweet in taste and mild in property as it receives cold water from greater yang as well as earth qi from greater yin. However, since Cebaiye (Chinese arborvitae twig and leaf) receives cold water from greater yang and the sovereign fire from lesser yin, it is bitter in taste and slightly warm in property. That explains why the leaf and fruit are different in taste and property.

70. 松 脂

松脂 气味苦甘温,无毒。主治痈疽恶疮,头疮白秃,疥瘙风气,安五脏,除热。久服轻身,不老延年。

松木之脂,俗名松香,处处山中有之。其木修耸多节,其皮粗厚有鳞,其叶有两鬣、五鬣、七鬣,其花蕊为松黄,结实状如猪心,木之余气结为茯苓。松脂入土,年深化成琥珀。其脂以通明如熏陆香颗者为胜,乃服食辟谷之品,神仙不老之妙药也。熬化滤过即为沥青。

松脂生于松木之中,禀木质而有火土金水之用。气味苦温,得火气也。得火气,故治肌肉之痈,经脉之疽,以及阴寒之恶疮。入土成珀,坚洁如金,裕金气也。裕金气,故治头疡白秃,以及疥瘙之风气。色黄臭香,味苦而甘,备土气也。备土气,故安五脏。木耐岁寒,经冬不凋,具水气也。具水气,故除热。久服则五运全精,故轻身,不老延年。

70. Songzhi〔松脂, pine oleoresin, Colophonium〕

It is bitter in taste, warm, sweet and non-toxic in property, and it is mainly used to treat welling-abscess and malign sore, white bald scalp sore, scabies and the pruritus due to wind qi, pacify the five zang-organs and relieve fever. Long-term taking of it will keep healthy, prevent aging and prolong life.

Songzhi (pine oleoresin), whose popular name is Songxiang [松香, rosin, Pini Resina], can be easily found everywhere in mountains. The tree is tall with a lot of knots; the bark is thick and rough with a lot of bud scales; the leaves may have two needles, five needles or seven needles; the flower pistil is yellow in color; the fruit looks like the pig heart; and the extraessence of the pine wood generates Fuling [伏苓, poria sclerotium, Wolfiporia Cocos]. The underearth Songzhi (pine oleoresin) will turn into Hupo [琥珀, amber, Succinum] over years. Songzhi (pine oleoresin) which is transparent and as big as mastiche is of better quality, and is an ideal product for fasting and pellet taking for longevity. It is a magic medicinal for immortality, and becomes pitch when it is boiled and filtered.

Growing in the pine wood, Songzhi (pine oleoresin) receives the property of wood with the effects of fire, earth, metal and water. It is bitter in taste and warm in property, as it gets fire qi. With fire qi, it can treat muscle abscess, meridian carbuncle and the severe sore due to yin cold. The underearth Songzhi (pine oleoresin) can turn into Hupo (amber) which is solid and clean like gold as it is abundant in metal qi. With metal qi, it can treat white bald scalp, scabies and the pruritus due to wind qi. Yellow in color with fragrance, it is bitter and sweet in taste, as it absorbs earth qi. With earth qi, it can pacify the five zang-organs. Absorbing water qi, the tree can tolerate cold and its leaves do not wither and fall all through the winter. With water qi, it can relieve fever. Long-term taking of it can strengthen the essence of five circuits, so it can keep healthy, prevent aging and prolong life.

71. 松 节 附

松节 附　气味苦温,无毒。主治百邪,久风,风虚脚痹,疼痛,酿酒,主脚软骨节风。《别录》附。

71. Songjie〔松节, knotty pine wood, Lignum Pini Nodi〕*supplement*

It is bitter in taste, warm and non-toxic in property, and it is mainly used to treat various pathogens, enduring wind impediment, the foot impediment due to wind deficiency and pain. Taking the liquor made from it can treat the joint-running wind with foot cartilages. Supplemented in *Ming Yi Bie Lu*〔《名医别录》, *Miscellaneous Records of Famous Physicians*〕.

72. 松 花 附

松花 附 别名松黄,气味甘温,无毒。主润心肺,益气,除风,止血,亦可酿酒。《本草纲目》附。

72. Songhua〔松花, pine pollen, Pini Pollen〕*supplement*

It is also known as Songhuang（松黄）. It is sweet in taste, and warm and non-toxic in property. It is mainly used to moisten the heart and the kidney, replenish qi, eliminate wind and staunch bleeding. It can also be made into liquor. Supplement in *Ben Cao Gang Mu*〔《本草纲目》, *Compendium of Materia Medica*〕

73. 茯 苓

茯苓 气味甘平,无毒。主治胸胁逆气,忧恚惊邪,恐悸。心下结痛,寒热,烦满,咳逆,口焦舌干,利小便。久服安魂养神,不饥延年。

茯苓生大山古松根下,有赤白二种。下有茯苓,则上有灵气如丝之状,山中人亦时见之。《史记·龟策传》作茯苓谓松之神灵,伏结而成。小者如拳,大者如斗,外皮皱黑,内质光白,以坚实而大者为佳。

茯苓,本松木之精华,借土气以结成,故气味甘平,有土位中央而枢机旋转之功。禀木气而枢转,则胸胁之逆气可治也。禀土气而安五脏,则忧恚惊恐悸之邪可平也。里气不和,则心下结痛。表气不和,则为寒为热。气郁于上,上而不下,则烦满咳逆,口焦舌干。气逆于下,交通不表,则小便不利。茯苓位于中土,灵气上荟,主内外旋转,上下交通,故皆治之。久服安肝藏之魂,以养心藏之

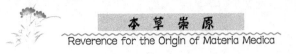

神。木生火也，不饥延年，土气盛也。

73. Fuling［伏苓, poria sclerotium, Wolfiporia Cocos］

It is sweet in taste, mild and non-toxic in property, and it is mainly used to cease the counterflow of qi from the chest and hypochondrium, alleviate anxiety, fright and palpitation, relieve the spasmatic pain in epigastrium, eliminate cold and heat, vexation and fullness, treat the coughing with dyspnea, dry mouth and tongue and disinhibit urination. Long-term taking of it will pacify the ethereal soul, nourish spirit, tolerate hunger, and prolong life.

Fuling (poria sclerotium) grows underneath the root of old pines in mountains, and it can be classified into two kinds: the red one and the white one. There are silk-like clouds of anima hanging around if there is Fuling (poria sclerotium) underneath, which is commonly seen in mountains. According to *Shi Ji · Gui Ce Zhuan*［《史记·龟策传》, *Historical Records · Biography of Guice*］, Fuling (poria sclerotium) is regarded as the sacred spirit of pines, which gets mature in summer. The smaller one is in size of fist and the bigger one in size of Dou (斗). Its skin is crinkled and black and the inside is smooth and white. The solid and big ones are of better quality.

Fuling (poria sclerotium) absorbs the essence of pine wood and gets ripen via earth qi, so it is sweet in taste and mild in property. It has the function of rotating qi movement because earth is in the centre. The counterflow of qi from the chest and hypochondrium will be treated due to the rotation of qi movement by receiving wood qi. It can pacify the five zang-organs because of receiving earth qi, so the pathogenic factors of anxiety, fright and palpitation will be expelled. There will be spasmatic pain in epigastrium without harmonious interior qi; there will be cold and heat without harmonious exterior qi; there will be vexation and fullness, coughing with dyspnea, dry mouth and tongue when qi stagnation is in the upper part without moving downward; there will be urine inhibition due to discoordination between the lung and the spleen and the qi counterflow in the lower part. Fuling (poria sclerotium) locates in center earth, and anima moves upward to get together to govern the rotation between the interior and the exterior and the coordination between the upper part and the lower part, so it can treat the diseases mentioned above. Long-term taking of it will pacify the ethereal soul stored in the liver and nourish the spirit stored in the heart. Wood generates fire, and it can make people tolerate hunger and prolong life due to the exuberance of earth qi.

74. 赤茯苓 附

赤茯苓 附　主破结气《药性本草》，泻心、小肠、膀胱湿热，利窍行水。《本草纲目》附。

74. Chifuling〔赤茯苓, red poria, Poria Rubra〕 *supplement*

It is mainly used to break qi stagnation *Yao Xing Ben Cao*〔《药性本草》, *Medicinal Properties of Materia Medica*〕, drain the dampness-heat of the heart, the small intestine, and the bladder, free orifices and disinhibit urination. Supplemented in *Ben Cao Gang Mu* 〔《本草纲目》, *Compendium of Materia Medica*〕.

75. 茯　神 附

茯神 附　气味甘平，无毒。主辟不祥，疗风眩、风虚、五劳、口干，止惊悸、多恚怒、善忘，开心益智，安魂魄，养精神。《别录》附。

离松木本体，不附根而生者。为茯苓。不离本体，抱根而生者，为茯神。虽分二种，总以茯苓为胜。

75. Fushen〔茯神, Indianbread with pine, Sclerotium Poriae Circum Radicem Pini〕 *supplement*

It is sweet in taste, mild and non-toxic in property, and it is mainly used to avoid ominous elements, treat wind dizziness, wind deficiency, five kinds of strain and dry mouth, relieve fright and palpitation, resentment and anger, and amnesia, soothe the heart and promote wisdom, pacify the ethereal soul and the corporeal soul, and cultivate the spirit. Supplemented in *Ming Yi Bie Lu*〔《名医别录》, *Miscellaneous Records of Famous Physicians*〕

Fuling (poria sclerotium) grows off the pine tree and detaches from its root, while Fushen (Indianbread with pine) grows on the tree and embraces the root. The former is always regarded of better quality than the latter although they belong to different two kinds.

76. 茯苓皮 附

茯苓皮 附　主治水肿肤胀,利水道,开腠理。《本草纲目》附。

76. Fulingpi [茯苓皮, poria skin, **Poriae Cutis**] *supplement*

It is mainly used to treat edema and anasarca, disinhibit water passage and open striae and interstice. Supplemented in *Ben Cao Gang Mu* [《本草纲目》, *Compendium of Materia Medica*].

77. 神 木 附

神木 附　主治偏风,口面喎斜,毒风筋挛,不语,心神惊掣,虚而健忘。《药性本草》附。

即茯神心内木也,又名黄松节。

愚谓:茯苓之皮与木,后人收用,各有主治,然皆糟粕之药,并无精华之气,不堪列于上品,只因茯苓而类载之于此。

77. Shenmu [神木, pinewood in poria, **Poriae Pini Radix**] *supplement*

It is mainly used to treat hemilateral wind, the deviation of the eyes and mouth, the muscular spasm due to wind toxin, aphonia, the panic attack of heart spirit, and the amnesia due to deficiency. Supplemented in *Yao Xing Ben Cao* [《药性本草》, *Medicinal Properties of Materia Medica*].

It is the wood inside Fushen [茯神, Indianbread with pine, Sclerotium Poriae Circum Radicem Pini], also known as Huangsongjie [黄松节, knotty pine wood, Pini Nodi Lignum].

Note by Gao Shishi (高世栻): The bark and wood of Fuling (poria sclerotium) are both inferior medicinals without essential qi though collected and used to treat some diseases by later generations. Therefore, they should not be classed as top grade and they are noted here just because they fall in the category of Fuling (poria sclerotium).

78. 蔓荆子

蔓荆子 气味苦,微寒,无毒。主治筋骨间寒热,湿痹拘挛,明目,坚齿,利九窍,去白虫。久服轻身耐老,小荆实亦等。

蔓荆生于水滨,苗高丈余,其茎小弱如蔓,故名蔓荆。春叶夏茂,六月有花,淡红色,九月成实,黑斑色,大如梧子而轻虚。一种木本者,其枝茎坚劲作科不作蔓,名牡荆,结实如麻子大,又名小荆实。

蔓荆多生水滨,其子黑色,气味苦寒,禀太阳寒水之气化,盖太阳本寒标热,少阴本热标寒。主治筋骨间寒热者,太阳主筋病,少阴主骨病,治太阳、少阴之寒热也。湿痹拘挛,湿伤筋骨也。益水之精,故明目。补骨之余,故坚齿。九窍为水注之气,水精充足,故利九窍。虫乃阴类,太阳有标阳之气,故去白虫。久服则筋骨强健,故轻身耐老。小荆实亦等,言蔓荆之外,更有一种小荆,其实与蔓荆之实功力相等,可合一而并用也。

78. Manjingzi〔蔓荆子, shrub chastetree fruit, Fructus Viticis〕

It is bitter in taste, slightly cold and non-toxic in property, and it is mainly used to treat the cold and heat between the sinews and bones, wind-dampness impediment and spasm, improve vision, strengthen the teeth, disinhibit nine orifices and kill white worms. Long-term taking of it will stay healthy and prevent aging. Xiaojingshi〔小荆实, small vitex fruit, Materia Medica Xiaojingshi〕has the same effects.

Manjing〔蔓荆, shrub chastetree, Fructus Viticis〕grows along the waterside. Its seedlings are around one Zhang in height. Its stems are as thin as the vine〔蔓, man in Chinese〕, for which it has got the name "Manjing". Its leaves grow out in spring and get lush in summer. The light red flowers blossom in the sixth lunar month and bear fruits in the ninth lunar month. The fruits are black in color, in size of a phoenix seed and light in weight. Another woody kind of it whose stems are very strong to bear branches rather than vines is known as Mujing〔牡荆, hemp-leaved vitex, Viticis Cannabifolii〕. Its fruit is as big as Mazi〔麻子, cannabis fruit, Cannabis Fructus〕, also known as Xiaojingshi (small vitex fruit).

Manjing (shrub chastetree) mostly grows along the waterside. Its fruit is black in color, bitter in taste and cold in property. It receives the qi transformation of cold water from greater yang, as greater yang pertains to the cold in root and to the heat in branch, while lesser yin pertains to the heat in root and to the cold in branch. In terms of the cold and heat between the sinews and bones, greater yang treats the diseases of the sinews and lesser yin treats the diseases of the bones, and then it is effective for the cold and heat of greater yang and lesser yin. Dampness impediment and spasm are caused by the dampness damage of the sinews and bones. It tonifies the water essence, so it can improve vision. It tonifies the extension parts of bones, so it can strengthen the teeth. The nine orifices are the regions where water qi infuses. With sufficient water essence, the nine orifices are thus nourished. The worms pertain to yin, and greater yang has the qi of branch yang, so it can kill white worms. Long-term taking of it can strengthen the sinews and bones, thus it can keep healthy and prevent aging. Xiaojingshi (small vitex fruit) has the same effects. There is the other kind of Xiaojing〔小荆, small vitex〕whose fruit has the same effects as that of Manjingzi (shrub chastetree fruit), so they can be used as one medicinal.

79. 小荆实 附

小荆实 附　气味苦温,无毒。主除骨间寒热,通利胃气,止咳逆,下气。《别录》附。

79. Xiaojingshi〔小荆实, small vitex fruit, Materi Medica Xiaojingshi〕 *supplement*

It is bitter in taste, warm and non-toxic in property, and it is mainly used to treat the cold and heat between the sinews and bones, tonify stomach qi, stop cough with dyspnea and descend qi. Supplemented in *Ming Yi Bie Lu* [《名医别录》, *Miscellaneous Records of Famous Physicians*].

80. 槐　实

槐实　气味苦寒,无毒。主治五内邪气热,止涎唾,补绝伤,火疮,妇人乳瘕,子脏急痛。

槐始出河南平泽,今处处有之。有数种,叶大而黑者,名欀槐。昼合夜开者,名守宫。槐叶细而青绿者,但谓之槐。槐之生也,季春五日而兔目,十日而鼠耳,更旬日而始规,再旬日而叶成,四五月间开黄花,六七月间结实作荚,连珠中有黑子,以子连多者为妙,其木材坚重,有青黄白黑色。《周礼》冬取槐檀之火。《淮南子》云:老槐生火。《天元主物薄》云:老槐生丹,槐之神异如此,其花未开时,炒过煎水,染黄甚鲜。陈藏器曰:子上房,七月收之,可染皂,近时用槐花染绿。

槐生中原平泽,花黄子黑,气味苦寒,木质有青、黄、白、黑色,老则生火生丹,备五运之全精,故主治五内邪气之热,五脏在内,故曰五内。邪气热,因邪气而病热也。肺气不能四布其水精,则涎唾上涌,槐实能止之。肝血不能渗灌于经脉,则经脉绝伤,槐实能补之。心火内盛,则为火疮。脾土不和则为乳瘕。肾气内逆,则子脏急痛。槐禀五运之气,故治肺病之涎唾,肝病之绝伤,心病之火疮,脾病之乳瘕,肾病之急痛,而为五内邪气之热者如此。

80. Huaishi [槐实, sophora fruit, Fructus Sophorae]

It is bitter in taste, cold and non-toxic in property, and it is mainly used to treat the pathogenic-qi heat in the five zang-organs, cease saliva and spittle, treat severe injury, scalded sore, the breast lump in woman and the urgent pain in uterus.

Firstly recorded to be growing in the lakes and pools of Henan (河南), the pogodatree now grows everywhere. There are several kinds. Those with big and black leaves are called Ranghuai(欀槐). Those with leaves that close in the day and open at night are called Shougong(守宫). Those with slender and green leaves are generally called Huai(槐). Its new leaves sprout out on the fifth day of the fifth lunar month, grow into the shape of the mouse's ear on the tenth day of the month, and begin to turn round in ten days and then take shape after another ten days. It blossoms with yellow flowers in the fourth and fifth lunar months and bear fruits and pods in the sixth and seventh lunar months. The pods look like connected beads, inside which there are black seeds. Those with more connected seeds in a pod are of better quality. Its wood is hard and heavy in texture, with the colors of green, yellow, white or black. *Zhou Li* [《周礼》, *Rites of Zhou*] says that the pagodatree wood can be used to make fire in winter. *Huai Nan Zi* [《淮南子》, *Huai Nan Tzu*] says that the old pagodatree wood can be used to make fire. *Kai Yuan Zhu Wu Bo* [《开元主物薄》, *Collection of Creatures in the Kaiyun Era*] says that the pagodatree is so magic that the old pagodatree can engender the inner exilir. Before blossom, fry them and decoct them in water. The decoction is very effective to dye fresh yellow. Chen Cangqi (陈藏器) said, "Its pods collected in the seventh lunar month can be used to dye things into black and lately people use its flowers to dye things into green."

The pagodatree grows in the pools and lakes of Zhongyuan (中原). Its flowers are yellow and its seeds are black. Its fruit is bitter in taste and cold in property. Its wood may be green, yellow, white or black in color. The old wood can be used to make fire or inner elixir. It obtains all the essence of the five circuits, so it can treat the pathogenic-qi heat in the five zang-organs. The five zang-organs are also known as five-nei [内, inner in English] as they are located in the inner of the body. The pathogenic qi is heat, so it can cause heat diseases. When lung qi fails to distribute its water essence, saliva and spittle will flow upward, which can be ceased by Huaishi (sophora fruit). When liver blood fails to flow to the meridians, there will be severe injury to the meridians, which can be nourished by Huaishi (sophora fruit). The exuberance of heart fire can cause scalded sore. The disharmony of the spleen and the stomach will cause breast lump in woman and the internal counterflow of kidney qi will cause the urgent pain in uterus. Huaishi (sophora fruit) receives the qi of the five circuits, so it can cease saliva and spittle due to the disease with the lung, treat the severe injury due to the disease with the liver, the scalded sore due to the disease with the heart, the breast lump in woman due to the disease with the spleen, and the urgent pain due to the disease with the kidney, all of which indicate the pathogenic-qi heat in the five zang-organs.

81. 槐 花 附

槐花 附 　气味苦平,无毒。主治五痔,心痛,眼赤,杀腹脏虫,及皮肤风热,肠风泻血,赤白痢。《日华本草》附。

81. Huaihua〔槐花, sophora flower, Flos Sophorae〕*supplement*

It is bitter in taste, mild and non-toxic in property, and it is mainly used to treat five kinds of hemorrhoids, heart pain, and the redness of the eyes, kill the worms in the abdomen, treat the wind-heat diseases with the skin, bloody stool and red and white dysentery. Supplemented in *Ri Hua Ben Cao*〔《日华本草》, *Rihuazi's Materia Medica*〕.

82. 槐 枝 附

槐枝 附 　气味苦平,无毒。主治洗疮,及阴囊下湿痒。八月断大枝,候生嫩蘖,煮汁酿酒,疗大风痿痹,甚效。《别录》附。

82. Huaizhi〔槐枝, sophora twig, Sophorae Ramulus〕*supplement*

It is bitter in taste, mild and non-toxic in property, and it is mainly used to treat the sores and damp itching beneath the scrotum. In the eighth lunar month, cut off the big branches. When the new sprouts grow out, decoct them to make liquor, which is very effective in treating the wilting and impediment due to severe wind. Supplemented in *Ming Yi Bie Lu*〔《名医别录》, *Miscellaneous Records of Famous Physicians*〕.

83. 槐 叶 附

槐叶 附 　气味苦平,无毒。主治煎汤,治小儿惊痫壮热,疥癣及疔肿。皮茎同用。《日华本草》附。

83. Huaiye〔槐叶, sophora leaf, Sophorae Folium〕 *supplement*

It is bitter in taste, and mild and non-toxic in property. Its decoction is mainly used to treat infantile fright epilepsy and high fever, scab, lichen and clove sores. Its bark and stem has the same effects. Supplemented in *Ri Hua Ben Cao*〔《日华本草》, *Rihuazi's Materia Medica*〕.

84. 槐　胶 附

槐胶 附　气味苦寒,无毒。主治一切风化涎痰,清肝脏风,筋脉抽掣,及急风口噤。《嘉祐本草》附。

84. Huaijiao〔槐胶, sophora resin, Sophorae Resina〕 *supplement*

It is bitter in taste, cold and non-toxic in property, and it is mainly used to treat various wind phlegms, the clear wind in the liver, and treat the convulsion of the muscles, tendons and clenched jaws due to acute wind stroke. Supplemented in *Jia You Ben Cao*〔《嘉祐本草》,*Materia Medica of the Jiayou Era*〕.

85. 干　漆

干漆　气味辛温,无毒。主治绝伤,补中,续筋骨,填髓脑,安五脏,五缓六急,风寒湿痹。生漆去长虫。久服轻身耐老。

漆树始出汉中山谷,今梁州、益州、广东、金州、歙州、陆州皆有。树高二三丈,干如柿,叶如椿,花如槐,实如牛奈子,木心色黄,六七月刻取滋汁,或以斧凿取干漆,不假日爆,乃自然干者,状如蜂房孔,孔间隔者为佳。

漆木生于西北,凿取滋汁而为漆,日曝则反润,阴湿则易干,如人胃府水谷所化之津液,奉心则化赤为血,即日曝反润之义也。入肾脏则凝结为精,即阴湿易干之义也。干漆气味辛温,先白后赤,生干则黑,禀阳明金精之质,而上奉于心,以资经脉,下交于肾,以凝精髓之药也。主治绝伤,资经脉也。补中,阳明居中土也。续筋骨者,治绝伤,则筋骨亦可续也。填髓脑者,凝精髓也。阳明水谷之精,滋灌五脏,故安五脏。驰纵曰缓,拘掣曰急,皆不和之意,五脏不和而驰纵,是为五缓,六腑不和而拘挈,是为六急。五缓六急,乃风寒湿之痹证,故曰风寒湿痹也。《素问·痹论》云:五脏皆有外合,六腑亦各有俞。皮肌脉筋骨之痹,各以其时,重感于风寒湿之气,则内舍五脏。五脏之痹,犹五缓也。风寒湿气中其俞,而食饮应之。循俞而入,各舍其腑。六腑之痹,犹六急也。是五缓六急,乃风寒湿痹也。生漆色白属金,金能制风,故生漆去长虫。久服则中土之精,四布运行,故轻身耐老。

85. Ganqi〔干漆, dried lacquer of true lacquertree, Resina Toxicodendri〕

It is pungent in taste, warm and non-toxic in property, and it is mainly used to treat severe damage, tonify the middle, invigorate the sinews and bones, enrich the brain, pacify the five zang-organs, treat the retardation of the five zang-organs, the contraction of the six fu-organs and the impediment due to wind, cold and dampness. Raw lacquer can kill roundworms. Long-term taking of it will keep healthy and prevent aging.

Firstly recorded to be growing in the mountain valleys of Hanzhong(汉中), Qishu〔漆树, Lacquer tree, Rhus verniciflua〕now grows in Liangzhou(梁州), Yizhou(益州), Guangdong(广东), Jinzhou(金州), Shezhou(歙州) and Luzhou(陆州). It is two or three Zhang in height, and its trunk looks like that of the persimmon tree; its leaves look like those of the toon tree; its flowers look like the sophora flowers and its fruits look like Niunaizi〔牛奈子, lanceolate codonopsis, Codonopsis Lanceolatae Radix〕. Its heartwood is yellow in color. In the sixth or seventh lunar month, carve it to get the thick juice or hew out the dried lacquer which gets dry naturally without being dried in the sun. It looks like beehives in shape and those with spaced holes are of better quality.

The lacquertree grows in the northwest. The dried lacquer is made after the thick juice is hewed out. It gets moistened with exposure to the sun while it is dried in the shade, which is similar to the fluids transformed from the grain and water in the stomach. The stomach offers the fluids to the heart which makes them red and transforms them into blood, indicating they get moistened in the sun. The fluids condense into essence in the kidney, indicating they get dried in the shade. Ganqi (dried lacquer of true lacquertree) is pungent in taste and warm in property. It is white in the early stage, turns red gradually and then turns black when it gets dried. Receiving the property of metal essence from yang brightness, it is a kind of medicinal that can tonify the heart in the upper part of the body so as to nourish meridians and flow downward to the kidney so as to congeal essence and marrow. It can nourish meridians, so it can treat severe damage. Since yang brightness locates in the center earth, it can tonify the middle. Since it can treat severe damage, it can invigorate the sinews and bones. Since it can congeal essence and marrow, it can enrich the brain. The essence of yang brightness transformed from the grain and water can tonify the five zang-organs, so it can pacify the five zang-organs. Convulsion means retardation and spasm means contraction means, both of which indicate disharmony. The disharmony of the five zang-organs leads to convulsion, which is the retardation of the five zang-organs; the disharmony of the six fu-organs leads to spasm, which is the contraction of the six fu-organs. The retardation of the five zang-organs and the contraction of the six fu-organs are both impediment due to wind, cold and dampness. Therefore, they are also known as wind-cold-dampness impediment. *Su Wen · Bi Lun* [《素问 · 痹论》, *Plain Questions · Discussion on Bi Syndrome*] says, " The five zang-organs are connected with certain parts of the body and the six fu-organs have their Back-Shu acupoints respectively. The impediments with the skin, muscles, sinews and bones are caused by the re-invasion of wind, cold and dampness in the corresponding seasons and then retained within the five zang-organs. " The impediments with the five zang-organs are just like the retardation of the five zang-organs. Wind, cold and dampness invade the body through these acupoints and intemperance in eating impairs the body inside. When the pathogenic factors invade the body through these acupoints, they eventually deepen into the fu-organs. The impediments with the six fu-organs are just like the contraction of the six fu-organs. That is why the retardation of the five zang-organs and the contraction of the six fu-organs are actually impediment due to wind, cold and dampness. The raw lacquer is white in color and pertains to metal. Since metal can restrain wind, the raw lacquer can kill roundworms. Long-term taking of it can transmit the essence of center earth all through the body, so it can keep healthy and prevent aging.

86. 黄　连

黄连　气味苦寒,无毒。主治热气,目痛,眦伤泣出,明目,肠澼,腹痛下痢,妇人阴中肿痛。久服令人不忘。

黄连始出巫阳山谷,及蜀郡大山之阳,今以雅州者为胜。苗高尺许,似茶丛生,一茎三叶,凌冬不凋,四月开花黄色,六月结实如芹子,色亦黄,根如连珠,形如鸡距,外刺内空。

黄连生于西蜀,味苦气寒,禀少阴水阴之精气。主治热气者,水滋其火,阴济其阳也。目痛、眦伤泣出者,火热上炎于目,则目痛而眦肉伤,眦肉伤则泣出。又曰:明目者,申明治目痛,眦伤泣出,以其能明目也。肠澼者,火热内乘于阴,夫热淫于内,薄为肠澼,此热伤阴分也。腹痛下痢者,风寒暑湿之邪伤其经脉,不能从肌腠而外出,则下行肠胃,致有肠痛下痢之证。黄连泻火热而养阴,故治肠澼腹痛下痢。妇人阴中肿痛者,心火协相火而交炽也。黄连苦寒,内清火热,故治妇人阴中肿痛。久服令人不忘者,水精上滋,泻心火而养神,则不忘也。大凡苦寒之药,多在中品下品,唯黄连列于上品者,阴中有阳,能济君火而养神也。少阴主水而君火在上,起冬不落叶。

凡物性有寒热温清燥润,及五色五味。五色五味以应五运,寒热温清燥润以应六气,是以上古司岁备物。如少阴君火,少阳相火司岁,则备温热之药。太阳寒水司岁,则备阴寒之药。厥阴风木司岁,则备清凉之药。太阴湿土司岁,则备甘润之药。阳明燥金司岁,则备辛燥之药。岐伯曰:司岁备物得天地之专精,非司岁备物则气散也。后世不能效上古之预备,因加炮制以助其力。如黄连水浸,附子火炮,即助寒水君火之火。后人不体经义,反以火炒黄连,尿煮附子。寒者热之,热者寒之,是制也,非制也。譬之鹰犬之力,在于爪牙。今束其爪,缚其牙,亦何贵乎鹰犬哉。

86. Huanglian〔黄连, coptis, Rhizoma Coptidis〕

It is bitter in taste, cold and non-toxic in property, and it is mainly used to treat heat qi, eye pain and epiphora due to canthus injury, improve vision, treat dysentery, the abdominal pain with diarrhea and swelling and the pain of the vulva. Long-term taking of it will strengthen memory.

Huanglian (coptis) was firstly recorded to be growing in the valleys of Wuyang (巫阳) and the sunny side of the mountains in Shujun (蜀郡). Today, those growing in Yazhou(雅州) are of better quality. Its seedlings are about one Chi in height like the thickly-grown tea bush, and each stalk has three leaves which do not wither even in cold winter. It blossoms with yellow flowers in the fourth lunar month, and it bears fruits like the yellow seeds of Qin [芹, cellery, Apii Herba] in the sixth lunar month. Its roots are like beads connected one another and the shape is like chicken feet with thorns on the surface and hollow inside.

Huanglian (coptis), firstly growing in Xishu (西蜀), is bitter in taste and cold in property. It receives the essence of water yin from lesser yin. It can treat heat qi because water can harmonize fire and yin can assist yang. Eye pain and epiphora due to canthus injury are caused by fire and heat flowing up to eyes, then eye pain leads to canthus injury, and canthus injury leads to epiphora. To improve vision is to treat eye pain and epiphora due to canthus injury. Dysentery is caused by fire and heat internally attacking yin, results in excessive interior heat attaching to the intestinal tract, which indicates heat damaging yin aspect. The abdominal pain with diarrhea is caused by the invasion of pathogen of wind cold and summerheat damp to meridians and the pathogen fails to emit from the interstice of the flesh but descends to the testines and stomach, resulting in the syndrome of abdominal pain with diarrhea. Huanglian (coptis) is effective in purging fire and heat and nourishing yin, so it can treat dysentery and abdominal pain with diarrhea. The swelling and pain of the vulva is caused by the interaction of heart fire and ministerial fire. Huanglian (coptis), bitter in taste and cold in property, can clear the internal fire and heat, and then it can treat the swelling and pain of the vulva. In terms of strengthening memory, if taking it for a long time, water essence ascends to nourish the upper part, purges the heart fire and nourishes the spirit, and then it strengthens memory. Most herbs which are bitter in taste and cold in property are classified as middle or low grade, while only Huanglian (coptis) is an exception and is classified as top grade because it has yang within yin and can assist sovereign fire to nourish the spirit. When lesser yin governs water and sovereign fire is in the upper, its leaves do not fall when winter comes.

All substances have different properties of being cold, hot, warm, clear, dry and moist, as well as five colors and five tastes. The five colors and five tastes correspond with five circuits and six properties with six qi, which is the ancestors' abidance of the rule of seasonal change in collecting and preparing herbs. For example, when the sovereign fire from lesser yin and the ministerial fire from lesser yang dominate, the drugs pertaining to warm and heat should be prepared. When the cold water from greater yang dominates, the drugs pertaining to yin cold should be prepared. When wind wood from reverting yin dominates, the drugs pertaining to clear and cool are prepared. When the damp earth from greater yin dominates, the drugs pertaining to moist and sweet should be prepared. When the dryness metal from yang brightness dominates, the drugs pertaining to dry and pungent should be prepared. Qibo (岐伯) said, "It is necessary to collect and prepare drugs according to the qi dominating in the year because they have absorbed the essence from the heaven and the earth, otherwise the property will not be pure." People later on could not exactly follow the ancestors to prepare the drugs so they process the drugs to strengthen their effects. For instance, soaking Huanglian (coptis) in water and processing Fuzi [附子, aconite, Aconiti Radix Lateralis Praeparata] with fire can strengthen the fire of cold water and sovereign fire. People later on, without thorough comprehension of what is described in *Huang Di Nei Jing* [《黄帝内经》, *Huangdi's Internal Classic*], incorrectly fried Huanglian (coptis) with fire and stew Fuzi (aconite) with urine. Processing the cold medicinal with heat while processing the heat medicinal with cold will limit the property of the medicinal, which doesn't correspond with the law. It is just like that the force of an eagle lies in its talons and the force of a dog lies in its fangs. Can the improper processed medicinal be better than the eagles and dogs whose talons and fangs are tied?

87. 蒲 黄

蒲黄 气味甘平,无毒。主治心腹、膀胱寒热,利小便,止血,消瘀血。久服轻身,益气力,延年神仙。

蒲,香蒲水草也,蒲黄乃香蒲花中之蕊屑,细若金粉,今药肆或以松花伪充，宜辨之。始出河东池泽，今处处有之，以秦州者为胜。春初生嫩叶，出水红白色，茸茸然。至夏抽梗于丛叶中，花抱梗端，如武士棒杵，故俚俗谓之蒲槌。

香蒲生于水中，色黄味甘，禀水土之专精，而调和其气血。主治心腹、膀胱寒热，利小便者，禀土气之专精，通调水道，则心腹、膀胱之寒热俱从小便出，而气机调和矣。止血，消瘀血者，禀水气之专精，生其肝木，则止新血，消瘀血，而血脉调和矣。久服则水气充足，土气有余，故轻身，益气力，延年神仙。

87. Puhuang [蒲黄, typha pollen, Pollen Typhae]

It is sweet in taste, mild and non-toxic in property, and it is mainly used to treat the cold and heat in the heart, abdomen and bladder, disinhibit urination, staunch bleeding and resolve blood stasis. Long-term taking of it will keep healthy, replenish qi and energy and prolong life like immortals.

The typha is a water plant and the typha pollen is the pistil pollen of its flowers. The typha pollen is as fine as the gold dust. Nowadays some drug stores use Songhua [松花, pine pollen, Pini Pollen] to fake Puhuang (typha pollen), so it is necessary to distinguish them. Originally growing in the lakes and pools of Hedong (河东), now the typha grows everywhere. Those growing in Qinzhou (秦州) are of better quality. It grows tender leaves in spring, red-white in color and in brushy shape when growing out of water. In summer, its stems sprout from leaves and its flowers grow out from the end of stems which look like the cudgel of the warrior. For that reason, it is commonly known as Puchui [蒲槌, typha cudgel].

The typha grows in water, yellow in color and sweet in taste. It receives the essence of water and earth, and it can harmonize qi and blood. It can treat the cold and heat in the heart, abdomen and bladder, and disinhibit urination because it receives the essence of earth qi to dredge and regulate the water passage, and thus heat in the heart, the abdomen and bladder can be dissipated through urination and the qi dynamic is harmonized consequently. It can staunch bleeding and resolve blood stasis because it receives the essence of water qi to engender liver wood, thus to staunch bleeding and resolve blood stasis and the blood and vessels will be harmonized consequently. Long-term taking of it can help keep sufficient water qi and abundant earth qi, so it can keep healthy, replenish qi and energy, and prolong life like immortals.

88. 菊 花

菊花 气味苦平,无毒。主治诸风头眩肿痛,目欲脱,泪出,皮肤死肌,恶风湿痹。久服利血气,轻身,耐老延年。

菊花处处有之,以南阳菊潭者为佳,菊之种类不一,培植而花球大者,只供玩赏。生于山野田泽,开花不起楼子,色只黄白二种,名茶菊者,方可入药,以味甘者为胜。古云:甘菊延令,苦菊泄人,不可不辨。《本经》气味主治,概茎叶花实而言,今时只用花矣。

菊花《本经》名节华,以其应重阳节候而华也。《月令》云:九月菊有黄花,茎叶味苦,花味兼甘,色有黄白,禀阳明秋金之气化。主治诸风头眩肿痛,禀金气而制风也。目欲脱泪出,言风火上淫于目,痛极欲脱而泪出。菊禀秋金清肃之气,能治风木之火热也。皮肤死肌,恶风湿痹,言感恶风湿邪而成风湿之痹证,则为皮肤死肌。菊禀金气,而治皮肤之风,兼得阳明土气,而治肌肉之湿也。周身血气,生于阳明胃府,故久服利血气轻身,血气利而轻身,则耐老延年。

88. Juhua〔菊花, flower of florists chrysanthemum, Flos Chrysanthemi〕

It is bitter in taste, mild and non-toxic in property, and it is mainly used to treat the wind dizziness of the head with swelling and pain, the eyes tending to prolapse, tearing, the numbness of skin like withered muscles, the aversion to wind and dampness impediment. Long-term taking of it will promote blood and qi, keep healthy, prevent aging and prolong life.

Juhua (flower of florists chrysanthemum) grows everywhere while those growing in the chrysanthemum ponds in Nanyang (南阳) are of the best quality. There are various types of Juhua (flower of florists chrysanthemum). Those cultivated with big flower bouquets are only for viewing. Only Chaju (茶菊), which grows in valleys, pools and fields, and only produces yellow or white flowers without bomb flowers, can be used as medicinal. Those with sweet taste are of better quality. As the old saying goes, the sweet chrysanthemum can prevent aging while the bitter chrysanthemum will make people fatigued, so it is necessary to distinguish the two. Its taste, property and effects put in *Shen Nong Ben Cao Jing* 〔《神农本草经》, *Shennong's Classic of Materia Medica*〕 generally refer to its stems, leaves, flowers and seeds, while nowadays only its flowers are used as medicinal.

In *Shen Nong Ben Cao Jing* 〔《神农本草经》, *Shennong's Classic of Materia Medica*〕, Juhua (flower of florists chrysanthemum) is named Jiehua 〔节华, festival boom〕, as it comes into boom in the time of the Double Ninth Festival. According to *Yue Ling* 〔《月令》, *The Phenology of Lunar Month*〕, it blossoms with yellow flowers in the ninth lunar month, and its stems and leaves are bitter in taste, and its flowers are bitter with sweetness in taste and yellow and white in color as it receives the qi transformation of autumn metal from yang brightness. It receives metal qi to restrain wind, so it can treat the wind dizziness of the head with swelling and pain. When wind fire ascends to invade eyes, it causes the eye prolapse due to distending pain and tearing. Having received the clear qi of autumn metal, it can restrain the fire heat of wind and wood. It can treat the numbness of skin like withered muscles and the aversion to wind and dampness impediment because the numbness of skin like withered muscles is caused by contraction of malign wind and dampness pathogen, resulting in wind and dampness impediment. Having received metal qi, it can expel the wind in the skin; with earth qi from yang brightness, it can expel the dampness in the muscles. Blood and qi all through the body are engendered in the stomach from yang brightness, so long-term taking of it will promote blood and qi, thus it can keep healthy, prevent aging and prolong life.

89. 茵陈蒿

茵陈蒿　气味苦平,微寒,无毒。主治风湿寒热邪气,热结黄疸。久服轻身益气,耐老,面白悦,长年。白兔食之仙。

　　茵陈蒿始出太山及丘陵坡岸上,今处处有之,不若太山者佳。苗似蓬蒿,其叶紧细,臭香如艾,秋后茎枯,终冬不死,至春因旧根而复生,故名茵陈。一种开花结实者,名铃儿茵陈。无花实者,名毛茵陈,入药以无花实者为胜。

《经》云:春三月,此为发陈,茵陈因旧苗而春生,盖因冬令水寒之气,而具阳春生发之机。主治风湿寒热邪气,得生阳之气,则外邪自散也。热结黄胆,得水寒之气,则内热自除也。久服则生阳上升,故轻身益气耐老。因陈而生新,故面白悦,长年。兔乃纯阴之物,喜阳春之气,故白兔食之而成仙。

89. Yinchenhao〔茵陈蒿, virgate wormwood, Artemisiae Scopariae Herba〕

It is bitter in taste, mild, slightly cold and non-toxic in property, and it is mainly used to treat the diseases caused by wind, dampness, cold, heat and pathogenic qi as well as the jaundice caused by heat accumulation. Long-term taking of it will keep healthy, replenish qi, prevent aging, brighten the complexion and prolong life. The white rabbit, after taking it, can become immortal.

Firstly recorded to be growing on the slope of Taishan Mountain（太山）and other hills, Yinchenhao（virgate wormwood）now grows everywhere, but not as good as that growing on Taishan Mountain（太山）. Its seedlings look like Penghaocai〔蓬蒿菜, garland chrysanthemum leaf, Chrysanthemi Coronarii Caulis et Folium〕and its leaves are condense and thin. It smells fragrant like Aiye〔艾叶, mugwort, Artemisiae Argyi Folium〕. It withers in autumn but does not die even after winter. In spring, the old root grows out again, so it is named Yinchen〔茵陈, chen means old in Chinese〕. The type that can bear flowers and fruits is called Ling'er Yinchen（铃儿茵陈）. The type that does not bear flowers and fruits is called Maoyinchen（毛茵陈）, which is better to be used as medicinal.

Huang Di Nei Jing〔《黄帝内经》, *Huangdi's Internal Classic*〕says, "In the three months of spring, all things on the earth begin to grow. The old seedlings of Yinchen（virgate wormwood）grow out as the qi of water cold in winter has the key to the growth and development of spring." With the qi of kidney-yang, the external pathogen will be dissipated, so it can treat the diseases caused by wind, dampness, cold, heat and pathogenic qi. Jaundice is caused by heat accumulation.

With qi of water cold, it can expel the internal heat. Long-term taking of it will make kidney-yang ascend, so it can keep healthy, replenish qi and prevent aging. The new is engendered by the old, so it can brighten the complexion and prolong life. The rabbit pertains to pure yin and it is fond of the qi of spring, so taking Yinchenhao (virgate wormwood) can help the white rabbit become immortal.

90. 天名精

天名精 气味甘寒,无毒。主治瘀血,血瘕欲死,下血,止血,利小便。久服轻身耐老。

天名精合根苗花实而言也,根名土牛膝,苗名活鹿草。实名鹤虱。所以名活鹿者,《异苑》云:宋元嘉中青州刘懵射一鹿,剖五藏以此草塞之,蹶然而起。懵怪而拔草便倒,如此三度,懵因密录,此草种之,治折伤愈多人,因以名之。始出平原川泽,今江湖间皆有之,路旁阴湿处甚多。春生苗,高二三尺,叶如紫苏叶而尖长,七月开黄白花,如小野菊,结实如茼蒿子,最黏人衣,狐气尤甚。炒熟则香,因名鹤虱,俗名鬼虱,其根黄白色,如牛膝而稍短,故名土牛膝。

鹿乃纯阳之兽,得此天名精而复活,盖禀水天之气而多阴精,故能治纯阳之鹿。主治瘀血,血瘕欲死,得水天之精气。阴中有阳,阳中有阴,故瘀久成瘕之积血,至欲死而可治,亦死而能生之义也。又曰:下血、止血者,申明所以能治瘀血血瘕欲死,以其能下积血,而复止新血也。水精之气,上合于天,则小便自利。久服则精气足,故轻身耐老。

90. Tianmingjing [天名精, carpesium, Carpesii Herba]

It is sweet in taste and cold in property, and it is mainly used to treat blood stasis, the severe lump due to blood stasis and bloody stool, staunch bleeding and disinhibit urination. Long-term taking of it will keep healthy and prevent aging.

Tianmingjing (carpesium) is a general name of its root, seedling, flower and seed. Its root is called Tuniuxi [土牛膝, native achyranthes, Achyranthis Radix]; its seedling is called Huolucao [活鹿草, deer resurrecting plant] and its seed is called Heshi [鹤虱, carpesium seed, Carpesii Fructus]. The name

Huolucao (deer resurrecting plant) derives from *Yi Yuan* [《异苑》, *Collection of Strange Stories*]: During Yuanjia Era of the Song Dynasty, a man named Liu Meng (刘憕) from Qingzhou (青州) once shot a deer. After removing the five zang-organs and stuff its body with this kind of plant, the deer suddenly got on its feet. With wonder, Liu Meng (刘憕) took out the plant, and then the deer fell down. And he did that for three times. Liu Meng (刘憕) noted it down and planted this herb and used it to treat fractures for many people. Thus this plant got the name Huolucao (deer resurrecting plant). Firstly recorded to be growing on the plains, in the mountains and on the marshes, it now grows everywhere besides rivers and lakes. Many can be found at the damp roadsides. It sprouts in spring and its seedlings are about two or three Chi in height. Its leaf, similar to that of Zisu [紫苏, perilla, Perillae Folium], is long and pointed. It blossoms with yellow and white flowers in the seventh lunar month, looking like small Yejuhua [野菊花, wild chrysanthemum flower, Chrysanthemi Indici Flos]. Its seed, looking like the seed of Tonghao [茼蒿, garland chrysanthemum, crowndaisy chrysanthemum], is easy to stick on clothes and has strong foxy smell. When it is stir-fried and cooked, it smells fragrant. Thus it is also known as Heshi [鹤虱, which means lice which tend to stick on clothes], or popularly known as Guishi (鬼虱). Its root is yellow-white in color, a little bit short like Niuxi [牛膝, achyranthes, Achyranthis Bidentatae Radix], so it is called Tuniuxi (native achyranthes).

The deer pertains to pure yang. It can be resurrected by Tianmingjing (carpesium) as the herb is abundant in yin essence due to receiving the qi of water and heaven, thus it can treat the deer that pertains to pure yang. It can treat blood stasis and the severe lump due to blood stasis because with the essence of water and heaven, it combines yin and yang in it, and it can treat the above-mentioned diseases, which also means it even can resurrect the dead. It can treat bloody stool and staunch bleeding, which means it can eliminate blood stasis and staunch the new bleeding, thus it can treat blood stasis and severe lump due to blood stasis. The qi of water essence is in accordance with the heaven upward, so urination will be promoted. Long-term taking of it can make essence sufficient, so it can keep healthy and prevent aging.

91. 鹤虱 ^附

鹤虱 ^附　气味苦辛，有小毒。主治蛔蛲虫。《唐本草》附。

鹤虱得天日之精气在上，故主杀阴类之蛔蛲。

91. Heshi［鹤虱，carpesium seed，Carpesii Fructus］ *supplement*

It is bitter and pungent in taste, and slightly toxic in property. It is mainly used to treat roundworm and pinworm. Supplemented in *Tang Ben Cao*［《唐本草》，*Tang Materia Medica*］.

It obtains the essence of the upper heaven and sun, so it can treat roundworm and pinworm that pertain to yin.

92. 土牛膝 ^附

土牛膝 ^附　又名杜牛膝，气味苦寒，主治吐血，牙痛，咽喉肿塞，诸骨哽咽。《新增》附。

天者阳也，下通水精，水者阴也，阴柔在下，故根名土牛膝。阳刚在上，故苗名活鹿，子名鹤虱，于命名之中，便有阴阳之义。

92. Tuniuix［土牛膝，native achyranthes，
Achyranthis Radix］ *supplement*

It is also known as Duniuxi（杜牛膝）. Bitter in taste and cold in property, it is mainly used to treat hematemesis, toothache, sore swollen throat and various bones stuck in the throat. Supplemented in *Xin Zeng*［《新增》，*New Supplement to Materia Medica*］

The heaven pertains to yang and interacts with water essence downward. Water pertains to yin. With yin in the lower part, the root of Tianmingjing［天名精，carpesium，Carpesii Herba］ is named Tuniuxi（native achyranthes）. With yang in the upper part, the seedling of Tianmingjing（carpesium）is named Huolu［活鹿草，deer resurrecting plant］, and its seed is named Heshi［鹤虱，carpesium seed，Carpesii Fructus］. The property of yin and yang is indicated in their names.

93．石龙刍

石龙刍　气味苦,微寒,无毒。主治心腹邪气,小便不利,淋闭风湿,鬼疰,恶毒。久服补虚羸,轻身,耳目聪明,延年。

石龙刍一名龙须草,近道水石处皆有之,生于缙云者佳,故又名缙云草。苗丛生直上,并无枝叶,状如棕心草。夏月茎端作小穗,开花结细实,赤色。吴人多栽莳之以织席。

石龙刍气味苦寒,生于水石间,得少阴水精之气化,故以龙名。又,龙能行泄其水精也,主治心腹邪气者,少阴水精之气,上交于心,则心腹之邪气可治也。小便不利,淋闭者,热邪下注而病淋,浊气不化而仍闭结,皆为小便不利。龙刍能启水精之气,上交于心,上下相交,则小便自利矣。又,少阴神气外浮,则能去风湿。少阴神气五内,则能除鬼疰也。又曰:恶毒者,言鬼疰之病,皆恶毒所为,非痈毒也。久服则水火相济,故能补虚羸而轻身。精神充足,故耳目聪明而延年。

93. Shilongchu [石龙刍, common rush herb, Herba Junci]

It is bitter in taste, slightly cold and non-toxic in property, and it is mainly used to treat the disease caused by the pathogenic qi in the heart and abdomen, dysuria, stranguria, wind-dampness, Guizhu [鬼疰, multiple infixation abscess] and the infectious disease. Long-term taking of it will tonify deficiency and emaciation, keep healthy, improve hearing and vision, and prolong life.

Shilongchu (common rush herb) is also known as Longxucao [龙须草, dragon's-whisker seaweed, Gracilaria]. It grows everywhere in the waters and among the rocks along the roadside. Those growing in Jinyun (缙云) are of good quality, so it is also called Jinyuncao (缙云草). Its seedlings grow straightly in cluster, without branches and leaves, in shape of Zongxincao [棕心草, manchurian beakgrain, Diarrhena Manshurica Maxim]. In summer, it grows small spikes on the end of its stems. It bears red and thin seeds after it blossoms. The people in Wu (吴) area used to plant it and weave straw mat with it.

Bitter in taste and cold in property, Shilongchu (common rush herb) grows among the waters and rocks. It receives the qi transformation of water essence from lesser yin, so it contains "Long"（龙, which means dragon in Chinese）in its name. Besides, the dragon can discharge water essence. When the qi of water essence from lesser yin ascends to interact with the heart, the disease caused by the pathogenic qi in the heart and abdomen can be treated. Dysuria is caused by the stagnation of turbid qi, and stranguria is caused by the descent of heat pathogen. Shilongchu（common rush herb）can activate the qi of water essence to ascend to interact with the heart. When the kidney interacts with the heart, urine is disinhibited. The spirit qi of lesser yin floating externally can dispel the wind dampness, and the spirit qi stored internally in the five zang-organs can expel Guizhu〔鬼疰, multiple infixation abscess〕. Besides, Guizhu〔鬼疰, multiple infixation abscess〕is a kind of infectious disease rather than a kind of abscess toxin. Long-term taking of it can make fire and water help each other, so it can supplement deficiency and emaciation and keep healthy. When the spirit is sufficient, people can hear and see better and live longer.

94. 车前子

车前子 气味甘寒,无毒。主治气癃,止痛,利水道小便,除湿痹。久服轻身耐老。

车前草《本经》名当道。《诗》名芣苢,好生道旁及牛马足迹中,故有车前当道,及牛遗马舄之名。江湖淮甸处处有之,春生苗叶,布地中,抽数茎作穗如鼠尾,花极细密,青色微赤。结实如葶苈子,赤黑色。

乾坤皆有动静,夫坤,其静也翕,其动也辟。车前好生道旁,虽牛马践踏不死,盖得土气之用,动而不静者也。气癃,膀胱之气癃闭也。气癃则痛,痛则水道之小便不利。车前得土气之用,土气行则水道亦行,而膀胱之气不癃矣。不癃则痛止,痛止则水道之小便亦利矣。土气运行,则湿邪自散,故除湿痹。久服土气升而水气布,故轻身耐老。《神仙服食经》云:车前,雷之精也,夫震为雷,为长男。《诗》言:采采芣苢,亦欲妊娠而生男也。

94. Cheqianzi〔车前子, seed of Asiatic plantain, Semen Plantaginis〕

It is sweet in taste, cold and non-toxic in property, and it is mainly used to treat qi block, relieve pain, disinhibit water passage and urination, and eliminate dampness impediment. Long-term taking of it can keep healthy and prevent aging.

In *Shen Nong Ben Cao Jing* [《神农本草经》, *Shennong's Classic of Materia Medica*], it is also called Dangdao (当道). And in *Shi Jing* [《诗经》, *The Book of Songs*], it is also called Fuyi (芣苢). It grows along the roadsides where the cows and horses have trod, for that reason it is also called Cheqian Dangdao (车前当道, which means the blocking the way ahead of carts in Chinese) and Niuyi Maxi (牛遗马舄, which means the footprint of cow and horseshoe in Chinese). It grows everywhere in Jianghu (江湖) and Huaidian (淮甸). In spring, it grows seedlings and leaves, spreading across the land. Its stems sprout out of the seedlings and leaves grow into spikes which look like mouse tails. Its flowers are thin and dense in shape, green with slightly red in color. Its fruit is like Tinglizi [葶苈子, pepperweed seed, Semen Lepidii Semen], black and red in color.

The heaven and the earth have their own movement. The earth is furling in static state and repelling in moving state. Cheqiancao [车前草, plantago, Plantaginis Herba] grows along the roadsides. It survives even after being trod by a cow or horse as it obtains the feature of earth qi which is moving instead of being static. Qi block, which means the qi of the bladder is blocked, causes pain and consequently inhibits the urination of waterway. Cheqianzi (seed of Asiatic plantain) has obtained the feature of earth qi. When earth qi moves, the water passage is disinhibited, and the qi in the bladder is not blocked and thus the pain is relieved and the urination of water passage is disinhibited. When earth qi moves, dampness pathogen is dissipated and dampness impediment is thus eliminated. Long-term taking of it can make earth qi ascend and water qi spread across the body, which can keep healthy and prevent aging. According to *Shen Xian Fu Shi Jing* [《神仙服食经》, *Canon of Immortals Diet*], Cheqianzi (seed of Asiatic plantain) is the essence of thunder and Zhen (震, one of the eight diagrams) refers to the thunder which comes into being when Emperor Fu (夫) shakes and also refers to the firstborn son. As is said in *Shi Jing* [《诗经》, *The Book of Songs*], the women gather Fuyi (芣苢) because they want to be pregnant and give birth to a boy.

95. 冬葵子

冬葵子 气味甘寒滑,无毒。主治五藏六腑寒热,羸瘦,五癃,利小便。久服坚骨,长肌肉,轻身延年。

葵菜处处有之,以八九月种者,覆养过冬,至春作子,谓之冬葵子。如不覆养,正月复种者,谓之春葵。三月始种,五月开红紫花者,谓之蜀葵。八九月开黄花者,谓之秋葵。葵种不一,此外尚有锦葵、黄葵、终葵、菟葵之名,花具五色及间色,更有浅深之不同。

葵花开五色,四季长生,得生长化收藏之五气,故治五藏六腑之寒热羸瘦。冬葵子覆养过冬,气味甘寒而滑,故治五癃。夫膀胱不利为癃。五为土数,土不运行,则水道闭塞,故曰五癃。治五癃,则小便自利。久服坚骨,得少阴之气也。长肌肉,得太阴之气也。坚骨长肌,故轻身延年。

95. Dongkuizi [冬葵子, seed of cluster mallow, Semen Malvae]

It is sweet in taste, cold, slippery and non-toxic in property, and it is mainly used to treat the diseases due to the cold and heat in the five zang-organs and six fu-organs, weakness and emaciation, and five kinds of stranguria and disinhibit urination. Long-term taking of it will strengthen the bones, promote the growth of the muscles, keep healthy and prolong life.

Kuicai [葵菜, mallow, Malva verticillata Linnaeus] grows everywhere and those planted in the eighth or ninth lunar month are covered for shelter from cold in winter and bear seeds in spring, which are called Dongkuizi (seed of cluster mallow). The uncovered mallow which will be replanted in the first lunar month is called Chunkui (春葵). Those planted in the third lunar month and blossoming with red and purple flowers in the fifth lunar month are called Shukui (蜀葵). Those blossoming with yellow flowers in the eighth or ninth lunar month are called Qiukui (秋葵). There is a variety of kinds of it. Besides those, there are also Jinkui (锦葵), Huangkui (黄葵), Zhongkui (终葵) and Tukui (菟葵), all of which blossom with flowers in one of five colors or their binary color, in different shades.

The mallow blossoms with flowers in five different colors and grows in four seasons. Obtaining five kinds of qi responsible for generation, growth, transformation, reaping and storage, it can treat the diseases due to the cold and heat in the five zang-organs and six fu-organs and weakness and emaciation. Covered for shelter from cold in winter, it is sweet in taste, cold and slippery in property, so it can treat five kinds of stranguria. Stranguria is caused by the inhibition of bladder. The number five corresponds with earth in the five elements. When earth movement stops, the water passage is blocked, which is called five kinds of stranguria. When the five kinds of stranguria are treated, urine is disinhibited. Since it has obtained the qi of lesser yin, long-term taking of it can strengthen the bones. Since it has obtained the qi of greater yin, it can promote the growth of the muscles. Since it can strengthen the bones and promote the growth of the muscles, it can keep healthy and prolong life.

96. 地肤子

地肤子　气味苦寒,无毒。主治膀胱热利小便,补中,益精气。久服耳目聪明,轻身耐老。

地肤子多生平泽田野,根作丛生,每窠有二三十茎,七月间开黄花,结子青白,晒干则黑,似初眠蚕沙之状。

地肤子气味苦寒,禀太阳寒水之气化,故主治膀胱之热而利小便。膀胱位居胞中,故补中而益水精之气。久服则津液滋灌,故耳目聪明,轻身耐老。

虞抟《医学正传》云:抟兄年七十,秋间患淋,二十余日,百方不效,后得一方,取地肤草,捣自然汁服之,遂通。至贱之物,有回生之功如此,是苗叶亦有功也。

96. Difuzi［地肤子, kochia, Kochiae Fructus］

It is bitter in taste, cold and non-toxic in property, and it is mainly used to resolve the heat in the bladder, disinhibit urination, tonify the middle and replenish essential qi. Long-term taking of it will improve hearing and vision, keep healthy and prevent aging.

Difuzi (kochia) mostly grows in the lakes, pools and fields. Its roots grow in clusters. Each Difuzi (kochia) has twenty or thirty stems. It blossoms with yellow flowers in the seventh lunar month. It bears green-white seeds which turn black after they are dried and look like Cansha 〔蚕沙, silkworm droppings, Bombycis Faeces〕 in initial dormancy.

Difuzi(kochia), bitter in taste and cold in property, has received the qi transformation of cold water from greater yang, so it can resolve the heat in the bladder and disinhibit urination. Since the bladder lies in the lower energizer, it can tonify the middle and replenish the qi of water essence. Long-term taking of it can make the liquids sufficient to nourish the whole body, thus to improve hearing and vision, keep healthy and prevent aging.

In *Yi Xue Zheng Zhuan* 〔《医学正传》, *The Orthodox Tradition of Medicine*〕, the author Yu Tuan（虞抟）said, "My elder brother, at the age of seventy, got stranguria in autumn. Within over twenty days, he tried more than a hundred formulas, but none of them was effective. Finally he tried this formula：collect Difucao 〔地肤草, kochia shoot, Kochiae Caulis et Folium〕, crush it to extract the juice, take the juice and the urine will be disinhibited." So common as it is, it has the magical treatment effect to save life, and its seedlings and leaves have similar effects.

97. 决明子

决明子气味咸平,无毒。主治青盲、目淫、肤赤、白膜、眼赤泪出。久服益精光,轻身。

决明子处处有之,初夏生苗,茎高三四尺,叶如苜蓿,本小末大,昼开夜合,秋开淡黄花五出,结角如细缸豆,长二三寸,角中子数十粒,色青绿而光亮,状如马蹄,故名马蹄决明,又别有草决明,乃青葙子也。

目者肝之窍,决明气味咸平,叶司开合,子色紫黑而光亮,禀太阳寒水之气,而生厥阴之肝木,故主治青盲、目淫、肤赤。青盲则生白膜,肤赤乃眼肤之赤,目淫则多泪,故又曰:白膜眼赤泪出也。久服则水精充溢,故益精光,轻身。

97. Juemingzi〔决明子, seed of sickle senna, Semen Cassiae〕

It is salty in taste, mild and non-toxic in property, and it is mainly used to treat optic atrophy, the disorder of the eyes, red or white retina, the redness of the eyes with tearing. Long-term taking of it will replenish the essence of the eyes and keep healthy.

Juemingzi（seed of sickle senna）grows everywhere. It sprouts in early summer, with stems of three or four Chi in height. Its leaf is like that of Muxu〔苜蓿, alfalfa, Medicaginis Herba〕, small in the leaf root and big in the tip. The leaves open in the daytime and close at night. It blossoms with light-yellow flowers five times in autumn. It bears pods which look like thin Jiangdou〔豇豆, cowpea, Vignae Sinensis Semen〕, two or three Cun in length. There are tens of grains of seeds in the pod and the seeds are green and bright in color. The pod is in horseshoe（"马蹄" in Chinese）shape, so it is called Mati Juming（马蹄决明）. There is another herb called Caojueming（草决明）, which is in fact Qingxiangzi〔青葙子, feather cockscomb seed, Semen Celosiae〕.

Eyes are the orifices of the liver. Juemingzi（seed of sickle senna）is salty in taste and mild in property. Its leaves open in the daytime and close at night. The seed, purple black and bright in color, receives the qi of cold water from greater yang and engenders the liver wood from reverting yin, so it can treat optic atrophy, the disorder of the eyes and redretina. The optic atrophy causes white retina, and red retina which means the retina is red. The disorder of the eyes causes tearing. So there is another saying that the white retina and the redness of the eyes will cause tearing. Long-term taking of it will make water essence sufficient, so it will replenish the essence of the eyes and keep healthy.

98. 茺蔚子

茺蔚子 气味辛甘,微温,无毒。主明目,益精,除水气。久服轻身。

茺蔚《本经》名益母,又名益明。《尔雅》名萑。今处处有之,近水湿处甚繁。春生苗如嫩蒿,入夏长三四尺,其茎方,其叶如艾,节节生穗,充盛蔚密,故名茺蔚。五月采穗,九月采子,每萼内有细子四粒,色黑褐。

茺蔚茎叶甘寒,子辛温。《本经》辛甘微温,概苗实而言也。茎方子黑,喜生湿地,禀水土之气化,明目益精,得水气也。除水气,土气盛也。久服则精气充尉,故轻身。

98. Chongweizi〔茺蔚子, motherwort fruit, Fructus Leonuri〕

It is pungent and sweet in taste, slightly warm and non-toxic in property, and it is mainly used to improve vision, replenish essence and eliminate water qi. Long-term taking of it will keep healthy.

In *Shen Nong Ben Cao Jing*〔《神农本草经》, *Shennong's Classic of Materia Medica*〕, Chongweizi (motherwort fruit) is called Yimu (益母) or Yiming (益明). In *Er Ya*〔《尔雅》, *On Elegance*〕, it is called Tui (蓷). Now it grows everywhere, and those growing on the waterside are exceptionally flourishing. In spring, it grows seedlings like tender Hao〔蒿, sweetwormwoodherb, Herba Artemisiae Annuae〕, which can grow to as tall as three or four Cun by early summer. Its stem is square, and its leaf is like Aiye〔艾叶, argywormwoodleaf, Folium Artemisiae Argyi〕. Ears grow out of the stem nodes, flush and dense, so it is called Chongwei (茺蔚, which means flush and dense in Chinese). Its ears are collected in the fifth lunar month and its fruits in the ninth lunar month. There are four fruits in one calyx, blackbrown in color.

The stem and leaf of Chongwei (motherwort) are sweet in taste and cold in property, and Chongweizi (motherwort fruit) is pungent in taste and warm in property. In *Shen Nong Ben Cao Jing*〔《神农本草经》, *Shennong's Classic of Materia Medica*〕, Chongwei (motherwort) is recorded to be pungent and sweet in taste and slightly warm in property regarding its plant and fruits. Its stems are square; its fruits are black, and it tends to grow in the wetland. Receiving the qi transformation of water and earth, it can improve vision and replenish essence by obtaining water qi. When water qi is eliminated, earth qi will be exuberant. So long-term taking of it will replenish essence, thus to keep healthy.

99．茺蔚茎叶花穗

茺蔚茎叶花穗　气味甘寒，微苦辛。主治隐疹，可作浴汤。

《诗》言：中谷有蓷，暵其干矣。益母草得水湿之精，能耐旱暵，滋养皮肤，故主治隐疹，可作浴汤。

茺蔚子明目益精而补肾，复除水气以健脾，故有茺蔚之名。益母草清热而解毒，凉血以安胎，故有益母之名。

李时珍曰：茺蔚子治妇女经脉不调，胎产，一切血气诸病妙品也。其根、茎、花、叶、实并皆入药，可同用。若治手足厥阴血分风热，明目，益精，调女人经脉，则单用茺蔚子为良。若治肿毒疮疡，消水行血，妇人胎产诸病，则宜并用为良。盖其根、茎、花、叶专于行，而子则行中有补故也。又曰：茎叶味辛而苦，花味微苦甘，根味甘，并无毒。

99. Chongwei Jingyehuasui〔茺蔚茎叶花穗, motherwort stem, leaf, flower and ear, Materia Medica Chongwei Jingyehuasui〕

They are sweet, slightly bitter and pungent in taste, cold in property, and they are mainly used to treat urticaria and can be used in bathing water.

Shi Jing〔《诗经》, *The Book of Songs*〕says that Tui（蓷）is found in a valley, which gets dried in the drought weather. Yimucao〔益母草, motherwort herb, Herba Leonuri〕, receiving the essence of water dampness, can endure drought and nourish the skin, so it can treat urticaria and can be used in bathing water.

Chongweizi〔茺蔚子, motherwort fruit, Fructus Leonuri〕can improve vision, replenish essence and tonify the kidney. It can also eliminate water qi to tonify the spleen, so it has got the name Chongweizi（motherwort fruit）. Yimucao（motherwort herb）can clear heat and remove toxin, cool the blood to calm fetus, so it is called Yimu（益母, which means to benefit mother in Chinese）.

Li Shizhen（李时珍）said, "Chongweizi（motherwort fruit）can treat the irregular meridians of women and facilitate childbirth. It is effective for various blood-qi-related diseases." Its root, stems, flowers, leaves and fruits are all used as medicinals and can be used in combination. To treat the wind heat in blood-aspect of hand and foot reverting yin, improve vision, replenish essence, regulate the meridians of women, it is better to use its fruits alone. To treat the swelling and toxin of sores, disperse water swelling, move the blood, and treat the childbirth-related diseases, it is better to use them in combination, as its root, stems, flowers and leaves are specially used for moving while its fruits can both move and nourish. He also said that its stems and leaves are pungent and bitter in taste, its flowers are slightly bitter and slightly sweet in taste, and its root is sweet in taste and non-toxic in property.

100. 丹　砂

丹砂　气味甘,微寒,无毒。主治身体五脏百病,养精神,安魂魄,益气明目,杀精魅邪恶鬼。永服通神明,不老,能化为汞。

　　丹砂又名朱砂,始出涪州山谷,今辰州、锦州及云南、波斯蛮獠洞中石穴内皆有,而以辰州者为胜,故又名辰砂。大者如芙蓉花,小者如箭镞,碎之作墙壁光明可鉴,成层可折,研之鲜红,斯为上品,细小者为米砂,淘土石中得者为土砂,又名阴砂,皆为下品。苏恭曰:形虽大而杂土石,又不若细而明净者佳。

　　水银出于丹砂之中,精气内藏,水之精也。色赤体坚,象合离明,火之精也。气味甘寒,生于土石之中,乃资中土,而得水火之精。主治身体五脏百病者,五脏之气,内归坤土,外合周身,丹砂从中土而达五脏之气,出于身体,则百病咸除。养精神者,养肾脏之精,心脏之神,而上下水火相交矣。安魂魄者,安肝脏之魂,肺藏之魄,而内外气血调和矣。调和其气,故益气。调和其血,故明目。上下水火相交,则精魅之怪,邪恶之鬼自消杀矣。久服则灵气充盛,故神明不老,内丹可成,故能化为汞。

100. Dansha [丹砂, cinnabar, Cinnabaris]

It is sweet in taste, slightly cold and non-toxic in property, and it is mainly used to treat all diseases in the five zang-organs, nourish essence and spirit, pacify the ethereal soul and corporeal soul, replenish qi, improve vision, expel the severe pathogenic factors like ghost and eliminate pathogenic qi. Long-term taking of it will invigorate spirit and mentality and prolong life. It can be transformed into

Shuiyin［水银, mercury, Hydrargyrum］.

　　Dansha (cinnabar) is also known as Zhusha (朱砂). Firstly recorded to be found in the valleys of Fuzhou (涪州), now it can be easily found in the stone caves of Chenzhou (辰州), Jinzhou (锦州), Yunnan (云南) and the south area such as Persia. Those growing in Chenzhou (辰州) are of better quality, so it is also called Chensha (辰砂). It can be as big as Furonghua［芙蓉花, cotton rose, Hibisci Mutabilis Flos］or as small as an arrowhead. Smash it to build wall, and the wall will be very bright. Those that can be peeled in different slices and turn red when ground are of the best quality. The small and thin ones are called Misha (米砂). Those got from washing earth and stones are called Tusha (土砂), also known as Yinsha (阴砂). Both of the latter two kinds are of inferior quality, as Sugong (苏恭) once said, "Big in size as they are, they are miscellaneous stones, not as good as the thin and bright ones."

Dansha (cinnabar) can be transformed into Shuiyin (mercury), where there is essential qi stored which is water essence. It is red in color and hard in texture. It is in accordance with Li (离, one of the eight diagrams) which refers to the light of fire, indicating it is fire essence. Sweet in taste and cold in property, it grows in the earth and stones, so it can tonify center earth and obtain water and fire essence. It can mainly treat all diseases in the five zang-organs because the qi of the five zang-organs returns internally to Kun (坤) earth and spreads out across the body. Dansha (cinnabar) can reach the qi of the five zang-organs from center earth and move out of the body, thus all diseases in the five zang-organs will be treated. It can nourish essence and spirit as it can nourish kidney essence and heart spirit, which will result in the interaction of water and fire in the upper and the lower. To pacify the ethereal soul and corporeal soul is to pacify the ethereal soul of the liver and the corporeal soul of the lung, thus the qi and blood of the inside and outside are harmonized. When qi is harmonized, qi can be replenished; when blood is harmonized, vision can be improved. When the water and fire in the upper and the lower are interacted, the severe pathogenic factors like ghost are expelled naturally. Long-term taking of it makes the spirit sufficient, so spirit and mentality can be invigorated, and the inner elixir can be cultivated, thus indicating it can be transformed into mercury.

101. 云 母

云母 气味甘平,无毒。主治身皮死肌,中风寒热,如在车船上,除邪气,安五脏,益子精,明目。久服轻身延年。

云母出太山山谷、齐山、庐山,及琅琊、北定山石间,今兖州云梦山及江州、淳州、杭越间,亦有生土石间,作片成层可析,明滑光白者为上。候云气所出之处,于下掘取即获,但掘时忌作声,此石乃云之根,故名云母,而云母之根,则阳起石也。

今时用阳起石者有之,用云母者甚鲜,故但存《本经》原文,不加诠释,后凡存《本经》而不诠释者,义俱仿此。

101. Yunmu〔云母, muscovite, Muscovitum〕

It is sweet in taste, mild and non-toxic in property, and it is mainly used to treat the numbness of the body and skin, wind stroke and vertigo feeling like staying in a cart or a ship caused by cold and heat, eliminate pathogenic qi, calm the five zang-organs, replenish fetal essence and improve vision. Long-term taking of it will keep healthy and prolong life.

Firstly recorded to be found in the valleys of Taishan Moutain(太山)and in the stones of Qishan Mountain(齐山), Lushan Mountain(庐山), Langya Mountain(琅琊山)and Beiding Mountain(北定山), now it can be easily found in Yunmeng Mountain(云梦山)of Yanzhou(兖州), and among the soil and stones of Jiangzhou(江州), Chunzhou(淳州)and Hangyue(杭越). Analyze it after peeling it into slices, and the smooth, bright and white ones are of good quality. Find the place(in the mountain)where clouds float out, dig the earth or stone and you can find it. Do dig it carefully and quietly as the stone is the root of cloud, so it gets the name Yunmu(云母), and its root is Yangqishi〔阳起石, actinolite, Actinolitum〕.

Nowadays Yangqishi（actinolite）is commonly used while Yunmu（muscovite）is rarely used. For that reason, the original text from *Shen Nong Ben Cao Jing*〔《神农本草经》, *Shennong's Classic of Materia Medica*〕is saved in this book without any notes. Hereinafter, any other original texts saved from *Shen Nong Ben Cao Jing* [《神农本草经》, *Shennong's Classic of Materia Medica*] without notes are also due to this reason.

102. 赤石脂

赤石脂 气味甘平,无毒。主治黄胆,泄痢,肠澼浓血,阴蚀,下血赤白,邪气痈肿,疽痔,恶疮,头疡疥瘙。久服补髓益气,肥健不饥,轻身延年,五色石脂,各随五色,补五脏。

《本经》概言五色石脂,今时只用赤白二脂。赤白二脂,赤中有白,白中有赤,总名赤石脂。不必如《别录》分为二也。始出南山之阳,及延州、潞州、吴郡山谷中,今四方皆有。此石中之脂,如骨之髓,故揭石取之以理腻粘舌缀唇者为上。

石脂乃石中之脂,为少阴肾脏之药。又,色赤象心,甘平属土。主治黄疸、泄痢、肠澼浓血者,脾土留湿,则外疸黄而内泄痢,甚则肠澼浓血。石脂得太阴之土气,故可治也。阴蚀下血赤白,邪气痈肿、疽痔者,少阴脏寒,不得君火之阳热以相济,致阴蚀而为下血赤白,邪气痈肿而为疽痔。石脂色赤,得少阴之火气,故可治也。恶疮、头疡、疥瘙者,少阴火热不得肾脏之水气以相滋,致火热上炎,而为恶疮之头疡疥瘙。石脂生于石中,得少阴水精之气,故可治也,久服则脂液内生,气血充盛,故补髓益气。补髓助精也,益气助神也,精神交会于中土,则肥健不饥,而轻身延年。《本经》概言五色石脂,故曰各随五色补五脏。

102. Chishizhi [赤石脂, red halloysite, Halloysitum Rubrum]

It is sweet in taste and mild in property, and it is mainly used to treat jaundice, diarrhea, the stool with pus and blood, genital erosion, the bloody stool with red and white elements, the welling-abscess and sore due to pathogenic qi, carbuncle, hemorrhoids, malign sore, head sore, scabies and pruritus. Long-term taking of it will tonify the marrow, replenish qi, fortify the body, tolerate hunger, keep healthy and prolong life. There are five colors of halloysites which correspond with the five colors, and thus they can respectively tonify the five zang-organs.

Shen Nong Ben Cao Jing [《神农本草经》, *Shennong's Classic of Materia*

Medica] gives a general introduction of five colors of halloysites, while only the white and red halloysite are used now. The red halloysite is touched with the white and vice versa, so they are generally called Chishizhi (red halloysite), and it is not necessary to name them separately like what has been done in *Ming Yi Bie Lu* [《名医别录》, *Miscellaneous Records of Famous Physicians*]. Firstly recorded to be found on the sunny side of Nanshan Mountain (南山) and in the valleys of Yanzhou (延州), Luzhou (潞州) and Wujun (吴郡), now it can be found everywhere. It is the mountain tallow in the stone, just like the marrow in the bone, so it can be got by uncovering the stone. Judging from its texture, the smooth ones which can stick to the tongue and lips are of good quality.

Chishizhi (red halloysite) is the mountain tallow in the stone. It is a medicinal that enters the kidney meridian of lesser yin. In addition, the red color symbolizes the heart. Sweet in taste and mild in property, it pertains to earth. It can treat jaundice, diarrhea, and the stool with pus and blood. When there is dampness in spleen earth, there will be jaundice outside, diarrhea inside and even severely, the stool with pus and blood. Chishizhi (red halloysite) obtains the earth qi from greater yin, so it can treat jaundice, diarrhea and the stool with pus and blood. Genital erosion, the bloody stool with red and white elements, the welling-abscess and sore due to pathogenic qi, carbuncle and hemorrhoids occur because the organs pertaining to lesser yin cannot assist each other for lack of yang heat from sovereign fire when cold invades them, thus causing genital erosion manifested as the bloody stool with red and white elements, and causing the welling-abscess and sore due to pathogenic qi manifested as carbuncle and hemorrhoids. Red in color, Chishizhi (red halloysite) obtains the fire qi from lesser yin, so it can treat those diseases. Malign sore, head sore, scabies and pruritus occur when there is no water qi of the kidney to nourish the fire heat of lesser yin, which causes fire heat to flame upward, resulting in malign sore, head sore, scabies and pruritus. Chishizhi (red halloysite) grows in stones and obtains the qi of water essence from lesser yin, so it can treat those diseases. Long-term taking of it can engender liquids inside and make qi blood sufficient, so it can tonify the marrow and replenish qi. Tonifying the marrow can promote essence, and replenishing qi can promote spirit. The interaction of essence and spirit in center earth can fortify the body and tolerate hunger, thus to keep healthy and prolong life. *Shen Nong Ben Cao Jing* [《神农本草经》, *Shennong's Classic of Materia Medica*] gives a general introduction of five colors of halloysites, so they are said to respectively tonify the five zang-organs in accordance with five colors.

103. 滑 石

滑石 气味甘寒,无毒。主治身热泄澼,女子乳难,癃闭,利小便,荡胃中积聚寒热,益精气。久服轻身耐饥,长年。

滑石一名液石,又名膋石,始出赭阳山谷及太山之阴,或掖北白山,或卷山,今湘州、永州、始安、岭南近道诸处皆有。初取柔软,久渐坚硬,白如凝脂,滑而且腻者佳。

滑石味甘属土,气寒属水,色白属金。主治身热泄澼者,禀水气而清外内之热也。热在外则身热,热在内则泄澼也。女子乳难者,禀金气而生中焦之汁,乳生中焦,亦水类也。治癃闭,禀土气而化水道之出也。利小便,所以治癃闭也。荡胃中积聚寒热,所以治身热泄澼也。益精气,所以治乳难也。久服则土生金而金生水,故轻身耐饥,长年。

103. Huashi [滑石, talc, Talcum]

It is sweet in taste, cold and non-toxic in property, and it is mainly used to treat fever, diarrhea, difficult lactation and ischuria, disinhibit urination, dispel the accumulation of cold and heat in the stomach and replenish essential qi. Long-term taking of it will keep healthy, tolerate hunger and prolong life.

Huashi (talc) is also called Yeshi (液石) or Liaoshi (膋石). Firstly recorded to be found in the mountain valleys of Zheyang (赭阳), on the shady side of Taishan Mountain (太山), or in Baishan Mountain (白山) of Yebei (掖北), or Juanshan Mountain (卷山), now it can be found everywhere in places nearby Xiangzhou (湘州), Yongzhou (永州), Shian (始安) and Lingnan (岭南). It is soft at the beginning, but will get hard with time going by. The smooth and fine ones as white as creamy are of good quality.

Its sweet taste pertains to earth, its cold property pertains to water, and its white color pertains to metal. Receiving water qi to clear the heat inside and outside, it can treat fever and diarrhea. The heat outside will cause fever, and the heat inside will cause diarrhea. To treat difficult lactation, it receives metal qi to engender the liquids in the middle energizer. Breast milk is engendered in the middle energizer and it is also a kind of water. To treat ischuria, it receives earth qi which transforms what is drained through the waterways. It can disinhibit urination, so it can treat ischuria. It can dispel the accumulation of cold and heat in the stomach, so it can treat fever and diarrhea. It can replenish essential qi, so it can treat difficult lactation. Long-term taking of it can make earth generate metal and make metal generate water, so it will keep healthy, tolerate hunger and prolong life.

104. 消 石

消石 气味苦寒,无毒。主治五脏积热,胃胀闭,涤去蓄结饮食,推陈致新,除邪气。炼之如膏。久服轻身。

消石又名火消,又名焰消。丹炉家用制五金八石,银工用化金银,军中用作烽燧火药,得火即焰起,故有火消、焰消之名。始出益州山谷及武都、陇西、西羌,今河北、庆阳、蜀中皆有,乃地霜也。冬间遍地生如白霜,扫取以水淋汁,煎炼而成,状如朴消,又名生消。再煎提过,或有锋芒如芒消,或有圭棱如马牙消,故消石亦有芒消、牙消之名,与朴消之芒牙同称,然水火之性则异也。

消石乃冬时地上所生白霜,气味苦寒,禀少阴、太阳之气化。盖少阴属冬令之水,太阳主六气之终。遇火能焰者,少阴上有君火,太阳外有标阳也。主治五脏积热,胃胀闭者,言积热在脏,致胃府之气胀闭不通。消石禀水寒之气,而治脏热。具火焰之性,而消胃胀也。涤去蓄结饮食,则胃府之胀闭自除。推陈致新,除邪气,则五脏之积热自散。炼之如膏,得阴精之体,故久服轻身。消石、朴消皆味盐性寒,《本经》皆言苦寒,初时则盐极而苦,提过则转苦为咸矣。

104. Xiaoshi [消石, niter, Nitrum]

It is bitter in taste, cold and non-toxic in property, and it is mainly used to

treat the accumulation of heat in the five zang-organs, relieve the distension and block of the stomach, remove the accumulation of undigested food, get rid of the stale to bring forth the fresh and eliminate pathogenic qi. It can be refined as paste, and long-term taking of it will keep healthy.

Xiaoshi (niter) is also called Huoxiao (火消) or Yanxiao (焰消). The alchemists use it to help make five metals of gold, silver, copper, iron and tin and refine eight stones of cinnabar, realgar, mica, hollow azurite, sulfur, halitum, niter and orpiment; the silversmiths use it to melt gold and silver; the soldiers use it as gunpowder for the beacon tower. Flames come out once it is ignited, so it is also called Huoxiao (火消) or Yanxiao (焰消). Firstly recorded to be found in the valleys of Yizhou (益州), and in Wudu (武都), Longxi (陇西) and Xiqiang (西羌), now it can be easily found in Hebei (河北), Qingyang (庆阳) and Shuzhong (蜀中) as the frost on the land. In winter, it exists everywhere like frost. Sweep the land to get it, filter it with water, decoct the water and you can get Xiaoshi (niter) which looks like Puxiao [朴消, niter, Sal Nitri], so it is also called Shengxiao (生消). Decocted again, it may have sharp edges like Mangxiao [芒消, sodium sulfate, Natrii Sulfa] or have smooth edges like Mayaxiao [马牙消, horse-tooth mirabilite, Natrii Sulfas Equidens], so it is also called Mangxiao (芒消) or Yaxiao (牙消). It shares the same name with Mangya (芒牙) of Puxiao (niter), but they differ in their properties as water or fire.

Xiaoshi (niter) is the white frost on the land in winter. Bitter in taste and cold in property, it receives the qi transformation from lesser yin and greater yang. Lesser yin pertains to winter water, and greater yang governs the ending of six qi. Flames come out once it is ignited as there is sovereign fire over lesser yin and there is branch yang outside greater yang. It can treat the accumulation of heat in the five zang-organs and relieve the distension and block of the stomach as the accumulation of heat in the five zang-organs leads to the distension and block of qi in the stomach. Xiaoshi (niter), receiving the qi of water cold, can purge heat in the five zang-organs. With the property of fire flames, it can relieve the distension of the stomach. It can remove the accumulation of undigested food, thus the distension and block of the stomach will be relieved. It gets rid of the stale to bring forth the fresh and eliminates pathogenic qi, and then the accumulation of heat in the five zang-organs is treated naturally. Refined as paste, it takes shape by obtaining yin essence, so long-term taking of it will keep healthy. Both Xiaoshi（niter）and Puxiao（niter）are salty in taste and cold in property while they are described as bitter in taste and cold in property in *Shen Nong Ben Cao Jing*［《神农本草经》, *Shennong's Classic of Materia Medica*］. The reason lies in that they are extremely salty and bitter at the beginning, and bitterness will transform to saltiness after they are refined.

105. 朴 消

朴消　气味苦寒,无毒。主治百病,除寒热邪气,逐六腑积聚结固留癖,能化七十二种石。炼饵服之,轻身神仙。

朴消始出益州山谷有咸水之阳,今西蜀青齐河东河北皆有。生于斥卤之地土,人刮扫煎汁,经宿结成,再煎提净,则结成白消,如冰如蜡。齐卫之消,底多而面上生细芒如锋,所谓芒消是也。川晋之消,底少而面上生牙,如圭角作六棱,纵横玲珑,洞彻可爱,所谓马牙消是也。

愚按:雪花六出,玄精石六棱,六数为阴,乃水之成数也。朴消、消石皆感地水之气结成,而禀寒水之气化,是以形类相同,但消石遇火能焰,兼得水中之天气。朴消只禀地水之精。不得天气,故遇火不焰也。所以不同者如此。有谓:冬时采取则为消石,三时采取则为朴消。有谓:扫取白霜则为消石,扫取泥汁则为朴消。有谓:出处虽同,近山谷者则为消石,近海滨者则为朴消。诸说不同,今并存之,以俟订正。

朴消禀太阳寒水之气化,夫太阳之气,本于水府,外行通体之皮毛,从胸膈而入于中土。主治百病寒热邪气者,外行于通体之皮毛也。外感百病虽多,不越寒热之邪气,治寒热邪气,则外感之百病皆治矣。逐六腑积聚结固留癖者,从胸膈而入于中土也,太阳之气,入于中土,则天气下交于地,凡六腑积聚结固留癖可逐矣。能化七十二种石者,朴消味咸,咸能软坚也。天一生水,炼饵服之,得先天之精气,故轻身神仙。

105. Puxiao［朴消, niter, Sal Nitri］

It is bitter in taste, cold and non-toxic in property, and it is mainly used to

treat all kinds of diseases, eliminate the cold and heat due to pathogenic qi, expel the accumulation of pathogenic factors in the six fu-organs and fixed lump and resolve seventy-two kinds of stones in the body. Taking elixirs made from it will keep healthy like immortals.

Firstly recorded to be found in the saline-alkali soil in the valleys of Yizhou (益州), now it can be easily found in Xishu (西蜀), Qingqi (青齐), Hedong (河东) and Hebei (河北). It grows in the saline-alkali soil. Collect and decoct it, Puxiao (niter) can be made after one night, decoct it again to refine, then Baixiao (白消) can then be made, looking like ice and wax. Those produced in Qi (齐) and Wei (卫), with more sediments and sharp edges on the surface, are called Xiaomang (消芒). Those produced in Chuan (川) and Jin (晋), with fewer sediments and teeth on the surface, like Guijiao (圭角) having six edges, and looking delicate, clear and ingenious from any angle, are called Mayaxiao (马牙消).

Note by Gao Shishi (高世栻): A snowflake has six petals, and Xuanjingshi [玄精石, selenite, Selenitum] has six edges. The number six pertains to yin, and it is also the number indicating the forming of water. Both Puxiao (niter) and Xiaoshi [消石, niter, Sal Nitri] come into being with the qi of earth water and receiving the qi transformation of cold water, so they look similar to each other, while Xiaoshi (niter) can burn once ignited as it also obtains the heaven qi of water. Puxiao (niter) cannot burn once ignited because it only receives the essence of earth water instead of heaven qi. That is the difference between them. There is a saying: The kind collected in winter is Xiaoshi (niter), and that collected in the other three seasons is Puxiao (niter). Another saying: That collected from white frost is Xiaoshi (niter), and that collected from the muddy water is Puxiao (niter). Another saying: Despite that they share the same source, that collected near valleys is Xiaoshi (niter), and that collected near shores is Puxiao (niter). Various sayings are kept in this book for correction.

Puxiao (niter) receives the qi transformation of cold water from greater yang. The qi of greater yang generates from the kidney, flows outside to the skin and hair of the body and enters center earth from the chest and diaphragm. It can treat all kinds of diseases and eliminate the cold and heat due to pathogenic qi, as it reaches the skin and hair of the body. All kinds of diseases contracted externally are caused by nothing more than the pathogenic qi of cold or heat. It can eliminate the cold and heat due to pathogenic qi, so it can treat all kinds of diseases contracted externally. It can expel the accumulation of pathogenic factors in the six fu-organs and fixed lump, because Puxiao (niter) can enter center earth from the chest and diaphragm. When the heaven qi from greater yang enters center earth, it interacts downward with earth, then the accumulation of pathogenic factors in the six fu-organs and fixed lump will be expelled. It can resolve seventy-two kinds of stones in the body as it is salty in taste, and saltiness can soften hardness. Heaven One (天一) generates water. When people take the elixir made from Puxiao (niter), they will obtain the essence of the earlier heaven, thus they can keep healthy like immortals.

106. 矾　石

矾石　气味酸寒,无毒。主治寒热泄痢白沃,阴蚀恶疮,目痛,坚骨齿。炼饵服之,轻身不老增年。

矾石始出河西山谷及陇西武都石门,今益州、晋州、青州、慈州、无为州皆有。一名湟石,又名羽湟、羽泽。矾有五种,其色各异,有白矾、黄矾、绿矾、皂矾、绛矾之不同。矾石,白矾也,乃采石敲碎煎炼而成。洁白光明者,为明矾。成块光莹如水晶者,为矾精。煎矾之法,采石数百斤,用水煎炼,其水成矾石之斤数不减,是石中之精气,假水而成矾,故有羽湟、羽泽之名。湟泽,水也,羽,聚也,谓聚水而成也。

矾石以水煎石而成,光亮体重,酸寒而涩,是禀水石之专精,能肃清其秽浊。主治寒热泄痢白沃者,谓或因于寒,或因于热,而为泄痢白沃之证。矾石清涤肠胃,故可治也。阴蚀恶疮者,言阴盛生虫,肌肉如蚀,而为恶疮之证,矾石酸涩杀虫,故可治也。以水煎石,其色光明,其性本寒,故治目痛。以水煎石,凝结成矾,其质如石,故坚骨齿。炼而饵服,得石中之精,补养精气,故轻身不老增年。

106. Fanshi〔矾石, alum, Alumen〕

It is sour in taste, cold and non-toxic in property, and it is mainly used to treat diarrhea and morbid leucorrhea due to cold and heat, genital erosion, malign sore and eye pain, and strengthen the bones and teeth. Taking elixirs made from it will keep healthy, prevent aging and prolong life.

Firstly recorded to be found in the valleys of Hexi（河西）and in Shimen（石门）and Wudu（武都）of Longxi（陇西）, now it can be easily found in Yizhou（益州）, Jinzhou（晋州）, Qingzhou（青州）, Cizhou（慈州）and Wuweizhou（无为州）. It is also called Huangshi（湟石）, Yuhuang（羽湟）and Yuze（羽泽）. There are five kinds of Fan（矾）in five colors of white, yellow, green, black and red, which are Baifan〔白矾, alum, Alumen〕, Huangfan〔黄矾, fibroferrite, Fibroferritum〕, Lüfan〔绿矾, melanterite, Melanteritum〕, Zaofan〔皂矾, melanterite, Melanteritum〕and Jiangfan〔绛矾, crimson melanterite, Melanteritum Rubrum〕. Fanshi（alum）is actually Baifan（alum）, made through collecting, cracking and refining stones. The smooth and bright kind is called Mingfan〔明矾, alum, Alumen〕. The kind agglomerated in lump as bright as crystal is called Fanjing（矾精）. The way to decoct Fan（矾）: collect hundreds of Jin of stones, decoct them with water, the decoction will turn into Fanshi（alum）and the weight remains the same as it is made by essential qi of stone with water, so it is also called Yuhuang（羽湟）and Yuze（羽泽）. Huang（湟）and Ze（泽）refer to water; Yu（羽）means converging, so its name indicates it is made by converging water.

Fanshi（alum）is made from decocting the stone with water. It is bright and heavy, sour and astringent in taste, and cold in property. Receiving the essence of water and stone, it can purify the filthy turbidity. Diarrhea and morbid leucorrhea are caused by cold or heat. Fanshi（alum）can clear the intestines and stomach, so it can treat the diarrhea and morbid leucorrhea due to cold and heat. Genital erosion and malign sore occur when excessive yin generates worms that will erode the muscles and flesh, resulting in malign sore. Fanshi（alum）, sour and astringent in taste, can kill worms, so it can treat genital erosion and malign sore.

It is bright when it is decocted with water, and it is cold in property, so it can treat eye pain. After decocting the stone with water, the decoction congeals into Fan （矾） which is the same as stone in property, so it can strengthen the bones and teeth. Elixirs made from it obtain the essence of the stone, so taking it can replenish essential qi, thus to keep healthy, prevent aging and prolong life.

107. 石　胆

石胆　气味酸辛寒，有小毒。主明目，治目痛，金疮诸痫痉，女子阴蚀痛，石淋寒热，崩中下血，诸邪毒气，令人有子。炼饵服之，不老。久服增寿神仙。

　　石胆《本经》名黑石，俗呼胆矾。始出秦川羌道山谷大石间，或羌里句青山，今信州铅山、嵩岳及蒲州皆有之，生于铜坑中，采得煎炼而成。又有自然生者，尤为珍贵。大者如拳，如鸡卵，小者如桃栗，击之纵横分解，但以火烧之成汁者，必伪也。涂于铁上及铜上烧之红者，真也。

　　胆矾气味酸辛而寒。酸，木也。辛，金也。寒，水也。禀金水木相生之气化。禀水气，故主明目，治目痛。禀金气，故治金疮诸痫痉，谓金疮受风，变为痫痉也。禀木气，故治女子阴蚀痛，谓土湿溃烂，女子阴户如虫啮缺伤而痛也。金生水，而水生木，故治石淋寒热，崩中下血，诸邪毒气，令人有子。夫治石淋寒热，崩中下血，金生水也。治诸邪毒气，令人有子，水生木也。炼饵服之不老，久服增寿神仙，得石中之精也。

107. Shidan ［石胆, chalcanthite, Chalcanthitum］

It is sour and pungent in taste, cold and slightly toxic in property, and it is mainly used to improve vision, treat eye pain, incised wound, the convulsion due to epilepsy, genital erosion and pain, urolithic stranguria, cold and heat and the hemorrhage with bloody stool, expel various pathogenic and toxic qi, and enable women to conceive babies. Taking elixirs made from it can prevent aging. Long-term taking of it will enable people to live as long as immortals.

In *Shen Nong Ben Cao Jing* ［《神农本草经》, *Shennong's Classic of Materia Medica*］, it is also called Heishi （黑石） and it is popularly called Danfan （胆矾）. Firstly recorded to be found among the huge stones in the mountain valleys in Qiangdao（羌道）of Qinchuan（秦川）or in Juqing Mountain（句青山）of Qiangli（羌里）, now it can be found in Qianshan Mountain（铅山）of Xinzhou（信州）, in Songyue（嵩岳）and Puzhou（蒲州）. Growing in the copper mine, it can be made through decocting and refining. Those growing naturally are especially precious. It can be as big as a fist or an egg, or as small as a walnut or chestnut. It will break into long blocks when hit. Those melting into juice when burnt with fire are fake. Those turning red after they are painted on iron and cooper and burnt with fire are authentic.

Shidan（chalcanthite）is sour and pungent in taste and cold in property. Sourness pertains to wood, pungency to metal and cold to water, so it receives the qi transformation from the mutual promotion of metal, water and wood. Receiving water qi, it can mainly improve vision and treat eye pain. Receiving metal qi, it can treat the incised wound and convulsion due to epilepsy when wind invades the incised wound, resulting in the convulsion due to epilepsy. Receiving wood qi, it can treat genital erosion and pain as earth dampness leads to ulceration, which makes the vaginal orifice hurt like being bitten by the insect. Metal generates water, and water generates wood, so Shidan（chalcanthite）can treat rolithic stranguria, cold and heat, the hemorrhage with bloody stool, expel various pathogenic and toxic qi and enable women to conceive babies. It can treat rolithic stranguria, cold and heat and the hemorrhage with bloody stool as metal generates water; it can expel various pathogenic and toxic qi and enable women to conceive babies as water generates wood. Taking elixirs made from it can prevent aging, and long-term taking of it will enable people to live as long as immortals as it obtains the essence of the stone.

108. 石钟乳

石钟乳 气味甘温，无毒。主治咳逆上气，明目，益精，安五脏，通百节，利九窍，下乳汁。

石钟乳一名虚中，一名芦石，一名鹅管石，皆取中空之意。石之津气钟聚成乳滴溜成石，故名石钟乳。今倒名钟乳石矣。出太山少室山谷，今东境名山石洞皆有，唯轻薄中通形如鹅翎管，碎之如爪甲，光明者为上。

石钟乳乃石之津液融结而成,气味甘温。主滋中焦之汁,上输于肺,故治咳逆上气。中焦取汁奉心,化赤而为血,故明目。流溢于中而为精,故益精。精气盛,则五脏和,故安五脏。血气盛,则百节和,故通百节。津液濡于空窍,则九窍自利。滋于经脉,则乳汁自下。

108. Shizhongru [石钟乳, stalactite, Stalactitum]

It is sweet in taste, warm and non-toxic in property, and it is mainly used to treat cough with dyspnea, descend adverse-rising qi, improve vision, replenish essence, pacify the five zang-organs, unobstruct all joints, disinhibit nine orifices and promote lactation.

It is also called Xuzhong (虚中), Lushi (芦石) and Eguanshi (鹅管石), all with the meaning of being hollow. The fluid and qi of stone congeals into emulsion droplet that drops and flows to form a stone, so it is called Shizhongru (stalactite), and now it is called the other way around as Zhongrushi (钟乳石). Firstly recorded to be found in the valleys of Taishan Mountain (太山) and Shaoshi Mountain (少室山), now it can be found in the stone caverns in the famous mountains in the East. The one, thin and light, hollow in the middle, in the shape of Elingguan (鹅翎管), like the claws and nails of animals when broken, and smooth and transparent, is of good quality. Shizhongru (stalactite), formed by the congealing of stone fluids, is sweet in taste and mild in property. It can nourish the fluids in the middle energizer which flow upward to the lung, so it can treat cough with dyspnea and descend adverse-rising qi. The middle energizer offers its fluids to the heart which makes them red and transforms them into blood, so it can improve vision. The fluids flow into the middle and transform into essence, so it can replenish essence. When essence is exuberant, the five zang-organs will be harmonized, so it can pacify the five zang-organs. When blood qi is exuberant, all joints will be harmonized, so it can unobstruct all joints. When the fluids moisten the nine orifices, the nine orifices will be disinhibited naturally. When the fluids nourish meridians, lactation will be promoted naturally.

109. 禹余粮

禹余粮 气味甘寒,无毒。主治咳逆,寒热烦满,下赤白,血闭,症瘕大热,炼饵服之,不饥,轻身延年。

　　禹余粮始出东海池泽及山岛中,今多出东阳泽州、潞州,石中有细粉如面,故曰余粮。李时珍曰:禹余粮乃石中黄粉,生于池泽,其生于山谷者,为太一余粮也。

仲祖《伤寒论》云:汗家重发汗,必恍惚心乱,小便已阴痛,宜禹余粮丸。全方失传,世亦罕用。

109. Yuyuliang [禹余粮, limonite, Limonitum]

It is sweet in taste, cold and non-toxic in property, and it is mainly used to treat cough with dyspnea, the vexation and fullness due to cold and heat, red and white dysentery, amenorrhea, abdominal mass and great heat. Taking the refined one will enable people to tolerate hunger, keep healthy and prolong life.

　　Firstly recorded to be found in the lakes and pools and on the mountains and islands in East Sea, now it is commonly found in Zezhou（泽州）and Luzhou（潞州）of Dongyang（东阳）. It is called Yuliang（余粮）because there is fine powder in the stone, just like flour. Li Shizhen（李时珍）said, "Yuyuliang（limonite）is the yellow powder in the stone, existing in lakes and pools. The one existing in the mountain valleys is called Taiyi Yuliang [太一余粮, limonite, Limonitum]."

In *Shang Han Lun* [《伤寒论》, *Treatise on Cold Damage*], Zhang Zhongjing（张仲景）said, "Diaphoretic is prohibited for those who have frequent perspiration. In case diaphoresis is adopted, the patient will become restless and illusive. After passing urine, he suffers urodynia. Yuyuliang Wan [禹余粮丸, limonite pill] is suitable in this case. The complete formula has been lost, so it is rarely used now."

110. 太一余粮

太一余粮 气味甘平,无毒。主治咳逆上气,症瘕,血闭,漏下,除邪气,肢节不利。久服耐寒暑,不饥,轻身,飞行千里,神仙。

陈藏器曰:太,大也。一,道也。大道之师,即理化神君,禹之师也,师尝服之,故有太一之名。陶弘景曰:《本草》有太一余粮、禹余粮两种,治体相同,而今世唯有禹余粮,不复识太一矣。李时珍曰:生池泽者,为禹余粮,生山谷者,为太一余粮,本是一物。晋宋以来,不分山谷池泽,通呼为太一禹余粮,义可知矣。

110. Taiyi Yuliang〔太一余粮,limonite,Limonitum〕

It is sweet in taste, mild and non-toxic in property, and it is mainly used to treat cough with dyspnea, descend adverse-rising qi, treat abdominal mass, amenorrhea, metrostaxis, the inhibited limb joints, and eliminate pathogenic qi. Long-term taking of it will enable people to tolerate cold, summer-heat and hunger, keep healthy, walk for thousands of Li like immortals flying in the sky.

Chen Cangqi(陈藏器)once said, "Tai(太)means greatness and Yi(一)refers to the Dao(道). The master of great Dao(道), Great Emperor of Law, is the teacher of Yu(禹)the Great. The master once tasted this herb, so it is called Taiyi(太一)." Tao Hongjing(陶弘景)said, "In *Shen Nong Ben Cao Jing*〔《神农本草经》, *Shennong's Classic of Materia Medica*〕, there are Taiyi Yuliang(limonite)and Yuyuliang〔禹余粮, limonite, Limonitum〕, which refers to the same medicinal. However, nowadays only Yuyuliang(limonite)is used while Taiyi Yuliang(limonite, Limonitum)is not recognized any longer." Li Shizhen(李时珍)once said, "Yuyuliang(limonite)grows in lakes and pools while Taiyi Yuliang(limonite)grows in mountain valleys. They are actually the same. Ever since the Jin and Song dynasties, regardless of whether growing in mountain valleys or pools and lakes, both of them are called Taiyi Yuyuliang(太一禹余粮)." So that's what we know about them.

111. 空 青

空青 气味甘酸寒,无毒。主治青盲,耳聋,明目,利九窍,通血脉,养精神,益肝气。久服轻身延年。

空青一名杨梅青,始出益州山谷及越隽山,今蔚兰、宣梓诸州有铜处,铜精熏则生空青,大者如拳如卵,小者如豆粒,或如杨梅。其色青,其中皆空,故曰空青。内有浆汁,为治目神药。不空无浆者,白青也。今方家以药涂铜物上,生青刮下,伪作空青,真者不可得。

111. Kongqing〔空青, globular azurite, Azurite〕

It is sour and sweet in taste, cold and non-toxic in property, and it is mainly used to treat bluish blindness and deafness, improve vision, disinhibit the nine orifices, free the blood and vessels, nourish spirit and replenish liver qi. Long-term taking of it will keep healthy and prolong life.

Kongqing (globular azurite), also known as Yangmeiqing (杨梅青), was firstly recorded to be found in the mountain valleys of Yizhou (益州) and Yuejun Mountain (越隽山), and now can be found in Weilan (蔚兰) and Xuanzi (宣梓) where it coexists with copper. It is produced by the fumigation of copper essence. It may be as big as a fist or an egg, or as small as a bean or a bayberry. It is green in color and hollow in the middle, thus called Kongqing (空青, means hollow and green). It contains juice inside which is very effective in treating the diseases with the eyes. The one that is not hollow and has no juice is called Baiqing (白青). Doctors now smear medicine on things made of copper, scrap off the aerugo and fake it as Kongqing (globular azurite). It is really very hard to get the genuine one.

112. 紫石英

紫石英 气味甘温,无毒。主治心腹咳逆邪气,补不足,女子风寒在子宫,绝孕,十年无子。久服温中,轻身延年。

紫石英始出太山山谷,今会稽、诸暨、乌程、永嘉、阳山、东莞山中皆有,唯太山者最胜。其色淡紫,其质莹澈,大小皆具五棱,两头如箭镞。

112. Zishiying〔紫石英,fluorite,Fluoritum〕

It is sweet in taste, warm and non-toxic in property, and it is mainly used to treat cough with dyspnea and the pathogenic qi in the heart and abdomen, tonify insufficiency and resolve the wind cold in the uterus that causes infertility for ten years. Long-term taking of it will warm the middle, keep healthy and prolong life.

Firstly recorded to be found in the valleys of Taishan Mountain（太山）, Zishiying（fluorite）now can be found in the mountains of Kuaiji（会稽）, Zhuji（诸暨）, Wucheng（乌程）, Yongjia（永嘉）, Yangshan（阳山）and Dongguan（东莞）. The one from Taishan Mountain（太山）is of the best quality. It is light purple in color, crystal clear in texture, with five edges no matter it is big or small, and its two ends look like arrowheads.

113. 白石英

白石英 气味甘,微温,无毒。主治消渴,阴痿不足,咳逆,胸膈间久寒,益气,除风湿痹。久服轻身长年。

白石英始出华阴山谷及太山,今寿阳、泽州、虢州、洛州山中俱有。大如指,长二三寸,六面如削,白莹如玉而有光,长五六寸,益佳。或问天地开辟,草木始生,后人分移莳植。故他处亦有。今土中所生之石,亦有始生,与他处之分何耶? 愚曰:草木金石虫鱼皆为物类,始生者开辟之初,物之先见也。他处者,生育之广,物之繁盛也。天气从东南而西北,则草木始生东南者,未始不生西北,西北虽生,不如东南之力也。地气从西北而东南,则金石之始生西北者,未始不生东南,东南虽生,不如西北之力也。而岂莳植移徙之谓哉。若以草木土石而异视之,何所见之不大也。

紫白石英,品类相同,主治亦不甚远。紫为木火之色,气味甘温,故治心腹、肾脏之寒。白为金方之色,气味甘,微温,亦治肾脏、胸膈之寒,而兼上焦之燥,此大体同而微异也。

113. Baishiying [白石英, crystobalite, Quartz album]

It is sweet in taste, slightly warm and non-toxic in property, and it is mainly used to treat consumptive thirst, the impotence due to insufficiency, cough with dyspnea and the frequent cold in the chest and diaphragm, replenish qi and eliminate wind-dampness impediment. Long-term taking of it will keep healthy and prolong life.

Firstly recorded to be found in the valleys of Huayin Mountain (华阴山) and Taishan Mountain(太山), Baishiying (crystobalite) now can be found in the mountains of Shouyang (寿阳), Zezhou (泽州), Guozhou (虢州) and Luozhou (洛州). It is as big as a finger, two or three Cun in length, with six smooth sides just like being cut by knives. It is as white and crystal clear as jade and shining. That with five or six Cun in length is of better quality. Plants came into being when the heaven was separated from the earth and people later on transplanted them, so they can now be found in other areas. Now, the stone growing out of soil also has its origin, so how do we tell the difference between it and the stones growing from other places? Note by Gao Shishi (高世栻): all creatures, including grasses, trees, metals, stones, insects and fish, that came into being at the beginning of the creation of the world, are the origins of later generations. Later, they spread and thrive in other places. Heaven qi ranges from the southeast to the northwest, so the plants that originally grew in the southeast may also grow in the northwest. Even if they grow in the northwest, they are not as vigorous as those growing in the southeast. Earth qi ranges from the northwest to the southeast, so the metals and stones that originally existed in the northwest may also exist in the southeast. Even if they exist in the southeast, they are not as vigorous as those existing in the northwest. So transplanting is not the only cause for the differences. Judging from different efficacy, tastes and properties of grasses, trees, soil and stones in different areas, how can we say there is no big difference?

Zishiying (fluorite) and Baishiying (crystobalite) are of the same family, so they are used to treat almost the same diseases. Purple is the color of the east and the south. Zishiying (fluorite) is sweet in taste and warm in property, so it can expel the cold in the heart, abdomen and kidney. White is the color of the west. Baishiying (crystobalite) is sweet in taste and slightly warm in property, so it can also treat the cold in the kidney, chest and diaphragm as well as dryness in the upper energizer. So their functions and the diseases treated by them are roughly the same with slight differences.

114. 龙 骨

龙骨 气味甘平,无毒。主治心腹鬼疰,精物老魅,咳逆,泄痢脓血,女子漏下,症瘕坚结,小儿热气惊痫。

晋地川谷及大山山岩,水岸土穴之中多有死龙之骨,今梁益、巴中、河东州郡山穴、水涯间亦有之骨。有雌雄骨,细而纹广者,雌也。骨粗而纹狭者,雄也。入药取五色具而白地碎纹,其质轻虚,舐之粘舌者为佳。黄白色者次之,黑色者下也。其质白重,而花纹不细者,名石龙骨,不堪入药,其外更有齿角,功用与龙骨相等。

鳞虫三百六十,而龙为之长,背有八十一鳞,具九九之数,上应东方七宿,得冬月蛰藏之精,从泉下而上腾于天,乃从阴出阳,自下而上之药也。主治心腹鬼疰、精物老魅者,水中天气,上交于阳,则心腹和平,而鬼疰精魅之阴类自消矣。咳逆者,天气不降也。泄痢脓血者,土气不藏也。女子漏下者,水气不升也。龙骨启泉下之水精,从地土而上腾于天,则阴阳交会。上下相和,故咳逆、泄痢漏下,皆可治也。土气内藏,则症瘕坚结自除,水气上升,则小儿热气惊痫自散,不言久服,或简脱也。

114. Longgu〔龙骨, dragon bone, Mastodi Ossis Fossilia〕

It is sweet in taste, mild and non-toxic in property, and it is mainly used to treat Guizhu〔鬼疰, multiple infixation abscess〕in the heart and abdomen, the pathogenic factors like ghost, cough with dyspnea, the diarrhea and dysentery with pus and blood, metrostaxis, the abdominal mass with hard lump, and the infantile fright epilepsy due to heat qi.

The bones of dead dragon were firstly recorded to be easily found in the river valleys of Jindi (晋地), among the mountain rocks, and in the soil holes by water, and now they are also found in the mountain caves and waters in the areas of Liangyi (梁益), Bazhong (巴中) and Hedong (河东). There are male and female dragon bones. Those that are thin with broad veins are female; those that are thick with narrow veins are male. For medical use, those in five colors and with fragmented veins on the white surface, light in weight, sticking to the tongue when licked are of good quality; the white-yellow ones are next to that, and the black ones are of the lowest grade. The one that is white and heavy and with broad veins is called Shilonggu (石龙骨), which cannot be used as medicinal. Its teeth and horns have the same effects as Longgu (dragon bone).

Among the three hundred and sixty kinds of animals with scales, the dragon ranks the top. It has eighty-one scales on its back, the number of which is the square of nine. The dragon corresponds with the seven stars in the east, obtains the essence stored in winter, and flies from the spring on the ground up to the sky, so its bone is a medicinal from yin to yang, and from the lower to the upper. It can treat the fatal tuberculosis in the heart and the abdomen and pathogenic factors like ghost because when the heaven qi of water interacts upward with yang, the heart and abdomen will be harmonized and Guizhu [鬼疰, multiple infixation abscess] and the pathogenic factors like ghost which pertain to yin will be eliminated naturally. Cough with dyspnea is caused when heaven qi cannot descend; the diarrhea and dysentery with pus and blood is caused when earth qi cannot be stored; metrostaxis is caused when water qi cannot ascend. Longgu (dragon bone) activates water essence below the spring, and rises to the sky from the earth, then yin and yang interact with each other. When the upper and the lower are harmonized, cough with dyspnea, the diarrhea and dysentery with pus and blood, and metrostaxis are treated. When earth qi is stored inside, the abdominal mass with hard lump will be eliminated naturally. When water qi ascends, the infantile fright epilepsy due to heat qi will be dissipated naturally. There is no record about the benefits of long-term taking of it probably because such record was lost in handing down the book.

115. 鹿 茸

鹿茸 气味甘温,无毒。主治漏下恶血,寒热,惊痫,益气,强志,发齿,不老。《本经》以白胶入上品,鹿茸入中品,今定俱入上品。

鹿游处山林,孕六月而生,性喜食龟,能别良草,卧则口鼻对尾闾,以通督脉。凡含血之物,肉最易长,筋次之,骨最难长。故人年二十骨髓方坚,唯麋鹿之角,自生至坚,无两月之久,大者至二十余斤,计一日夜须生数两。凡骨之生无速于此,故能补骨血,益精髓。又,头者,诸阳之会,上钟于茸,故能助阳。凡用必须鹿茸,今麋鹿并用,不可不别。

鹿性纯阳,息通督脉,茸乃骨精之余,从阴透顶,气味甘温,有火土相生之义。主治漏下恶血者,土气虚寒,则恶血下漏。鹿茸禀火气而温土,从阴出阳,下者举之,而恶血不漏矣。寒热惊痫者,心为阳中之太阳,阳虚则寒热。心为君主而藏神,神虚则惊痫。鹿茸阳刚渐长,心神充足,而寒热惊痫自除矣。益气强志者,益肾脏之气,强肾藏之志也。生齿不老者,齿为骨之余,从其类而补之,则肾精日益,故不老。

115. Lurong〔鹿茸,velvet deerhorn,Cervi Cornu Pantotrichum〕

It is sweet in taste, warm and non-toxic in property, and it is mainly used to treat the metrostaxis with malign blood, cold and heat and fright epilepsy, replenish qi, strengthen memory, promote the growth of the teeth and prevent aging. In *Shen Nong Ben Cao Jing* 〔《神农本草经》, *Shennong's Classic of Materia Medica*〕, Baijiao〔白胶, antler glue, Colla Cornus Cervi〕was classified as the top grade and Lurong (velvet deerhorn) as the medium grade, while today they are both classified as the top grade.

The deer live in the mountain forests and give birth after six months of pregnancy. Fond of eating the turtle, they can identify good grass. When they lie down, their mouth and nose will face their coccyxes directly so that their governor vessels are dredged. For all the creatures with blood, the growth of the flesh is the fastest, and the sinews and bones are the slowest. So human beings will not have strong bone marrows until they are twenty years old. The only exception is the deerhorn which will be strong in less than two months since it grows out. The big one can weigh over twenty Jin, growing on average several Liang each day. No animal with bones can grow as fast as that, so Lurong (velvet deerhorn) can tonify bones and nourish blood and replenish essence and marrow. Besides, the head is the joint of various kinds of yang which gather in the horn, so it can assist yang. Only the horns of deer can be used as medicinal, but now the horns of elks are also used, so it is necessary to distinguish them from each other.

The deer pertains to pure yang; its governor vessels are connected with its mouth and nose, and its horns are the surplus part of bone essence, growing out of the head from yin (kidney essence). It is sweet in taste and warm in property, indicating the mutual generation of fire and earth. It can treat the metrostaxis with malign blood because it is caused by the deficiency-cold of earth qi. Lurong (velvet deerhorn) receives fire qi to warm earth, conducts yang from yin and leads yang to moving upward from yin, so it can staunch the metrostaxis with malign blood. The heart is the greater yang among yang, and cold and heat are caused by yang deficiency. The heart is the sovereign that stores spirit, and fright epilepsy is caused by spirit deficiency. Lurong (velvet deerhorn) can make yang qi grow gradually and make heart spirit sufficient, so cold and heat and fright epilepsy can be treated naturally. That it can replenish qi and strengthen memory means it can replenish kidney qi and strengthen the mind stored in the kidney. It can promote the growth of the teeth and prevent aging because the teeth are the surplus part of the bones; the kidney governs the bones which is of the same species with Lurong (velvet deerhorn), so it can replenish kidney essence, thus to prevent aging.

116. 鹿角胶

鹿角胶 气味甘平,无毒。主治伤中,劳绝,腰痛,羸瘦,补中,益气,妇女血闭无子,止痛,安胎。久服轻身延年。

鹿角胶原名白胶,以鹿角寸截,米泔浸七日令软,再入急流水中浸七日,刮去粗皮,以东流水,桑柴火煮七日,旋旋添水,取汁沥净,加无灰酒熬成膏,冷则胶成矣。

鹿茸形如萌栗,有初阳方生之意。鹿角形如剑戟,具阳刚坚锐之体,水熬成胶,故气味甘平,不若鹿茸之甘温也。主治伤中劳绝者,中气因七情而伤,经脉因劳顿而绝。鹿胶甘平滋润,故能治也。治腰痛羸瘦者,鹿运督脉,则腰痛可治矣。胶能益髓,则羸瘦可治矣。补中者,补中焦。益气者益肾气也。治妇人血闭无子者,鹿性纯阳,角具坚刚,胶质润下,故能启生阳,行瘀积,和经脉而孕子也。止痛安胎者,更和经脉而生子也。久服则益阴助阳,故轻身延年。

116. Lujiaojiao［鹿角胶, deer-horn glue, Colla Corni Cervi］

It is sweet in taste, mild and non-toxic in property, and it is mainly used to treat the damage to the middle, severe strain, lumbago and emaciation, tonify the middle, replenish qi, treat amenorrhea and infertility, relieve pain and calm fetus. Long-term taking of it will keep healthy and prolong life.

Lujiaojiao (deer-horn glue), originally known as Baijiao (白胶), can be processed in this way: Cut it into parts with the length of one Cun, soak them in rice water for seven days to soften it, then soak it in fast-flowing water for seven days, scrape off the rough skin, put it in east-flowing water and boil it with the fire of mulberry wood for seven days, add in water gradually, drain off the water, add in Wuhuijiu［无灰酒, limeless wine, Vinum Sine Calce］to decoct it into paste which will turn into glue when cooling off.

The deerhorn looks like the newly grown Lizi［栗子, chestnut, Castaneae Semen］, indicating the meaning of newly generated yang qi. The antler, like sword in shape, is strong, hard and sharp in texture. Decocted into paste with water, it is sweet in taste and mild in property, unlike the sweet taste and warm property of Lurong［鹿茸, velvet deerhorn, Cervi Cornu Pantotrichum］. The qi in the middle is damaged by seven emotions, and meridians become exhausted due to overstrain. Lujiaojiao (deer-horn glue) is sweet in taste, mild and moist in property, so it can treat the damage to the middle and severe strain. It can treat lumbago and emaciation because the deer can move the governor vessel, and then lumbago can be treated. It can replenish marrow, so emaciation can be treated. To tonify the middle is to tonify the middle energizer and to replenish qi is to replenish kidney qi. It can treat amenorrhea and infertility because the deer pertains to pure yang. Its horn is hard and strong, and the deer-horn glue is moist in nature and has the effect of descending, so it can activate kidney yang, move stasis, and harmonize the meridian to assist women to get pregnant. To relieve pain and calm fetus can further harmonize the meridian to assist women to give birth. Long-term taking of it can nourish yin and assist yang, so it can keep healthy and prolong life.

117. 鹿 角

鹿角 气味咸温,无毒。主治恶疮痈肿,逐邪恶气,留血在阴中,除少腹血痛,腰脊痛,折伤恶血,益气。《别录》附。

鹿角功力与茸、胶相等,而攻毒破泄,行之瘀逐邪之功居多,较茸、胶又稍锐焉。

117. Lujiao〔鹿角, antler, Cornu Cervi〕

It is salty in taste, warm and non-toxic in property, and it is mainly used to treat malign sores, carbuncle and swelling, expel pathogenic and malign qi, eliminate the retention of blood stasis in the genitals, relieve the blood pain in the lesser abdomen and pain in the lumbar spine, eliminate the malign blood due to fracture and replenish qi. Supplemented in *Ming Yi Bie Lu*〔《名医别录》, *Miscellaneous Records of Famous Physicians*〕.

Lujiao (antler) has the same action as Lurong〔鹿茸, velvet deerhorn, Cervi Cornu Pantotrichum〕 and Lujiaojiao〔鹿角胶, deer-horn glue, Colla Corni Cervi〕. It is mainly used to attack toxin, treat diarrhea, move stasis and expel pathogen. In these respects, it is more effective than the other two.

118. 牛 黄

牛黄 气味苦平,有小毒。主治惊痫寒热,热盛狂痉,除邪逐鬼。

牛黄生陇西及晋地之特牛胆中,得之须阴干百日使燥,无令见日月光。出两广者,不甚佳。出川蜀者,为上。凡牛有黄,身上夜视有光,眼如血色,时时鸣吼，恐惧人。又好照水，人以盆水承之，伺其吐出，乃喝而迫之，黄即堕下水中。大者如鸡子黄，小者如龙眼核，重叠可揭，轻虚气香，有宝色者佳，如黄土色者下也。人喝取者为上，杀取者次之。李时珍曰：牛之黄，牛之病也。因其病在心及肝胆之间凝结成黄，故能治心及肝胆之病。但今之牛黄皆属杀取，苦寒有毒，虽属上品，服之无益也。

牛黄，胆之精也。牛之有黄，犹狗之有宝，蚌之有珠，皆受日月之精华而始成。无令见日月光者，恐复夺其精华也。牛属坤土，胆具精汁，禀性皆阴，故气味苦平，而有阴寒之小毒。主治惊痫寒热者，得日月之精而通心主之神也。治热盛狂痓者，禀中精之汁而清三阳之热也。除邪者，除热邪，受月之华，月以应水也。逐鬼者，逐阴邪，受日之精，日以应火也。牛黄有毒，不可久服，故不言也。

李东垣曰：中风入脏，始用牛黄，更配脑麝，从骨髓透肌肤，以引风出。若风中于府，及中经脉者，早用牛黄，反引风邪入骨髓，如油入面，不能出矣。愚谓：风邪入脏，皆为死证，虽有牛黄，用之何益。且牛黄主治皆心家风热狂烦之证，何会入骨髓而治骨病乎？脑麝从骨髓透肌肤，以引风出，是辛窜透发之药。风入于脏，脏气先虚，反配脑麝，宁不使脏气益虚而真气外泄乎？如风中腑及中经脉，正可合脑、麝而引风外出，又何致如油入面而难出耶。东垣好为臆说，后人不能参阅圣经，从而信之，致临病用药畏首畏尾，六腑经脉之病留而不去，次入于脏，便成不救，斯时用牛黄、脑麝，未见其能生也。李氏之说恐贻千百世之祸患，故不得不明辩极言，以救其失。

118. Niuhuang ［牛黄，bovine bezoar，Bovis Calculus］

It is bitter in taste, mild and non-toxic in property, and it is mainly used to treat fright epilepsy, cold and heat, the mania and convulsion due to exuberant heat, and expel the pathogen and pathogenic factors like ghosts.

Niuhuang (bovine bezoar) grows in the gallbladder of the bull in Longxi (陇西) and Jindi (晋地). To get it, it is necessary to dry the gallbladder in the shade over a hundred days in avoidance of both sunlight and moonlight. That produced in Guangdong (广东) and Guangxi (广西) is not of good quality. That produced in Chuanshu (川蜀) is of better quality. The bull with bezoar is luminous at night, has blood-colored eyes, roars from time to time, and is afraid of people. It prefers looking in the water, and people put a basin of water before the bull waiting for it to spit out the bezoar. Shout at it loudly, and then the bezoar will be spat out and fall into the water. It can be as big as egg yolk or as small as the seed of Lonyan〔龙眼, longan, Longan Arillus Recens〕. It is in the layers which can be undraped, and it is light and fragrant. The one in golden color is of good quality and the one in ocher color is of poor quality. The one got through yelling at the bull is of good quality and that got through killing the bull is next to the former. Li Shizhen（李时珍）said, "The bull having a bezoar indicates that it suffers from a disease. The disease lies between its heart and its liver and gallbladder, and congeals into the bezoar, so Niuhuang（bovine bezoar）can treat the diseases related to the heart, liver and gallbladder. Nowadays, all the bezoars are got through killing the bull, which is bitter in taste, cold and toxic in property. Although it is ranked the top grade, it has no benefit to people."

Niuhuang（bovine bezoar）is the essence of the gallbladder. The bezoar is to bull what Goubao〔狗宝, dog's stomach calculus, Canis Stomachi Calculus〕is to dog and what pearl is to mussel, all of which are formed with the absorption of the essence of the sun and the moon. If exposed to the sun and the moon, they may lose the essence again. The bull pertains to Kun（坤）earth and its gallbladder contains essential liquids, both of which pertain to yin, so Niuhuang（bovine bezoar）is bitter in taste and mild in property with the slight toxin of yin cold. It can treat fright epilepsy and cold and heat because it obtains the essence of the sun and the moon so as to connect the spirit governed by the heart. It can treat the mania and convulsion due to exuberant heat because it receives the liquids of center essence so as to clear the heat of triple yang. That it can expel pathogen means it can expel heat pathogen because it absorbs the essence of the moon which corresponds with water. That it can expel pathogenic factors like ghosts means it can expel yin pathogen because it absorbs the essence of the sun which corresponds with fire. Niuhuang（bovine bezoar）is toxic in property and should not be taken for a long term, so it is not necessary to say a lot about it.

Li Dongyuan（李东垣）said, " To treat the wind stroke in the zang-organs, at first Niuhuang（bovine bezoar）was used in combination with Longnao〔龙脑, borneol, Borneolum〕and Shexiang〔麝香, musk, Moschus〕to expel the wind from the bone marrow to the skin. If the wind attacks the fu-organs and meridians, using Niuhuang (bovine bezoar) too early will, on the contrary, lead the wind pathogen into the bone marrow, like the oil into powder, and it cannot be expelled." Note by Zhang Zhicong (张志聪): Wind pathogen attacking the zang-organs is a deadly disease which cannot be cured even if Niuhuang (bovine bezoar) is used. Besides, it is mainly used to treat the wind heat mania and the vexation of people suffering from heart disease, how can it enter the bone marrow to treat bone diseases? Longnao (borneol) and Shexiang (musk) which expel wind from the bone marrow to the skin are a kind of medicinal effective in promoting out the thrust and effusion with dissipating acridity. Wind entering the zang-organs will cause the qi deficiency in the zang-organs while Longnao (borneol) and Shexiang (musk) are used to treat it. How will it not aggravate the deficiency and cause the outward discharge of genuine qi? If wind attacks the fu-organs and meridians, the combination of Niuhuang (bovine bezoar), Longnao (borneol) and Shexiang (musk) will work quite well to expel the wind out. How can it lead to the situation that the wind is hard to be expelled, just like the oil in powder? Therefore, the above comments made by Li Dongyuan (李东垣) are just his subjective speculation, and people later on believed him without referring to the medical canons, which caused them to be overcautious when prescribing medicine in treating diseases. The disease in the six fu-organs and meridians cannot be cured and when the disease attacks the zang-organs, it turns out deadly. By then, using Niuhuang (bovine bezoar) in combination with Longnao (borneol) and Shexiang (musk) may not save the patient. What Li Dongyuan (李东垣) said may be harmful and misleading for thousands of years, so I have to clarify his mistakes here for remedy.

119. 阿 胶

阿胶 气味甘平,无毒。主治心腹内崩,劳极洒洒如疟状,腰腹痛,四肢酸疼,女子下血,安胎,久服轻身益气。

山东兖州府,古东阿县地有阿井,汲其水煎乌驴皮成胶,故名阿胶。此清济之水,伏行地中,历千里而发现于此井,济居四渎之一,内合于心,并有官舍封禁，发煮胶以供天府，故真胶难得，货者多伪。其色黯绿，明净不臭者为真，俗尚黑如漆。故伪造者，以寻常之水煎牛皮成胶，搀以黑豆汁，气臭质浊，不堪入药。

《本草乘雅》云：东阿井在山东兖州府阳谷县，东北六十里，即古之东阿县也。《水经注》云：东阿井大如轮，深六七丈，水性下趋，质清且重，岁常煮胶以贡。煮法必取乌驴皮刮净去毛，急流水中浸七日，入瓷锅内渐增阿井水煮三日夜，则皮化，滤清再煮稠粘，贮盆中乃成耳。冬月易干，其色深绿且明亮轻脆，味淡而甘，亦须陈久，方堪入药。设用牛皮及黄明胶并杂他药者，慎不可用。

余尝逢亲往东阿煎胶者，细加询访，闻其地所货阿胶，不但用牛马诸畜杂皮，并取旧箱匣坏皮及鞍辔靴屧，一切烂损旧皮皆充胶料。人间尚黑，则入马料、豆汁以增其色。人嫌秽气，则加樟脑等香，以乱其气，然美恶犹易辨也。今则作伪者，日益加巧，虽用旧皮浸洗日久，臭秽全去，然后煎煮，并不入豆汁及诸般香味，俨与真者相乱。人言真胶难得，真胶未尝难得，特以伪者杂陈并得，真者而亦疑之耳。人又以胶色有黄有黑为疑者，缘冬月所煎者，汁不妨嫩，入春后嫩者，难于坚实，煎汁必老。嫩者色黄，老者色黑，此其所以分也。昔人以光如墅漆，色带油绿者为真，犹未悉其全也。又谓：真者拍之即碎，夫拍之即碎，此唯极陈者为然，新胶安得有此。至谓真者，绝无臭气，夏月亦不甚湿软，则今之伪者，未尝不然，未可以是定美恶也。又闻古法先取狼溪水以浸皮，后取阿井水以煎胶，狼溪发源于洪范泉，其性阳，阿井水之性阴，取其阴阳相配之意，火用桑薪煎炼四日夜而后成。又谓：烧酒为服胶者所最忌，尤当力戒。此皆前人所未言者，故并记之。

阿胶乃滋补心肺之药也。心合济水，其水清重，其性趋下，主清心主之热而下交于阴。肺合皮毛，驴皮主导肺气之虚而内入于肌。又，驴为马属，火之畜也，必用乌驴，乃水火相济之义。崩，堕也，心腹内崩者，心包之血，不散经脉，下入于腹而崩堕也。阿胶益心主之血，故治心腹内崩。劳极，劳顿之极也。洒洒如疟状者，劳极气虚，皮毛洒洒如疟状之先寒也。阿胶益肺主之气，故治劳极洒洒如疟状。夫劳极，则腰腹痛。洒洒如疟状，则四肢痠痛。心腹内崩，则女子下血也。心主血，肺主气，气血调和，则胎自安矣。滋补心肺。故久服轻身益气。

按：《灵枢·经水》篇云：手少阴外合于济水，内属于心。隐庵心合济水之说，盖据此也。李中梓谓：《内经》以济水为天地之肝，故阿胶入肝功多，当是误记耳。

119. Ejiao〔阿胶, ass hide glue, Asini Corii Colla〕

It is sweet in taste, mild and non-toxic in property, and it is mainly used to treat the bleeding in the heart and abdomen, the severe consumptive diseases with chills like malaria, the pain in the lumbus and abdomen, the aching pain of the four limbs, and vaginal bleeding and calm fetus. Long-term taking of it can keep healthy and replenish qi.

In ancient Donge（东阿）County of Yanzhou（兖州）, Shandong（山东）Province, there is a well named E（阿）. Draw the water out of the well, use the water to decoct the black donkey's hide into paste, and then Ejiao（ass hide glue）is made. Made with water from E（阿）Well, it is called Ejiao（阿胶）. The water, out of Jishui River（济水）, flows underground for a thousand Li to this well. Jishui River（济水）is one of the four great rivers and corresponds to the heart. The authorities block the well, and then only they can decoct Ejiao（ass hide glue）with the water to supply the royal storeroom. Therefore, the genuine Ejiao（ass hide glue）is rare and that for sale is mostly fake. It is dark-green in color. That clean and bright without odor is genuine. That as black as paint is commonly highly regarded, so the fake one is made by decocting cowhide with common water and adding in black bean sauce. Smelly and turbid, the fake one can not be used as medicinal.

According to Ben Cao Cheng Ya〔《本草乘雅》, Explanation on Materia Medica from Four Aspects〕, Donge（东阿）Well is located sixty Li in the northeast of Yanggu（阳谷）County of Yanzhou（兖州）, Shandong（山东）Province, which is the ancient Donge（东阿）County. According to Shui Jing Zhu〔《水经注》, Commentary on the Waterways Classic〕, Donge（东阿）Well is as wide as vehicle wheel, with six or seven Zhang in depth. The water tends to go downward in property. Clear in quality and large in density, the water is used to decoct Ejiao（ass hide glue）for annual tribute. The decoction method: scrap and dehair the black donkey's hide, soak it in fast-flowing water for seven days, put it in a porcelain pot, gradually add water from E（阿）Well to decoct it for three days and nights. When the donkey's hide melts, filter it and decoct it again to make it thick and viscous, put it in a basin, then Ejiao〔ass hide glue〕is made. It is easy to dry in winter. It is dark-green in color, bright and crisp, bland but slightly sweet in taste. Only after being laid aside for a long time can it be used as medicinal. Do not use that made with cowhide, Huangmingjiao〔黄明胶, oxhide glue, Bovis Gelatinum Corii〕, and the mixture of other medicinals.

I once met a person who went to Donge（东阿）in person to decoct Ejiao（ass hide glue）. The careful inquiry revealed that the one sold there is faked with not only the hides of cows, horses and other livestock, but also the rotten leather from the old box and suitcases as well as saddles, bridles, boots, shoes, and all other worn and old leather. Since that in black color is highly recognized, fodder and bean sauce are added to enhance the color. To lessen the odor, spices like Zhangnao〔樟脑, camphor, Camphora〕are added in it to confuse the smell, but it is still easy to distinguish if the quality is good or not. Today, the method to fake it is more delicate: soak the worn leather for a longer time to clear off the odor, and then decoct it without adding bean sauce and other spices, thus almost making the fake like the genuine. It is said that the genuine Ejiao（ass hide glue）is hard to get. Actually, to get the genuine is not so hard, but the fake is mixed with the genuine, thus making the genuine also under question. People also doubt the one yellow or black in color. The reason lies in that the decoction of Ejiao（ass hide glue）in winter should be tender. If that decocted in spring is tender, it is not easy to get firm, so it should be slightly over-decocted in spring. The tender one is yellow and the over-decocted is black in color, that is the difference. People used to regard that as bright as black paint and brilliant green in color as the genuine, but it is not a complete understanding. One more saying: the genuine breaks into pieces once patted. However, the true reason lies in that it happens only to the old one and never in the case of the new one. As for the saying that the genuine Ejiao（ass hide glue）has by no means any odor, and does not become moist and soft in summer; however, the fake Ejiao（ass hide glue）today is no exception to that. Therefore, this is not the rule to distinguish whether the quality is good or not. I also heard that the ancient method is to soak the hide in water of Langxi

（狼溪）River and then decoct it with water from E（阿）Well. Langxi（狼溪）River, whose water is yang in property, originates from Hongfan（洪范）Spring. However, the water from E（阿）Well is yin in property. So the ancient method has the intention of combining yin and yang. Decoct the hide with mulberry wood fire for four days and nights, and then Ejiao（ass hide glue）is made. Another saying: taking Ejiao（ass hide glue）with the white liquor is a taboo which should be strictly avoided. All of the sayings have never been mentioned before, so they are all together noted here.

Ejiao（ass hide glue）is effective in tonifying the heart and the lung. The heart corresponds with the water from Jishui River（济水）, which is clear in property and large in density and tends to go downward in property. So it can mainly clear the heat governed by the heart and interact with yin downward. The lung corresponds to the skin and hair, so the donkey's hide can remove the deficiency of lung qi and connect the muscles inside. Additionally, the donkey, the genus of Equus, is an animal pertaining to fire. To make Ejiao（ass hide glue）, it is necessary to use the black donkey, so as to achieve the effect of water and fire assisting each other. Bleeding means the falling of blood. The bleeding in the heart and abdomen is caused when the blood of pericardium can not spread to collaterals, and then flows downward into the abdomen and thus causes metrorrhagia. Ejiao（ass hide glue）can tonify the blood governed by the heart, so it can treat the bleeding in the heart and abdomen. Severe consumption refers to extreme exhaustion and deficiency. The severe consumptive disease with chills like malaria means that severe consumptive disease and qi deficiency causes the shivering of the skin and hair, resulting in chills, like the feeling of cold as the initial symptom of malaria. Ejiao（ass hide glue）can replenish the qi governed by the lung, so it can treat the severe consumptive disease with chills. Severe consumptive disease leads to the pain in the lumbus and abdomen. The chills like malaria lead to the aching pain of the four limbs. The bleeding in the heart and abdomen leads to the vaginal bleeding. The heart governs the blood and the lung governs qi. When the blood and qi are harmonized, the fetus is calmed. It can tonify the heart and the lung, so long-term taking of it can keep healthy and replenish qi.

Note by Gao Shishi（高世栻）：According to *Ling Shu · Jing Shui* [《灵枢·经水》, *Miraculous Pivot · The Channel Rivers*], the channel of hand lesser yin corresponds to Jishui River（济水）outside and pertains to the heart inside. That is why Zhang Yin'an（张隐庵）said，"The heart corresponds to Jishui River（济水）." Li Zhongzi（李中梓）said，"In *Huang Di Nei Jing* [《黄帝内经》, *Huangdi's Internal Classic*], Jishui River（济水）is regarded as the liver of the heaven and earth, so Ejiao（ass hide glue）is more effective in entering the liver." What he said is a misdescription.

120. 麝 香

麝香 气味辛温,无毒。主辟恶气,杀鬼精物,去三虫蛊毒,温疟,惊痫。久服除邪,不梦寤魇寐。

麝形似獐而小,色黑,常食柏叶及蛇虫,其香在脐,故名麝脐香。李时珍曰:麝之香气远射,故谓之麝香。生阴茎前皮内,别有膜袋裹之,至冬香满,入春满甚,自以爪别出覆藏土内,此香最佳,但不易得。出羌夷者多真,最好,出隋郡、义阳、晋溪诸蛮中者亚之。出益州者,形扁多伪。凡真香,一子分作三四子,刮取血膜,杂以余物裹以四足膝皮而货之。货者又复为伪,用者辨焉。

凡香皆生于草木,而麝香独出于精血。香之神异者也,气味辛散温行。主辟恶气者,其臭馨香也。杀鬼精物,去三虫蛊毒者,辛温香窜,从内透发,而阴类自消也。温疟者,先热后寒,病藏于肾。麝则香生于肾,故治温疟。惊痫者,心气昏迷,痰涎壅滞。麝香辛温通窍,故治惊痫。久服则腑脏机关通利,故除邪,不梦寤魇寐。

120. Shexiang [麝香, musk, Moschus]

It is pungent in taste, warm and non-toxic in property, and it is mainly used to dispel malign qi, expel the strange pathogenic factors like ghosts, eliminate the parasitic toxin due to three kinds of worms, and treat malaria and fright epilepsy. Long-term taking of it will eliminate pathogens and avoid being awakened by nightmares.

The musk deer looks like river deer in shape but smaller. Black in color, it feeds on Baiye〔柏叶, arborvitae leaf, Platycladi Cacumen〕, snakes and worms. The musk grows from its umbilicus (which is called "脐" in Chinese), thus called Sheqixiang (麝脐香). Li Shizhen (李时珍) said, "It is called Shexiang (musk) because its smell spreads very far." Growing in the foreskin of the penis, it is wrapped by musk pod. The musk grows to fill the sac by winter and is too full to be held in spring. The musk deer takes the musk out with its paws and hides it in the earth. This kind of musk is of the best quality, but it is hard to get. The one produced in Qiangyi (羌夷) is mostly genuine and of the best quality. The one produced in the southern areas like Suijun (隋郡), Yiyang (义阳) and Jinxi (晋溪) is next to that. The one produced in Yizhou (益州) is flat in shape and mostly fake. For the genuine ones, divide one musk into three or four parts and scrape the blood membrane, mix it with other things and wrap them with the fur of deer's four hoofs, which can be sold as goods. However, there are some fake musk goods. So it is necessary to distinguish them from the genuine ones before using them.

Almost all fragrance is generated from plants and only the musk from essence and blood, which is miraculous. The musk is pungent in taste, so it is effective in dissipating and it is warm in property, so it is effective in moving. It can mainly dispel pathogenic qi because it smells fragrant. It can expel the strange pathogenic factors like ghosts and eliminate the parasitic toxin due to three kinds of worms because with pungent taste, warm property and penetrating fragrance, it can promote the outthrust and effusion from interior, thus to eliminate the yin factors mentioned above. It can treat the worm malaria hidden in the kidney with the symptom of fever first and then chills because Shexiang (musk) is born in the kidney. Fright epilepsy is caused by coma due to the deficiency of heart qi, phlegm and fluid retention and congestion. Shexiang (musk), pungent in taste and warm in property, can relieve orifices, so it can treat fright epilepsy. Long-term taking of it can dredge and lubricate the valves of the zang-fu organs, so it can eliminate pathogen and avoid being awakened by nightmares.

121. 龟 甲

龟甲 气味甘平,无毒。主治漏下赤白,破症瘕痎疟,五痔,阴蚀,湿痹,四肢重弱,小儿囟不合。久服轻身不饥。

龟凡江湖间皆有之,近取湖州、江州,交州者为上。甲白而厚,其色分明,入药最良。有出于水中者,有出于山中者,入药宜用水龟。古时上下甲皆用,至日华子只用下板,而后人从之。陶弘景曰:入药宜生龟炙用。日华子曰:腹下曾灼十通者,名败龟板,入药良。吴球曰:先贤用败龟板补阴,借其气也。今人用钻过及煮过者,性气不存矣。唯灵山诸谷,因风堕自败者最佳。田池自败者次之。人打坏者又次之。愚谓:龟通灵神而多寿,若自死者,病龟也。灼过者,灵性已过。唯生龟板炙用为佳。

介虫三百六十,而龟为之长,龟形象离,其神在坎,首入于腹,肠属于首,是阳气下归于阴,复通阴气上行之药也。主治漏下赤白者,通阴气而上行也。破症瘕者,介虫属金,能攻坚也。痎疟,阴疟也。阳气归阴,则阴寒之气自除,故治痎疟。五痔、阴蚀者,五痔溃烂缺伤,如阴虫之蚀也。阳入于阴,则阴虫自散。肠属下者,则下者能举,故五痔阴蚀可治也。湿痹四肢重弱者,因湿成痹,以致四肢重弱。龟居水中,性能胜湿,甲属甲胃,质主坚强,故湿痹而四肢之重弱可治也。小儿囟不合者,先天缺陷,肾气不充也。龟藏神于阴,复使阴出于阳,故能合囟。久服则阴平阳秘,故轻身不饥。《本经》只说龟甲,后人以甲熬胶,功用相同,其质稍滞。甲性坚劲,胶性柔润,学者以意会之,而分用焉,可也。

121. Guijia [龟甲, tortoise shell, Testudinis Plastrum]

It is sweet in taste, mild and non-toxic in property, and it is mainly used to treat the red and white vaginal discharge in women, abdominal mass, malaria, five kinds of hemorrhoids, genital erosion, dampness impediment, the heaviness and weakness of the four limbs and infantile metopism. Long-term taking of it will keep healthy and make people feel no hunger.

Tortoise can be found everywhere in lakes and rivers, and those found near Huzhou (湖州), Jiangzhou (江州) and Jiaozhou (交州) are of better quality. Those whose shells are white and thick and clear in color are the best for medicinal use. Tortoises can grow in waters or in mountains, but those growing in waters are more appropriate for medicinal use. The upper and lower shell were both used in ancient times, and Ri Huazi (日华子) only used the lower shell and people later on followed suit ever since. Tao Hongjing (陶弘景) said, "For medicinal use, it is appropriate to broil the living tortoise." Ri Huazi (日华子) said, "The lower shell under the abdomen that has been burnt ten times is called Baiguiban [败龟板, tortoise plastron, Testudinis Plastrum], which is better for medicinal use." Wu Qiu (吴球) said, "The wise ancestors used Baiguiban (tortoise plastron) to tonify yin, which was using its qi for purpose. Nowadays, people use those that have been drilled or boiled but its property and qi have actually lost. Those from tortoises growing in the mountain valleys of Lingshan Mountain (灵山) and air slaked after tortoises die naturally are of the best quality. Those from tortoises growing in fields and ponds and spoiled after tortoises dying naturally are next to it. Those processed by people and spoiled after they eat the tortoises are of the lowest quality among the three." Note by Gao Shishi (高世栻): the tortoise can communicate with deities so it lives a long life. Those dying naturally die of sickness. For those who have been burnt, their spirituality has lost. So only the boiled shell of living tortoise is good for medicinal use.

Among the three hundred and sixty kinds of crustaceans, the tortoise ranks the first. The tortoise looks like Li (离) in the Eight Diagrams and its spirit lies in Kan (坎) in the Eight Diagrams. Its head hides in the abdomen and the intestines pertain to the head, which means it is a kind of medicinal which can make yang qi go downward to yin and lead yin qi to go upward. It can treat the red and white vaginal discharge in women just because it can lead yin qi to go upward. It can treat abdominal mass as crustacean pertains to metal so it can attack hard things. Malaria is related to yin. When yang qi goes to yin, the qi of cold yin is dispelled naturally, so it can treat malaria. Five kinds of hemorrhoids and genital erosion refer to ulceration and open injury due to five kinds of hemorrhoids that are like being eroded by worms. When yang enters yin, the yin worms will be dispelled naturally. The intestines, located in the lower part of the body, pertains to yin and can lead yang to move upward from yin, so five kinds of hemorrhoids and genital erosion can be treated. Dampness causes impediment and then leads to the heaviness and weakness of the four limbs. The tortoise lives in water, so it can restrict dampness; its shell protects its body like an armour and is hard in property, so it can treat dampness impediment, and the heaviness and weakness of the four limbs. Infantile metopism is a born defect caused by the deficiency of kidney qi. The tortoise stores spirit in yin and can return yin to yang, so it can make the fontanel closed. Long-term taking of it can make yin at peace and yang compact, which can keep healthy and make people feel no hunger. *Shen Nong Ben Cao Jing* [《神农本草经》, *Shennong's Classic of Materia Medica*] only talks about Guijia (tortoise shell), but people later on also used its shell to decoct the glue which has the same effect but is slightly stagnant in property. The shell is hard and the glue is soft in texture, so learners should have an insightful understanding of it and use their different effects respectively.

122. 牡 蛎

牡蛎 气味咸平,微寒,无毒。主治伤寒寒热,温疟洒洒,惊恚怒气,除拘缓,鼠瘘,女子带下赤白。久服强骨节,杀邪鬼延年。

> 牡蛎出东南海中,今广闽、永嘉、四明海旁皆有之,附石而生,磈礌相连如房,每一房内有肉一块,谓之蛎黄,清凉甘美,其腹南向,其口东向,纯雄无雌,故名曰牡,粗大而坚,故名曰蛎。

牡蛎假海水之沫,凝结而成形,禀寒水之精,具坚刚之质。太阳之气,生于水中,出于肤表,故主治伤寒寒热,先热后寒,谓之温疟。皮毛微寒,谓之洒洒。太阳之气,行于肌表,则温疟洒洒可治也。惊恚怒气,厥阴肝木受病也。牡蛎南生东向,得水中之生阳,达春生之木气,则惊恚怒气可治矣。生阳之气,行于四肢,则四肢拘缓自除。鼠瘘乃肾脏水毒,上淫于脉。牡蛎味咸性寒,从阴泄阳,故除鼠瘘。女子带下赤白,乃胞中湿热下注。牡蛎禀水气而上行,阴出于阳,故除带下赤白。具坚刚之质,故久服强骨节。纯雄无雌,故杀邪鬼。骨节强而邪鬼杀,则延年矣。

122. Muli [牡蛎, oyster shell, Concha Ostreae]

It is salty in taste, mild, slightly cold and non-toxic in property, and it is mainly used to treat the cold damage with aversion to cold and heat, the warm malaria with chills, fright, resentment and anger, contracture, scrofula, and the red and white vaginal discharge in women. Long-term taking of it will strengthen joints, dispel the pathogenic factors like ghost and prolong life.

Firstly recorded to be growing in the seas of the southeast, it now can be found on the seasides of Guangmin (广闽), Yongjia (永嘉) and Siming (四明). They grow attaching themselves to stones, unevenly connected like houses. Within each house, there is a piece of flesh, called Lihuang (蛎黄), which is cool and delicious. Its abdomen faces the south and its mouth faces the east. There is only male one but no female one, so there is Mu (牡) in its name; it is coarse, big and hard, so Li (蛎) is in its name.

Muli (oyster shell) comes into being from congealing the foam of seawater. It receives the essence of cold water, and it is hard in property. The qi of greater yang originates from water and flows in the fleshy exterior, so it can mainly treat the cold damage with aversion to cold and heat. Warm malaria means suffering from fever first followed by aversion to cold. The skin and hair feel slightly the aversion to cold, resulting in shivering and chills. The qi of greater yang flows in the fleshy exterior, so the warm malaria with chills can be treated. Fright, resentment and anger are caused when the liver wood from reverting yin is damaged. Muli (oyster shell) grows in the south and faces the east, so it obtains the kidney yang of water and reaches the wood qi of spring resuscitation, so it can treat fright, resentment and anger. When the qi of kidney yang flows to the four limbs, the contracture in the four limbs is treated naturally. Scrofula is caused by the excessive water toxin in the kidney affecting the upper meridians. Muli (oyster shell), salty in taste and cold in property, can drain yang from yin, so it can treat scrofula. The red and white vaginal discharge in women is the dampness and heat flowing downward from the uterus. Muli (oyster shell) receives water qi, makes it move upward, and makes yin go upward from yang, so it can treat the red and white vaginal discharge in women. It is hard in texture, so long-term taking of it can strengthen joints. There is only male one but no female one, so it can dispel the pathogenic factors like ghost. When joints are strengthened and the pathogenic factors like ghost are dispelled, life is prolonged.

123. 桑螵蛸

桑螵蛸 气味咸甘平,无毒。主治伤中、疝瘕、阴痿,益精,生子,女子血闭腰痛,通五淋,利小便水道。

螵蛸,螳螂子也。在桑树作房,粘于枝上,故名桑螵蛸。是兼得桑皮之津气也。其粘在他树上者,不入药用。螳螂两臂如斧,当难不避,喜食人发,能翳叶捕蝉,一前一却。其房长寸许,大如拇指,其内重重相隔,隔中有子,其形如蛆卵,至芒种节后,一齐生出,约有数百枚。月令云:仲夏螳螂生是也。

《经》云:逆夏气,则太阳不长。又云:午者,五月,主右足之太阳。螳螂生于五月,禀太阳之气而生,干则强健,其性怒升。子生于桑,又得桑之金气,太阳主寒水,金气属阳明,故气味咸甘。主治伤中,禀桑精而联属经脉也,治疝瘕,禀刚锐而疏通经脉也。其性怒升,当辙不避,具生长迅发之机,故治男子阴痿,而益精生子。女子肝肾两虚,而血闭腰痛。螳螂捕蝉,一前一却,乃升已而降,自然之理,故又通五淋,利小便水道。

123. Sang Piaoxiao［桑螵蛸, **mantis egg-case**, Ootheca Mantidis］

It is salty and sweet in taste, mild and non-toxic in property, and it is mainly used to treat the damage to the middle, hernia and movable abdominal mass, replenish essence, help women to conceive babies, treat the amenorrhea and lumbago in women and five kinds of stranguria, and disinhibit urination and water passage.

Piaoxiao［螵蛸, mantis egg-case］is the egg capsule of mantis. It is called Sang Piaoxiao（桑螵蛸）because it is formed on mulberry（桑）tree and attached to the branches thus to receive the essential qi of mulberry bark. Those attached to other trees can not be used as medicinal. With the arms like axes in shape, mantises never flinch from difficulties. They like eating humans' hair and catch the cicada by hiding behind leaves, then moving forward and backward. The egg-case is a little over one Cun in length, as big as the thumb. Inside it are different layers of compartments which contain eggs that look like those of maggot in shape. After the Grain in Ear day, they grow out together, over a hundred in number. According to *Yue Ling*［《月令》, *The Phenology of Lunar Month*］, mantises are born in midsummer.

According to *Huang Di Nei Jing* [《黄帝内经》, *Huangdi's Internal Classic*], if against summer qi, greater yang can not generate. One more saying: Wu (午), the fifth lunar month, governs the greater yang of the right foot. The mantis is born in the fifth lunar month by receiving the qi of greater yang. The movement of the heaven is full of power and the heaven has the nature of rising. Its egg grows on mulberry branches and receives the metal qi of mulberry. Greater yang governs cold water and metal qi pertains to yang brightness, so it is salty and sweet in taste. It can treat the damage to the middle as it receives mulberry essence to connect meridians. It can treat hernia and movable abdominal mass as it receives the properties of hardness and sharpness, thus to dredge meridians. Like the heaven, it also has the nature of rising. It does not flinch from difficulties and has the key to growth and development, so it can treat the impotence in men, replenish essence and help women to conceive babies. Deficiency in the liver and kidney causes the amenorrhea and lumbago in women. When the mantis catches the cicada, it moves forward and then backward, which corresponds to the natural law of ascending and descending, so it can treat five kinds of stranguria and disinhibit urination and water passage.

124. 蜂 蜜

蜂蜜 气味甘平,无毒。主治心腹邪气,诸惊痫痓,安五脏诸不足,益气补中,止痛,解毒,除众病,和百药。久服强志轻身,不饥不老,延年神仙。

蜂居山谷,蜜从石岩下流出者,名石蜜。蜂居丛林,蜜从树木中流出者,名木蜜,皆以色白如膏者佳。若人家作桶,收养割取者,是为家蜜,此蜜最胜。春分节后,蜂采花心之粉,置之两髀而归,酝酿成蜜。如遇牡丹、兰蕙之粉,或负于背,或戴于首归,以供王蜂。王所居层叠如台,有君臣之义。寒冬无花,深藏房内,即以酿蜜为食,春暖花朝后,复出采花也。

草木百卉,五色咸具,有五行之正色,复有五行之间色,而花心只有黄白二色,故蜜色有黄白也。春夏秋集采群芳,冬月退藏于密,得四时生长收藏之气,吸百卉五色之精。主治心腹邪气者,甘味属土,滋养阳明中土,则上下心腹之正气自和,而邪气可治也。诸惊痫痓,乃心主神气内虚,蜂蜜花心酿成,能和心主之神,而诸惊痫痉可治也。安五脏诸不足者,花具五行,故安五脏之不足。益气补中者,气属肺金,中属胃土,蜂采黄白金土之花心,故益气补中也。止痛解毒者,言蜂蜜解毒,故能止痛也。除众病,和百药者,言百药用蜂蜜和丸,以蜂蜜能除众病也,久服强志,金生水也。轻身不饥,土气盛也。轻身不饥,则不老延年,神仙可冀。

124. Fengmi〔蜂蜜,honey,Mel〕

It is sweet in taste, mild and non-toxic in property, and it is mainly used to expel the pathogenic qi in the heart and abdomen, treat various fright, epilepsy and convulsion, tonify the insufficiency of the five zang-organs, replenish qi and tonify the middle, relieve pain, resolve toxin, treat various diseases and harmonize various medicinals. Long-term taking of it will improve memory, tolerate hunger, keep healthy and prolong life like immortals.

For the bees living in mountain valleys, Fengmi (honey) that flows downward from rocks is called Shimi (石蜜). For the bees living in forests, Fengmi (honey) that flows from trees is called Mumi (木蜜). Among both of the two kinds, that white in color and in paste shape is of good quality. That cut off to be collected in buckets made by beekeepers is called Jiami (家蜜), which is of the best quality. After the Spring Equinox, bees collect pollen, place it between two thighs and go back to the hive to make it into Fengmi (honey). In the case of the pollen of peony or orchid, they carry it on the back or head and go back to give it to the queen bee. The storey inhabited by the queen bee is laid in the form of a platform to differentiate it as the monarch and her subjects. In cold winter when there is no flower, they hide in the hive and feed on Fengmi (honey) they have made. By spring, when it gets warm and flowers begin to blossom, they come out to collect pollen.

Various plants and flowers have all the five colors, in pure color or in binary colors of the five elements. However, the stamen or pistil has only two colors of yellow and white, so Fengmi (honey) is yellow or white in color. Bees collect pollen from various flowers in spring, summer and autumn, and hibernate in hive in winter. Therefore, Fengmi (honey) obtains the qi of generating and storing in the four seasons and the essence of five colors from various flowers. It can expel the pathogenic qi in the heart and abdomen as the sweet taste pertains to earth that can nourish center earth from yang brightness, then the healthy qi up in the heart and down in the abdomen are harmonized and pathogenic qi is expelled. It can treat various fright, epilepsy and convulsion caused by the deficiency of spirit qi governed by the heart as Fengmi (honey) is made from the flower pollen of the stamen or pistil, which is also called Huaxin (花心, which means flower heart), then the spirit governed by the heart is quieted and various fright, epilepsy and convulsion can be treated. It can tonify the insufficiency of the five zang-organs as flowers possess all the five elements. It can replenish qi and tonify the middle as qi pertains to kidney metal and the middle pertains to stomach earth. Bees collect the flower pollen of the stamen or pistil that is yellow and white in color and pertains to metal and earth in property, so it can replenish qi and tonify the middle. It can relieve pain and resolve toxin as Fengmi (honey) can resolve toxin thus to relieve pain. It can treat various diseases and harmonize various medicinals as it is used to make pills out of various medicinals so as to treat various diseases. Long-term taking of it will improve memory as metal generates water. It can tolerate hunger as earth qi is exuberant. It can keep healthy and tolerate hunger, so it can prevent aging and prolong life, and it can even make people live like immortals.

125. 蜜　蜡

蜜蜡　气味甘,微温,无毒,主治下痢脓血,补中,续绝伤金疮,益气,不饥耐老。

蜜蜡乃蜜脾底也,取蜜后将底炼过,滤入水中候凝,取之即成蜡矣。今人谓之黄蜡,以其生自蜜中,故名蜜蜡。黄蜜之底,其色则黄,白蜜之底,其色则白,但黄者多,而白者少,故又名黄蜡。汪机《本草会编》:一种虫白蜡,乃是小虫,所作其虫食冬青树汁,叶涎粘嫩茎上,化为白脂,至秋刮取,以水煮溶,滤置冷水中,则凝聚成块,此虫白蜡也,与蜜蜡之白者不同。

蜂采花心,酿成蜜蜡,蜜味甘,蜡味淡,禀阳明太阴土金之气,故主补中益气。蜜蜡味淡,今曰甘者,淡附于甘也。主治下痢脓血,补中,言蜜蜡得阳明中土之气,治下痢脓血,以其能补中也。续绝伤金疮,益气,言蜜蜡得太阴金精之气,续金疮之绝伤,以其能益气也。补中益气,故不饥耐老。

125. Mila [蜜蜡, beeswax, Cera Flava]

It is sweet in taste, slightly warm and non-toxic in property, and it is mainly used to relieve the diarrhea with pus and blood, tonify the middle, treat the fracture of the bones and sinews caused by incised wound, replenish qi, tolerate hunger and prevent aging.

Mila (beeswax) is the semidents of Fengmi [蜂蜜, honey, Mel]. After refining Fengmi (honey), filter it in water to make it congeal and the conglomeration is Mila (beeswax). Today people call it Huangla (黄蜡) and also call it Mila (蜜蜡) as it is collected from Fengmi (honey). The semidents of yellow Fengmi (honey) is yellow in color and that of white Fengmi (honey) is white in color, and since yellow color is the majority, Mila (beeswax) is also called Huangla (黄蜡). According to *Ben Cao Hui Bian* [《本草会编》, *A Collection of Materia Medica*] written by Wang Ji (汪机), there is Chongbaila [虫白蜡, insect wax, Cera Chinensis Cera] made by a small insect which eats the sap of Dongqing [冬青, Chinese ilex, Ilicis Chinensis] and spits on the tender stem. The spit turns into resin. Scrape off the resin in autumn, make it melt by boiling it in water, filter it and place it in cold water, and then it congeals into lump, which is Chongbaila (insect wax), different from white Mila (beeswax).

Mila (beeswax) is made from Fengmi (honey) collected from pollen by bees. Fengmi (honey) is sweet in taste while Mila (beeswax) is bland in taste. Receiving the qi of earth and metal from yang brightness and greater yin, Mila (beeswax) can tonify the middle and replenish qi. Mila (beeswax) is bland in taste and today it is also said to be sweet in taste as the bland taste is subject to sweetness. It can relieve the diarrhea with pus and blood and tonify the middle as it receives the qi of center earth from yang brightness to tonify the middle so as to relieve the diarrhea with pus and blood. It can treat the fracture of the bones and sinews caused by incised wound and replenish qi as it receives the qi of metal essence from greater yin to replenish qi so as to treat fractured bones and sinews caused by incised wound. Since it can tonify the middle and replenish qi, it can tolerate hunger and prevent aging.

卷中　本经中品

Volume 2　Medium-Grade Medicinals

126. 玄 参

玄参　气味苦,微寒,无毒。主治腹中寒热积聚,女子产乳余疾,补肾气,令人明目。

　　玄参近道处处有之,二月生苗,七月开花,八月结子黑色,其根一株五七枚,生时青白有腥气,曝干铺地下,久则黑也。

玄乃水天之色,参者参也,根实皆黑。气味苦寒,禀少阴寒水之精,上通于肺,故微有腥气。主治腹中寒热积聚者,启肾精之气,上交于肺,则水天一气,上下环转,而腹中之寒热积聚自散矣。女子产乳余疾者,生产则肾脏内虚,乳子则中焦不足,虽有余疾,必补肾和中。玄参滋肾脏之精,助中焦之汁,故可治也。又曰补肾气,令人明目者,言玄参补肾气,不但治产乳余疾,且又令人明目也。中品治病,则无久服矣,余俱仿此。

126. Xuanshen［玄参, figwort root, Radix Scrophulariae］

It is bitter in taste, slightly cold and non-toxic in property, and it is mainly used to resolve the accumulation of cold and heat in the abdomen, remove postpartum blood stasis, replenish kidney qi and improve vision.

　　It grows everywhere in the places nearby. It sprouts in the second lunar month, blossoms in the seventh and bears black seeds in the eighth. One root bears five to seven Xuanshen (figwort root). The raw one is blue-green in color and stinky in smell, which will turn black over time when it is laid on the ground and dried.

Xuan (玄), dark black, is the color of integrating the water and the sky. Shen (参) refers to a ginseng-like herb. Both the roots and the seeds of Xuanshen (figwort root) are black. Bitter in taste and cold in property, it receives the essence of cold water from lesser yin and moves upward to connect the lung, thus it has a slightly stinky smell. It can mainly resolve the accumulation of cold and heat in the abdomen by activating kidney essence qi to interact upward with the lung, resulting in the integrating of the water and the sky, which can then circulate up and down, and the accumulation of cold and heat can therefore be naturally resolved. It can remove postpartum blood stasis as the delivery of a baby will cause internal kidney deficiency, and lactation will cause the insufficiency of the middle energizer. It is necessary to tonify the kidney and harmonize the middle when suffering from postpartum blood stasis. Xuanshen (figwort root) can nourish kidney essence and assist the middle energizer to produce fluids, thus it is effective for removing postpartum blood stasis. It can also replenish kidney qi and improve vision. It can replenish kidney qi, which can not only remove postpartum blood stasis, but also improve vision. As a kind of medium-grade herb, do not take it for a long time to treat diseases, which is also applicable to other medium-grade herbs.

127. 丹 参

丹参 气味苦,微寒,无毒。主心腹邪气,肠鸣幽幽如走水,寒热积聚,破症除瘕,止烦满,益气。

　　丹参出桐柏川谷太及山,今近道处处有之。其根赤色。大者如指,长尺余,一苗数根。

　　丹参、玄参,皆气味苦寒,而得少阴之气化,但玄参色黑,禀少阴寒水之精,而上通于天,丹参色赤,禀少阴君火之气,而下交于地,上下相交,则中土自和。故玄参下交于上,而治腹中寒热积聚,丹参上交于下,而治心腹邪气,寒热积聚。君火之气下交,则土温而水不泛溢,故治肠鸣幽幽如走水。破症除瘕者,治寒热之积聚也。止烦满益气者,治心腹之邪气也,夫止烦而治心邪,止满而治腹邪,益正气所以治邪气也。

127. Danshen [丹参, salvia root, Radix Salviae Simplicifoliae]

It is bitter in taste, slightly cold and non-toxic in property, and it is mainly used to eliminate the pathogenic qi in the heart and abdomen, treat borborygmus sounding like running water, resolve the accumulation of cold and heat, disperse abdominal mass, relieve vexation and fullness, and replenish qi.

Originally growing in the valleys of Tongbai (桐柏) and Taiji Mountain (太及山), now it grows everywhere in the places nearby. Its root is red in color, and the big one is as big as a finger and as long as one Chi. One Danshen (salvia root) generally has several roots.

Bitter in taste and cold in property, both Danshen (salvia root) and Xuanshen [玄参, figwort root, Radix Scrophulariae] obtain the qi transformation from lesser yin. Black in color, Xuanshen (figwort root) receives the essence of cold water from lesser yin and flows upward to the heaven; red in color, Danshen (salvia root) receives the qi of sovereign fire from lesser yin and interacts downward with the earth, thus the middle and the earth become naturally harmonized with the interaction upward and downward. Xuanshen (figwort root) can resolve the accumulation of cold and heat in the abdomen by interacting with the upper from the lower. Danshen (salvia root) can eliminate the pathogenic qi in the heart and abdomen and resolve the accumulation of cold and heat by interacting with the lower from the upper. When the qi of sovereign fire interacts with the lower, the earth will get warm, and water will not overflow, thus borborygmus sounding like running water can be treated. Dispersing abdominal mass is to resolve the accumulation of cold and heat. Relieving vexation and fullness and replenishing qi are to eliminate the pathogenic qi in the heart and abdomen. Specifically, relieving vexation is to eliminate the pathogenic qi in the heart, and stopping fullness is to eliminate the pathogenic qi in the abdomen. Therefore, replenishing healthy qi can eliminate pathogenic qi.

128. 紫 参

紫参 气味苦寒,无毒。主治心腹积聚,寒热邪气,通九窍、大小便。

紫参《本经》名牡蒙,出河西及冤句山谷,今河中晋解齐及淮蜀州郡皆有之。苗长一二尺,茎青而细,叶似槐叶,亦有似羊蹄者。五月开细白花,似葱花,亦有红紫,而似水荭者。根淡紫黑色,如地黄状,肉红白色,内浅皮深,三月采根,火炙干便成紫色。又云六月采,晒干用。

《金匮》泽漆汤方,用紫参。本论云:咳而脉沉者,泽漆汤主之。《纲目集解》云:古方所用牡蒙,皆为紫参,而陶氏又以王孙为牡蒙,今用亦希。因《金匮》方有紫参,故存于此。

128. Zishen [紫参, Chinese sage herb, Herba Salviae Chinesnsis]

It is bitter in taste, cold and non-toxic in property, and it is mainly used to treat abdominal mass and cold-heat diseases caused by pathogenic qi, relieve the nine orifices, disinhibit urination and purge defecation.

It is mentioned as Mumeng (牡蒙) in *Shen Nong Ben Cao Jing* [《神农本草经》, *Shennong's Classic of Materia Medica*]. Originally growing in the valleys of Hexi (河西) and Yuanju (冤句), now it grows in Hezhong (河中), Jin (晋), Xie (解), Qi (齐), Huai (淮) and Shu (蜀). It has two-Chi-tall seedlings and a thin blue-green stem. Some leaves are similar to Huaiye [槐叶, sophora leaf, Sophorae Folium], and some are similar to those of Yangti [羊蹄, root of Japanese dock, Radix Rumicis]. It blossoms in the fifth lunar month with small white flowers similar to Conghua [葱花, scallion flower, Allii Fistulosi Flos]. It also blossoms with red-purple flowers similar to those of Shuihong [水荭, herb of prince's feather, Herba Polygoni Orientalis]. Its root is slightly purple-black similar to that of Dihuang [地黄, rehmannia, Radix Rehmanniae], which shades from red externally to white internally. Its root collected in the third lunar month turns purple when stir-fried and dried. According to another record, the root collected in the sixth lunar month is dried for future use.

It is used in Zeqi Tang [泽漆汤, Sun Spurge Decoction] in *Jin Gui Yao Lüe* [《金匮要略》, *Synopsis of the Golden Chamber*], which records that the decoction is adopted to treat cough and deep pulse. *Ben Cao Gang Mu Ji Jie* [《本草纲目集解》, *The Grand Compendium of Materia Medica Collected and Analysed*] says that Mumeng (牡蒙) used in the ancient formulas is indeed Zishen (Chinese sage herb), but Tao Hongjing (陶弘景) also called Mumeng (牡蒙) Wangsun (王孙), which is rarely used now. It is retained here, because it is used in the formulas recorded in *Jin Gui Yao Lüe* [《金匮要略》, *Synopsis of the Golden Chamber*].

129. 白前根 附

白前根 附　气味甘,微温,无毒。主治胸胁逆气,咳嗽上气,呼吸欲绝。《别录》附。

陶弘景曰,白前出近道,根似细辛而大,色白,不柔易折。苏恭曰:苗高尺许,其叶似柳,或似芫花,根长于细辛,白色生洲渚沙碛之上,不生近道,俗名石蓝,又名嗽药。马志曰:根似白薇、牛膝辈。陈嘉谟曰:似牛膝粗长坚直,折之易断者,白前也。似牛膝细短柔软,折之不断者,白薇也。近道俱有,形色颇同,以此别之,大致差误。

寇宗奭曰:白前能保定肺气,治嗽多用,以温药相佐使尤佳。李时珍曰:白前色白而味微辛甘,手太阴药也。长于降气,肺气壅实而有痰者宜之。若虚而长哽气者,不可用。张仲景治咳而脉浮者,泽漆汤中亦用之。愚以泽漆汤方有紫参,复有白前,故因紫参而附白前于此也。白前虽《别录》收入中品,而仲祖方中先用之,则弘景亦因古方录取,但出处不若《本经》之详悉,学人须知之。

129. Baiqiangen [白前根, willowleaf rhizome, Rhizoma Cynanchi Stauntonii] *supplement*

It is sweet in taste, slightly warm and non-toxic in property, and it is mainly used to descend the adverse-rising qi in the chest and ribs, treat cough with dyspnea and relieve suffocation. Supplemented in *Ming Yi Bie Lu* [《名医别录》, *Miscellaneous Records of Famous Physicians*].

Tao Hongjing (陶弘景) said, "It grows in the places nearby. White in color and bigger in size, its root looks like that of Xixin [细辛, manchurian wildginger, Herba Asari], which is brittle and easily broken." Su Gong (苏恭) said, "It is over one Chi tall, with its leaves similar to Liuye [柳叶, willow leaf, Salicis Folium] or to those of Yuanhua [芫花, lilac daphne flower bud, Flos Genkwa]. White in color, its root is longer than that of Xixin (manchurian wildginger), which grows on the marsh and sand rather than in the places nearby. It is popularly called Shilan (石蓝) or Souyao (嗽药)." Ma Zhi (马志) said, "Its root is similar to that of Baiwei [白薇, blackend swallowwort root, Radix Cynanchi Atrati] and that of Niuxibei [牛膝辈,

achyranthes, Achyranthis Bidentatae Radix]." Chen Jiamo (陈嘉谟) said, "If the root similar to that of Niuxi [牛膝, achyranthes, Achyranthis Bidentatae Radix] is thick, long, straight and easily broken, it is actually that of Baiqian (willowleaf rhizome). If the root similar to that of Niuxi (achyranthes) is thin, short, soft and not easily broken, it is actually that of Baiwei (blackend swallowwort root). Both herbs grow in the places nearby and are very similar in shape and color. If they are distinguished by the method mentioned above, there will be fewer mistakes."

Kou Zongshi (寇宗奭) said, "Baiqian (willowleaf rhizome) can protect and stabilize lung qi and is usually used to treat cough. It works more effectively when using the medicinal of warm property as assistant and guide." Li Shizhen (李时珍) said, "Baiqian (willowleaf rhizome), white in color, slightly pungent and sweet in taste, is a medicinal entering the hand greater yin meridian. It is effective in descending qi and is suitable for treating lung qi obstruction with phlegm. It is not suitable for treating deficiency with long panting." Zhang Zhongjing (张仲景) used Zeqi Tang [泽漆汤, Sun Spurge Decoction] which includes it to treat cough with floating pulse. I think that Zishen [紫参, Chinese sage herb, Herba Salviae Chinesnsis] is used in the formula of the decoction, which includes Baiqian (willowleaf rhizome) as well, thus Baiqian (willowleaf rhizome) is supplemented here after the entry Zishen (紫参). Although it is collected in *Ming Yi Bie Lu* [《名医别录》, *Miscellaneous Records of Famous Physicians*] as a medium-grade herb, it has already been used in the formula by Zhang Zhongjing (张仲景). Tao Hongjing (陶弘景) collected it because of the discovery of its usage in the ancient formulas, but the description of its origin in his book is not as detailed as that in *Shen Nong Ben Cao Jing* [《神农本草经》, *Shennong's Classic of Materia Medica*], which should be kept in mind by learners.

130. 当 归

当归　气味苦温,无毒。主治咳逆上气,温疟寒热洗洗在皮肤中,妇人漏下绝子,诸恶疮疡金疮,煮汁饮之。

当归始出陇西川谷及四阳黑水,今川蜀、陕西诸郡皆有。春生苗,绿叶青茎,七八月开花,似莳萝娇红可爱,形圆象心,其根黑黄色,今以外黄黑,内黄白,气香肥壮者为佳。

当归花红根黑,气味苦温,盖禀少阴水火之气。主治咳逆上气者,心肾之气上下相交,各有所归,则咳逆上气自平矣。治温疟寒热洗洗在皮肤中者,助心主之血液从经脉而外充于皮肤,则温疟之寒热洗洗然,而在皮肤中者,可治也。治妇人漏下绝子者,助肾脏之精气从胞中而上交于心包,则妇人漏下无时,而绝子者,可治也。治诸恶疮疡者,养血解毒也。治金疮者,养血生肌也。凡药皆可煮饮,独当归言煮汁饮之者,以中焦取汁变化而赤,则为血。当归滋中焦之汁以养血,故曰煮汁。谓煮汁饮之,得其专精矣。《本经》凡加别言,各有意存,如术宜煎饵,地黄作汤,当归煮汁,皆当体会。

130. Danggui〔当归, Chinese angelica, Radix Angelicae Sinensis〕

It is bitter in taste, warm and non-toxic in property, and it is mainly used to relieve cough with dyspnea, descend adverse-rising qi, treat warm malaria with chills and fever in the skin causing shivering, cure the infertility caused by metrostaxis, resolve various severe sores, ulcers and incised wound. Boil it and take the decoction.

Firstly recorded to be growing in the valleys of Longxi（陇西）and in Heishui（黑水）of Siyang（四阳）, now it grows everywhere in Chuanshu（川蜀）and Shaanxi（陕西）. It sprouts in spring with green leaves and a blue-green stem. It blossoms in the seventh and eighth lunar month with lovely and red flowers similar to those of Shiluo〔莳萝, dill, Anethi Caulis et Folium〕. The flowers are round, which are similar to the hearts in shape. It has black-yellow roots. The one with a yellow-black exterior, a yellow-white interior, a fragrant smell and rich flesh is of better quality.

Bitter in taste and warm in property, it receives the qi of water and fire from lesser yin with red flowers and black roots. It can mainly treat cough with dyspnea and descend adverse-rising qi. Heart qi and kidney qi interact with each other up and down and play their respective roles, thus cough with dyspnea can be naturally treated, and adverse-rising qi can be naturally descended. It can treat warm malaria with chills and fever in the skin causing shivering. It can assist the blood governed by the heart to flow outward from the meridians to fortify the skin, and warm malaria with chills and fever in the skin causing shivering can therefore be cured. It can treat the infertility caused by metrostaxis. It can assist the essential qi of the kidney to move upward from the uterus to interact with the pericardium, and the infertility caused by irregular metrostaxis can therefore be treated. It can treat various severe sores and ulcers, for it can nourish blood and resolve toxin. It can cure incised wound, for it can nourish the blood and promote granulation. Herbs can all be decocted and taken, but this process is exclusively mentioned in the record of Danggui (Chinese angelica). The middle energizer absorbs the essence of juice and transforms it into red fluid, which is then blood. Danggui (Chinese angelica) can nourish the essence of the middle energizer to nurture the blood, which is why the decocting process is exlusively mentioned here. Decoct it to make juice, take the juice and obtain its essence. In *Shen Nong Ben Cao Jing* [《神农本草经》, *Shennong's Classic of Materia Medica*], the supplemented words all have their special meanings, for example, Baizhu [白术, white atractylodes rhizome, Rhizoma Atractylodis Macrocephala] is suitable to be decocted and made into cakes, Dihuang [地黄, rehmannia, Radix Rehmanniae] to be decocted to make soup, and Danggui (Chinese angelica) to be decocted to make juice, which should all be completely understood.

131. 芍 药

芍药　气味苦平,无毒。主治邪气腹痛,除血痹,破坚积,寒热,疝瘕,止痛,利小便,益气。

　　芍药始出中岳山谷,今白山、蒋山、茅山、淮南、杨州、江浙、吴松处处有之,而园圃中多莳植矣。春生红芽,花开于三月四月之间,有赤白二色,又有千叶、单叶、楼子之不同,入药宜用单叶之根,盖花薄则气藏于根也。开赤花者,为赤芍,开白花者,为白芍。

初之气,厥阴风木。二之气,少阴君火。芍药春生红芽,禀厥阴木气而治肝。花开三四月间,禀少阴火气而治心。炎上作苦,得少阴君火之气化,故气味苦平。风木之邪,伤其中土,致脾络不能从经脉而外行,则腹痛。芍药疏通经脉,则邪气在腹而痛者,可治也。心主血,肝藏血,芍药禀木气而治肝,禀火气而治心,故除血痹。除血痹,则坚积亦破矣。血痹为病,则身发寒热。坚积为病,则或疝或瘕。芍药能调血中之气,故皆治之。止痛者,止疝瘕之痛也。肝主疏泄,故利小便。益气者,益血中之气也。益气则血亦行矣。

芍药气味苦平,后人妄改圣经,而曰微酸。元明诸家相沿为酸寒收敛之品,凡里虚下利者,多用之以收敛,夫性功可以强辩,气味不可诬传,试将芍药咀嚼,酸味何在?又谓:新产妇人忌用芍药,恐酸敛耳。夫《本经》主治邪气腹痛,且除血痹寒热,破坚积疝瘕,则新产恶露未尽正宜用之。若里虚下利,反不当用也。

又谓:白芍、赤芍各为一种,白补赤泻,白收赤散,白寒赤温,白入气分,赤入血分,不知芍药花开赤白,其类总一。李时珍曰:根之赤白,随花之色也。卢子由曰:根之赤白,从花之赤白也,白根固白,而赤根亦白,切片,以火酒润之,覆盖过宿,白根转白,赤根转赤矣。今药肆中一种赤芍药,不如何物草根,儿医、疡医多用之。此习焉而不察,为害殊甚。愚观天下之医,不察《本经》,不辨物性,因讹传讹,固结不解,咸为习俗所误,宁不悲哉。

131. Shaoyao [芍药, peony, Paeoniae Radix]

It is bitter in taste, mild and non-toxic in property, and it is mainly used to expel pathogenic qi, relieve abdominal pain, eliminate blood impediment, disperse hard mass, treat the diseases of cold and heat, resolve hernia and movable abdominal mass, relieve pain, disinhibit urination and replenish qi.

Firstly recorded to be growing in the valleys of Zhongyue (中岳), now it grows everywhere in Baishan Mountain (白山), Jiangshan Mountain (蒋山), Maoshan Mountain (茅山), Huainan (淮南), Yangzhou (杨州), Jiangzhe (江浙) and Wusong (吴松). It is usually planted in the garden. It grows red seedlings in spring and blossoms between the third and fourth lunar months with red or white flowers. It has many flower forms, such as Qianye (double flowered peony), Danye (single flowered peony), Qilou (bomb flowered peony), etc. It is suitable to use the roots of single flowered peonies as medicinal, for qi is stored in their roots because of few petals. Those with red flowers are Chishao [赤芍, red peony root, Radix Paeoniae Rubra], and those with white flowers are Baishao [白芍, debark peony root, Radix Paeoniae Alba].

The initial stage of qi is the wind wood of reverting yin. The second stage of qi is the sovereign fire of lesser yin. Shaoyao (peony) grows red seedlings in spring and can treat the diseases of the liver by receiving wood qi from reverting yin. It blossoms in the third and fourth lunar month, and it can treat the diseases of the heart by receiving fire qi from lesser yin. Fire characterized by flaring up is manifested as the bitter taste. It obtains the qi transformation of sovereign fire from lesser yin, thus it is bitter in taste and mild in property. The pathogen of wind wood damages center earth, which makes the spleen collateral unable to flow outward through the meridians, resulting in abdominal pain. Shaoyao (peony) can dredge the meridians, thus it can relieve the pain caused by pathogenic qi invading the abdomen. The heart governs the blood, and the liver stores the blood. Shaoyao (peony) can treat the diseases of the liver by receiving wood qi and those of the heart by receiving fire qi, thus it can eliminate blood impediment. Blood impediment is eliminated, and hard mass can then be dispersed. Blood impediment is accompanied by cold and heat. Hard mass is manifested as hernia or movable abdominal mass. Shaoyao (peony) can regulate blood qi, thus it can treat the above diseases. Relieving pain is to relieve the pain of hernia and movable abdominal mass. The liver governs the free flow of qi, thus it can disinhibit urination. Replenishing qi is to replenish blood qi, and promote the circulation of the blood.

Shaoyao (peony) is bitter in taste and mild in property, but people later on distorted the classics, saying that it is slightly sour in taste. Scholars in the Yuan Dynasty and the Ming Dynasty continued to follow this view, believing that it is sour in taste, cold and astringent in property and using it to treat the diarrhea due to interior deficiency by astringing intestinal qi. The property and actions can be defended by sophistry, but the taste cannot be rumored. After chewing it, you will ask a question: Is it sour in taste? It is stated that women who have just given birth should not use it for fear of its sour taste and astringency. *Shen Nong Ben Cao Jing* [《神农本草经》, *Shennong's Classic of Materia Medica*] records that Shaoyao (peony) can expel pathogenic qi, relieve abdominal pain, eliminate blood impediment with cold and heat, disperse hard mass and resolve hernia and movable abdominal mass, thus it is exactly suitable to use Shaoyao (peony) for the women who have just given birth with lochiorrhea. It is not suitable to use it for the people suffering from the diarrhea caused by interior deficiency.

It is also stated that Baishao (debark peony root) and Chishao (red peony root) are two different kinds. Baishao (debark peony root) can tonify, and Chishao (red peony root) can purge; the former is astringent, and the latter is dispersive; the former is cold in property, and the latter is warm in property; the former enters the qi aspect, and the latter enters the blood aspect. People are not clear about the fact that although Shaoyao (peony) can blossom with red or white flowers, both of them pertain to the same family. Li Shizhen (李时珍) said, "The root color depends on the flower color." Lu Ziyou (卢子由) said, "The root color depends on the flower color. The root of Baishao (debark peony root) is white, and the root of Chishao (red peony root) is also white. Slice their roots, soak them in alcohol overnight, and the root of Baishao (debark peony root) is still white while that of Chishao (red peony root) turns red." Currently, drug stores sell a kind of so-called Chishao (red peony root) with no idea of its origin, which is usually used by the pediatricians and doctors in charge of sores and wounds. Having been used to it, they are not aware of its problems, which does harm a lot. In my humble opinion, doctors have not completely studied *Shen Nong Ben Cao Jing* [《神农本草经》, *Shennong's Classic of Materia Medica*] or distinguished the properties of medicinals, which will result in the circulation of erroneous reports. Bad old practices die hard. Isn't it sad that all these things are wronged by customs?

132. 芎 劳

芎劳　气味辛温,无毒。主治中风入脑头痛,寒痹,筋挛缓急,金疮,妇人血闭无子。

芎劳今关陕、川蜀、江南、两浙皆有,而以川产者为胜,故名川芎。清明后宿根生叶,似水芹而香,七八月开碎白花,结黑子。川芎之外,次则广芎,外有南芎,只可煎汤沐浴,不堪入药。川芎之叶,名蘼芜,可以煮食,《本经》列于上品。

芎劳气味辛温,根叶皆香,生于西川,禀阳明秋金之气化。名芎劳者,乾为天,为金,芎,芎䓖也。劳,穷高也。皆天之象也。主治中风入脑头痛者,芎劳禀金气而治风,性上行而治头脑也。寒痹筋挛缓急者,寒气凝结则痹,痹则筋挛缓急,驰纵曰缓,拘挛曰急。芎劳辛散温行,不但上彻头脑而治风,且从内达外而散寒,故寒痹筋挛,缓急可治也。治金疮者,金疮从皮肤而伤肌肉,芎劳禀阳明金气,能从肌肉而达皮肤也。治妇人血闭无子者,妇人无子,因于血闭,芎劳禀金气而平木,肝血疏通,故有子也。

沈括《笔谈》云:川芎不可久服、单服,令人暴死。夫川芎乃《本经》中品之药,所以治病者也,有病则服,无病不宜服。服之而病愈,又不宜多服。若佐补药而使之开导,久服可也。有头脑中风寒痹筋挛之证,单用可也。遂以暴死加之,谓不可久服、单服,执矣。医执是说,而不能圆通会悟,其犹正墙而立也与。

132. Xiongqiong〔芎劳, Sichuan lovage rhizome, Rhizoma Ligustici Chuanxiong〕

It is pungent in taste, warm and non-toxic in property, and it is mainly used to treat the headache caused by the invasion of pathogenic wind into the brain, cold impediment, muscular spasm and convulsion, incised wound and the infertility caused by amenorrhea.

It now grows in Guanshan (关陕), Chuanshu (川蜀), Jiangnan (江南) and Liangzhe (两浙), and those growing in Sichuan (四川) are of better quality, thus it is called Chuanxiong (川芎). Its perennial roots begin to grow leaves after Pure Brightness (清明), which are fragrant and similar to those of Shuiqin〔水芹, water dropwort, Oenanthes Javanicae Herba〕. It blossoms with small white flowers in the seventh and eighth lunar months and bears black fruits. As for the quality, Chuanxiong (川芎) is followed by Guangxiong (广芎), and Guangxiong (广芎) is followed by Nanxiong (南芎). Both of them can only be decocted for bathing, not for medical uses. The leaves of Chuanxiong (川芎) are called Miwu〔蘼芜, chuanxiong leaf, Chuanxiong Folium〕, which can be cooked for eating and is listed as a top-grade herb in *Shen Nong Ben Cao Jing*〔《神农本草经》, *Shennong's Classic of Materia Medica*〕.

Pungent in taste and warm in property, it grows in Xichuan (西川) with fragrant roots and leaves and receives the qi transformation of autumn metal from yang brightness. It is called Xiongqiong (Sichuan lovage rhizome). Qian (乾, one of the eight diagrams) refers to the heaven and pertains to metal. Xiong (芎) is fornix. Qiong (劳) means being extremely high. All of them are the manifestations of the heaven. It can mainly treat the headache caused by the invasion of pathogenic wind into the brain, for it can treat the diseases caused by wind by receiving metal qi and treat those of the brain through its property of flowing upward. It can treat cold impediment, muscular spasm and convulsion. The stagnation of cold qi can cause impediment, and impediment can cause muscular spasm and convulsion. Convulsion means retardation, and spasm means contraction. Xiongqiong (Sichuan lovage rhizome) has the effect of dissipating and moving with its pungent taste and warm property, thus it can not only treat the diseases caused by wind by flowing upward to the brain, but also dissipate cold by penetrating from the inside to the outside. The above diseases can therefore be treated. It can treat incised wound, which can penetrate the skin to injure the muscles. It receives qi from yang brightness, thus it can reach the skin through the muscles. It can treat the infertility caused by amenorrhea, for it can balance wood by receiving metal qi. Thus, the liver blood is activated, and infertility can then be treated.

Shen Kuo (沈括) said in *Meng Xi Bi Tan* [《梦溪笔谈》, *Brush Talks from Dream Brook*], "Chuanxiong (川芎) cannot be taken for a long time or alone. If so, it will cause sudden death." Chuanxiong (川芎) is listed as a medium-grade herb in *Shen Nong Ben Cao Jing* [《神农本草经》, *Shennong's Classic of Materia Medica*]. Thus, take it when suffering from diseases, and vice versa. People can recover by taking it, but it is not suitable to take it excessively. It can have the dredging effect when it is used together with assisted tonic, thus it is possible to take it for a long time. It can be used alone to treat wind stroke, cold impediment and muscular spasm. Thus, it is one-sided to say that Chuanxiong (川芎) cannot be taken for a long time or alone for fear of the imposed sudden death. The obstinacy in following the statement and inability to grasp flexibly what the classics say can be regarded as ignoranance.

133. 牡 丹

牡丹 气味辛寒,无毒。主治寒热中风,瘈疭惊痫,邪气,除症坚瘀血,留舍肠胃,安五脏,疗痈疮。

牡丹始出蜀地山谷及汉中,今江南、江北皆有,而以洛阳为盛。冬月含苞紫色,春初放叶,三月开花有红白黄紫及桃红、粉红、佛头青、鸭头绿之色。有千叶、单叶、起楼、平头种种不一,入药唯取野生红白单叶者之根皮用之。单瓣则专精在本,其千叶五色异种,只供玩赏之品。千叶者,不结子,唯单瓣者,结子黑色,如鸡豆子大,子虽结仍在根上发枝分种,故名曰牡色红入心,故名曰丹。

牡丹根上生枝,皮色外红紫,内粉白,命名曰牡丹,乃心主血脉之药也,始生西北,气味辛寒,盖禀金水相生之气化。寒热中风,瘈疭惊痫。邪气者,言邪风之气,中于人身,伤其血脉,致身发寒热,而手足瘈疭,面目惊痫。丹皮禀金气而治血脉之风,故主治也。症坚瘀血留舍肠胃者,言经脉之血,不渗灌于络脉,则留舍肠胃,而为症坚之瘀血,丹皮辛以散之,寒以清之,故主除焉。花开五色,故安五脏,通调血脉,故疗痈疮。

133. Mudan [牡丹, moutan, Cortex Moutan Radicis]

It is pungent in taste, cold and non-toxic in property, and it is mainly used to treat cold-heat diseases and wind stroke, resolve tugging and slackening and fright epilepsy, cure the diseases caused by pathogenic qi, eliminate abdominal mass and blood stasis remaining in the intestines and stomach, harmonize the five zang-organs and cure abscess.

Firstly recorded to be growing in the valleys in Shu (蜀) area and in Hanzhong (汉中), now it grows both in Jiangnan (江南) and Jiangbei (江北). It is planted in a large number in Luoyang (洛阳). It comes into bud in purple in the eleventh lunar month and into leaf in the early spring. It blossoms in different colors, such as red, white, yellow, purple, peach, pink, ultramarine and green, in the third lunar month. It has many flower forms, such as Qianye (double flowered moutan), Danye (single flowered moutan),

Qilou (bomb flowered moutan), Pingtou (anemone flowered moutan), etc. Only the roots and barks of single Mudan (moutan) in red and white can be used as medicinal. The essence of single Mudan (moutan) is exclusively stored in its roots, and the double one can be in five colors and in different kinds, which is only for viewing. The double one does not bear fruits, and only the single one can bear black fruits, as big as Jidouzi [鸡豆子, gordon euryale seed, Semen Euryales]. Though it has borne seeds, it can still sprout on its roots, and the sprout will grow into the branch to be planted, thus it is called Mu [牡, male]. Its red color extends to the center of the flower, thus it is called Dan [丹, red].

It branches from the root, with its root bark being red-purple outside and pink-white inside. It is a medicinal entering the heart which governs the blood vessels. Pungent in taste and cold in property, it originally grew in the northwest. It receives the qi transformation from the mutual generation of metal and water. Danpi [丹皮, tree peony root bark, Cortex Moutan Radicis] can mainly treat cold-heat diseases and wind stroke, and resolve tugging, slackening and fright epilepsy. The qi of the pathogenic wind invades the human body and damages the blood vessels, resulting in cold and heat of the body, tugging and slackening of the hands and feet as well as the fright epilepsy of the face. Danpi (tree peony root bark) can dispel the wind of the blood vessels by receiving metal qi, thus it can treat the above diseases. The blood of the meridians remains in the intestines and stomach instead of flowing into the collateral vessels, resulting in abdominal mass and blood stasis. Danpi (tree peony root bark) has the dissipating effect with its pungency and the clearing effect with its cold, thus it can mainly eliminate abdominal mass and blood stasis. Mudan (moutan) blossoms with flowers in five colors, thus it can harmonize the five zang-organs. It can dredge and regulate the blood vessels, thus it can cure abscess.

134. 地　榆

地榆　气味苦微寒,无毒。主治妇人产乳痉病,七伤,带下,五漏,止痛,止汗,除恶肉,疗金疮。

地榆处处平原川泽有之,宿根在土,三月生苗,初生布地,独茎直上,高三四尺,叶似榆叶而狭长如锯齿状,其根外黑里红,一名玉豉,又名酸赭。

地榆一名玉豉,其臭兼酸,其色则赭,故《别录》又名酸赭,盖禀厥阴木火之气,能资肝脏之血也。主治妇人产乳痓病者,谓产后乳子,血虚中风而病痓。地榆益肝藏之血,故可治也。七伤者,食伤,忧伤,饮伤,房室伤,饮伤,劳伤,经络营卫气伤,内有干血,身皮甲错,两目黯黑也。地榆得先春之气,故能养五脏而治七伤。带下五漏者,带漏五色,或如青泥,或如红津,或如白涕,或如黄瓜,或如黑衃血也。止痛者,止妇人九痛,一阴中痛,二阴中淋痛,三小便痛,四寒冷痛,五月经来时腹痛,六气满来时足痛,七汗出阴中如虫啮痛,八胁下皮肤痛,九腰痛。地榆得木火之气,能散带漏下之瘀,而解阴凝之痛也。止汗者,止产后血虚汗出也。除恶肉,疗金疮者,生阳气盛,则恶肉自除,血气调和,则金疮可疗。

134. Diyu〔地榆，garden burnet root，Radix Sanguisorbae〕

It is bitter in taste, slightly cold and non-toxic in property, and it is mainly used to treat postpartum convulsion, seven damages and leucorrhea diseases with five colors, cease pain, stop sweating, eliminate malign flesh and cure incised wound.

It grows everywhere on the plains and in the mountains and swamps. Its perennial root remains in the earth and sprouts in the third lunar month. Its newly-grown seedlings spread on the ground, and its stems grow straight upward to three or four Chi tall. Its leaves, similar to Yuye〔榆叶, dwarf elm leaf, Ulmi Pumilae Folium〕, are long, narrow and serrated. Its root is black outside and red inside. It is also called Yuchi（玉豉）and Suanzhe（酸赭）.

It is also called Yuchi（玉豉）. It is sour in smell and reddish-brown in color, thus it is also called Suanzhe（酸赭）in *Ming Yi Bie Lu*〔《名医别录》, *Miscellaneous Records of Famous Physicians*〕. It receives the qi of wood and fire from reverting yin, thus it can nourish the blood of the liver. It can mainly treat postpartum convulsion, which is caused by blood deficiency and wind stroke during lactation. Diyu（garden burnet root）can nourish the blood of the liver, thus it can treat the above disease. Seven damages are the damages caused by unregulated eating, anxiety, unregulated drinking, sexual intemperance, hunger, overstrain and impaired meridians, nutrient qi and defensive qi, resulting in blood stasis, scaly skin and dark circles. Diyu (garden burnet root) can nourish the five zang-organs and treat seven damages by obtaining qi from the early spring. The leucorrhea diseases with five colors are manifested as the diseases in five colors and forms, which are like blue-green mud, red fluid, white snivel, yellow pulp and black coagulated blood. Ceasing pain is to cease nine types of women's pain, including the pain of the vulva, strangury, painful urination, the pain caused by cold, the abdominal pain during menstruation, the foot pain caused by qi fullness, the pain as painful as being bitten by insects caused by vulva sweating, the skin pain in the rib-side and lumbago. It obtains the qi of wood and fire, thus it can disperse the stasis caused by leukorrhea and remove the congealing pain in the vulva. Stopping sweating is to stop the sweating caused by postpartum blood deficiency. It can eliminate malign flesh and cure incised wound, because exuberant kidney-yang qi can lead to the elimination of malign flesh, and the harmony of qi and blood can lead to the treatment of incised wound.

135. 紫 草

紫草 气味苦寒,无毒。主治心腹邪气,五疸,补中,益气,利九窍。

　　紫草出砀山山谷及襄阳、南阳、新野所在皆有,人家或种之。苗似兰香,赤茎青节,二月开花紫白色,结实白色,春社前后采根阴干,其根头有白毛如茸,根身紫色,可以染紫。

　　紫乃苍赤之间色,紫草色紫,得火气也。苗似兰香,得土气也。火土相生,能资中焦之精汁,而调和其上下,故气味苦寒,主治心腹之邪气。

　　疸者,干也,津液干枯也。五疸者,惊疸、食疸、气疸、筋疸、骨疸也。紫草禀火土之气,滋益三焦,故治小儿之五疸。补中者,补中土也。益气者,益三焦之气也。九窍为水注之气,补中土而益三焦,则如雾如沤如渎,水气环复,故利九窍。

135. Zicao [紫草, arnebia root, Radix Arnebiae]

It is bitter in taste, cold and non-toxic in property, and it is mainly used to

treat the pathogenic qi in the heart and abdomen and five kinds of infantile malnutrition, tonify the middle, replenish qi and disinhibit the nine orifices.

It grows in the valleys of Dangshan Mountain (砀山) and everywhere in Xiangyang (襄阳), Nanyang (南阳) and Xinye (新野), which is planted by farmers. Its seedlings are similar to those of Lanxiang [兰香, basil, Basilici Herba]. It has a red stem with blue-green nodes. It blossoms with purple-white flowers in the second lunar month and bears white fruits. Collect its roots and dry them in the shade around Spring Sacrifice Day (春祉). The tip of its root is covered with white hair, which looks like downy grass. Its root is purple, which can be used to dye things purple.

Purple is a color intermediate between green and red. Zicao (arnebia root) is purple in color, thus it obtains fire qi. Its seedlings are similar to those of Lanxiang (basil), thus it obtains earth qi. The mutual generation of fire and earth can nourish the essence of the middle energizer and harmonize the upper energizer and the lower energizer. Thus, bitter in taste and cold in property, it can mainly treat the pathogenic qi in the heart and abdomen.

Infantile malnutrition means dryness, exhausted body fluid. There are five kinds of it: infantile malnutrition involving heart, infantile malnutrition due to improper feeding, infantile malnutrition involving qi, infantile malnutrition involving sinew, and infantile malnutrition involving bones. Zicao (arnebia root) can nourish the triple energizer by receiving fire qi and earth qi, thus it can treat five kinds of infantile malnutrition. Tonifying the middle is to tonify center earth. Replenishing qi is to replenish the qi of the triple energizer. The nine orifices are the regions where water qi infuses. Since Zicao (arnebia root) can tonify center earth and benefit the triple energizer, it can therefore disinhibit the nine orifices, with the upper energizer serving as sprayer, the middle energizer as fermentor and the lower energizer as drainer, resulting in the cycle of water qi.

136. 泽 兰

泽兰 气味苦,微温,无毒。主治金疮,痈肿,疮脓。

泽兰始出汝南诸大泽旁,今处处有之,多生水泽下湿地,叶似兰草,故名泽兰。茎方色青节紫，叶边有锯齿，两两对生，节间微香，枝叶间微有白毛，七月作萼色纯紫，开花紫白色，其根紫黑色。

泽兰本于水，而得五运之气，故主治三因之证。生于水泽，气味苦温，根萼紫黑，禀少阴水火之气也。茎方叶香，微有白毛，边如锯齿，禀太阴土金之气也。茎青节紫，叶生枝节间，其茎直上，禀厥阴之木气也。主治金疮痈肿疮脓者，金疮乃刀斧所伤，为不内外因之证。痈肿乃寒邪客于经络，为外因之证，疮脓乃心火盛而血脉虚，为内因之证。泽兰禀五运而治三阴之证者如此。

136. Zelan〔泽兰，hirsute shiny bugleweed herb，Herba Lycopi〕

It is bitter in taste, slightly warm and non-toxic in property, and it is mainly used to treat incised wound, abscess and sore with pus.

Firstly recorded to be growing near various lakes in Runan (汝南), now it grows everywhere. It mostly grows on the marshland, with its leaves similar to those of Lancao〔兰草, fortune eupatorium herb, Herba Eupatorii〕, thus it is called Zelan (hirsute shiny bugleweed herb). It has a square blue-green stem with purple nodes. It has serrated leaves with opposite leaf arrangements. It is slightly fragrant between nodes. There is fine white hair between branches and leaves. It blossoms with purple-white flowers in the seventh lunar month, with its calyx being purple and its roots purple-black.

Its root grows in water, thus it can obtain the qi from five circuits, which enables it to treat the diseases of three types of cause. Growing in water, bitter in taste, warm in property, it has purple-black roots and calyxes and receives the qi of water and fire from lesser yin. It also receives the qi of earth and metal from greater yin with a square stem and fragrant leaves, which have serrated edges and are covered with fine white hair. It has a square blue-green stem with purple nodes, has leaves growing between branches and receives wood qi from reverting yin. It can mainly treat incised wound, abscess and sore with pus. Incised wound is caused by a knife or an axe, which is the disease of the non-internal and non-external cause. Cold pathogen invades the meridians, resulting in abscess, which is the one of the external cause. The exuberance of heart fire and the deficiency of the blood vessel can cause sore with pus, which is the one of the internal cause.

Zelan (hirsute shiny bugleweed herb) can treat the diseases of three types of cause by receiving the qi of five circuits.

137. 茜草根

茜草根　气味苦寒,无毒。主治寒湿风痹、黄疸、补中。《别录》云:治蛊毒,久服益精气,轻身。

茜草《诗》名茹藘,《别录》名地血,一名染绯草,又名过山龙,一名西天王草,又名风车草。始出乔山山谷及山阴谷中,东间诸处虽有而少,不如西间之多,故字从西。十二月生苗,蔓延数尺,方茎中空有筋,外有细刺,数寸一节,每节五叶,七八月开花,结实如小椒,中有细黑子,其根赤色。《周礼》庶氏掌除蛊毒,以嘉草攻之,嘉草者,蘘荷与茜也。主蛊为最,故《别录》用治蛊毒。

茜草发于季冬,根赤子黑,气味苦寒,禀少阴水火之气化。方茎五叶,外有细刺,又禀阳明金土之气化。主治寒湿风痹者,禀少阴火气而散寒,阳明燥气而除湿,阳明金气而制风也。得少阴之水化,故清黄疸。《周礼》主除蛊毒,故补中,中土调和,则蛊毒自无矣。《素问》治气竭肝伤,血枯经闭,故久服益精气,轻身。

《素问·腹中论》岐伯曰:病名血枯者,此得之年少时,有所大脱血,若醉入房中,气竭肝伤,故月事衰少不来。帝曰:治以何术? 岐伯曰:以四乌鲗骨,一藘茹,二物并合之,丸以雀卵,大如小豆,以五丸为后饭,饮以鲍鱼汁,利肠中及伤肝也。藘茹当作茹藘,即茜草也。《本经》下品中有蔄茹。李时珍引《素问》乌鲗骨藘茹方注解云:《素问》蔄茹,当作茹藘,而蔄与藘音同字异也。愚谓:乌鲗骨方,当是茜草之茹藘,非下品之蔄茹也。恐后人疑而未决,故表正之。

137. Qiancaogen [茜草根, madder, Rubiae Radix]

It is bitter in taste, cold and non-toxic in property, and it is mainly used to treat the impediment diseases due to cold, dampness and wind, resolve jaundice and tonify the middle. *Ming Yi Bie Lu* [《名医别录》, *Miscellaneous Records of Famous Physicians*] says, "It can eliminate parasitic toxin. Long-term taking of it can replenish essential qi and keep healthy."

It is mentioned as Rulü (茹蔍) in *Shi Jing* [《诗经》, *The Book of Songs*] and Dixue (地血) in *Ming Yi Bie Lu* [《名医别录》, *Miscellaneous Records of Famous Physicians*]. It is also called Ranfeicao (染绯草), Guoshanlong (过山龙), Xitian Wangcao (西天王草) and Fengchecao (风车草). Firstly recorded to be growing in the valleys of Qiaoshan Mountain (乔山) and in Shanyin Mountain (山阴山), now it grows everywhere in the east in smaller quantity compared with that in the west, thus the Chinese character "西" (west) is used in its name. It sprouts in the twelfth lunar month, with its vines stretching to several Chi wide. Its stem is square and hollow, with fibers inside and fine thorns outside. There are several inches between its nodes, each of which has five leaves. It blossoms in the seventh and eighth lunar months. It bears fruits as small as those of Huajiao [花椒, pricklyash peel, Pericarpium Zanthoxyli], with fine black seeds inside. It has red roots. *Zhou Li* [《周礼》, *Rites of Zhou*] records that an official who worked as Shushi (庶氏), a title whose responsibility was in charge of eliminating parasitic toxin, used Jiacao (嘉草) to eliminate the toxin. Jiacao (嘉草) are Ranghe [襄荷, Japanese ginger, Zingiberis Miogae Rhizoma] and Qiancao [茜草, madder, Rubiae Radix], which are the most effective herbs for parasitic toxin, thus the action of eliminating parasitic toxin is included in *Ming Yi Bie Lu* [《名医别录》, *Miscellaneous Records of Famous Physicians*].

Bitter in taste and cold in property, it sprouts in winter with red roots and black seeds. It receives the qi transformation of water and fire from lesser yin. It has a square stem, has five leaves on each node with fine thorns outside and receives the qi transformation of metal and earth from yang brightness. It can mainly treat the impediment diseases due to cold, dampness and wind, because it can dissipate cold by receiving the fire qi from lesser yin, eliminate dampness by receiving the dryness qi from yang brightness and control wind by receiving the metal qi from yang brightness. It receives the water transformation of lesser yin, thus it can treat jaundice. *Zhou Li* [《周礼》, *Rites of Zhou*] says that Qiancaogen (madder) can mainly eliminate parasitic toxin, and tonify the middle. Center earth is harmonized, and parasitic toxin can then be eliminated. *Su Wen* [《素问》, *Plain Questions*] says that it can treat the liver impairment caused by the exhaustion of qi and treat the amenorrhea caused by the exhaustion of blood, thus long-term taking of it can replenish essential qi and keep healthy.

In *Fuzhong Lunpian* [《素问·腹中论》, *Discussion on the Abdominal Disorders*], Qibo（岐伯）answered, "The disease is called amenorrhea. It is caused by massive loss of blood when the patient is young, or by having intercourse after drinking liquor, which will exhaust qi and impair the liver, resulting in scanty menstruation or even amenorrhea." Huangdi（黄帝）asked, "How do we treat it?" Qibo（岐伯）answered, "Mix four cuttlefish bones, one Lüru（藘茹）with sparrows' eggs to make pills as large as Xiaodou [小豆, black gram, Phaseoli Mungo Semen]. Take five pills each time before meals and drink some abalone soup to smooth the intestines and nourish the impaired liver." Lüru（藘茹）is Rulü（茹藘）, which is actually Qiancao（茜草）. Lüru（藘茹）is classified as a low-grade herb in *Shen Nong Ben Cao Jing* [《神农本草经》, *Shennong's Classic of Materia Medica*]. Li Shizhen（李时珍）said that Lüru（藘茹）in *Su Wen* [《素问》, *Plain Questions*] is Rulü（茹藘）since Lü（藘）and Lü（蘆）are homophones by citing the annotation of Wuzeigu Lüru Fang（乌鲗骨藘茹方, Cuttlefish Bone Madder Formula）in *Su Wen* [《素问》, *Plain Questions*]. In my humble opinion, Rulü（茹藘）in Wuzeigu Fang [乌鲗骨方, Cuttlefish Bone Formula] is Qiancao（茜草）rather than Lüru（藘茹）, a low-grade herb. I would like to make it clear here for fear that people later on will remain doubtful.

138. 秦 艽

秦艽 气味苦平,无毒。主治寒热邪气,寒湿风痹,肢节痛,下水,利小便。

秦艽出秦中,今泾州、鄜州、岐州、河陕诸郡皆有。其根土黄色,作罗纹交纠左右旋转。李时珍曰:以左纹者良,今市肆中或左或右,俱不辨矣。

秦艽气味苦平,色如黄土,罗纹交纠,左右旋转,禀天地阴阳交感之气,盖天气左旋右转,地气右旋左转,左右者,阴阳之道路。主治寒热邪气者,地气从内以出外,阴气外交于阳,而寒热邪气自散矣。治寒湿风痹,肢节痛者,天气从外以入内,阳气内交于阴,则寒湿风三邪,合而成痹,以致肢节痛者,可愈也。地气运行则水下,天气运行则小便利。

138. Qinjiao〔秦艽, largeleaf gentian root, Radix Gentianae Macrophyllae〕

It is bitter in taste, mild and non-toxic in property, and it is mainly used to disperse cold and heat as well as pathogenic qi, treat cold-dampness diseases, wind impediment and the pain of the limbs and joints, precipitate water and disinhibit urination.

Originally growing in Qinzhong（秦中）, now it grows in Jingzhou（泾州）, Fuzhou（鄜州）, Qizhou（岐州）and Heshan（河陕）. Its roots are earthy yellow and intertwine with each other horizontally. Li Shizhen（李时珍）said, "Those whose roots intertwine left are of good quality. Those whose roots intertwine either left or right coexist in the markets. Both of them can be used as medicinal without careful examination."

Bitter in taste and mild in property, its roots are earthy yellow and intertwine with each other horizontally. It receives qi from the interaction between yin in the earth and yang in the heaven. Heaven qi ascends left and descends right, and earth qi ascends right and descends left. Left and right stand for the routes of yin and yang along which they are ascending and descending. It can mainly disperse cold and heat as well as pathogenic qi. Earth qi（yin qi）moves out of the body and interacts with yang qi（heaven qi）externally, thus cold and heat as well as pathogenic qi can be naturally dispersed. It can treat cold-dampness diseases, wind impediment and the pain of the limbs and joints. Heaven qi（yang qi）enters the body and interacts with yin qi（earth qi）internally, thus the pain of the limbs and joints, which is caused by the impediment resulting from three kinds of pathogen, i. e., cold, dampness and wind, can be treated. Water can be precipitated when earth qi circulates well, and urination can be disinhibited when heaven qi circulates well.

139. 防　己

防己　气味辛平,无毒。主治风寒温疟热气,诸痫,除邪,利大小便。

防己《本经》名解离,以生汉中者为佳,故名汉防己。江南诸处皆有,总属一种,因地土不同,致形有大小,而内之花纹皆如车辐。所谓木防己者,谓其茎梗如木,无论汉中他处皆名木防己,即通草,名木通之义。非出汉中者,名汉防己,他处者,名木防己也。上古诸方,皆云木防己汤,是木防己,乃其本名,生汉中佳,故后人又有汉防己之称,其茎蔓延如葛,折其茎一头吹之,气从中贯,俨如木通,其根外白内黄,破之黑纹四布,故名解离。

防己气味辛平,色白纹黑,禀金水相生之气化。其茎如木,木能防土,己者土也,故有防己之名。主治风寒温疟热气者,风寒之邪,藏于肾脏,发为先热后寒之温疟。温疟者,热气有余之疟也。《经》云:温疟者,先热后寒,得之冬中于风寒,此病藏于肾。防己启在下之水精而输转于外,故治风寒温疟热气也。诸痫除邪者,心包受邪,发为牛马猪羊鸡诸痫之证。防己中空藤蔓,能通在内之经脉,而外达于络脉,故治诸痫除邪也。利大小便者,土得木而达,木防其土,土气疏通,则二便自利矣。

愚按:防己气味辛平,茎空藤蔓,根纹如车辐,能启在下之水精而上升,通在内之经脉而外达,故《金匮要略》云:膈间支饮,其人喘满,心下痞坚,面色黧黑者,其脉沉紧,得之数十日,医吐下之,不愈,木防己汤主之。又云:风水脉浮身重,汗出恶风者,防己黄芪汤主之。皮水为病,四肢肿,水气在皮肤中,四肢聂聂动者,防己茯苓汤主之。《千金方》治遗尿小便涩,三物木防己汤主之。而李东垣有云:防己乃下焦血分之药,病在上焦气分者,禁用。试观《金匮》诸方所治之证,果在气分乎?血分乎?抑在上焦乎?下焦乎?盖防己乃行气通上之药,其性功与乌药、木通相类,而后人乃以防己为下部药,不知何据。东垣又云:防己大苦寒,能泻血中湿热,比之于人,则险而健者也,幸灾乐祸,能为乱阶,然善用之,亦可敌凶突险,此瞑眩之药也。故圣人存而不废噫。神农以中品之药为臣,主通调血气,祛邪治病,无毒有毒,斟酌其宜,随病而用。如防己既列中品,且属无毒,以之治病,有行气清热之功。险健为乱之说,竟不知从何处得来,使后人遵之如格言,畏之若毒药,非先圣之罪人乎。东垣立言,多属臆说,盖其人富而贪名,又无格物实学。李时珍乃谓千古而下,唯东垣一人,误矣。嗟嗟!安得伊耆再治世,更将经旨复重宣。

139. Fangji〔防己, fourstamen stephania root, Radix Stephaniae Tetrandrae〕

It is pungent in taste, mild and non-toxic in property, and it is mainly used to treat wind-cold diseases, warm malaria and the diseases caused by heat qi, eliminate epilepsy, disperse pathogen, purge defecation and disinhibit urination.

It is mentioned as Jieli（解离）in *Shen Nong Ben Cao Jing* [《神农本草经》, *Shennong's Classic of Materia Medica*], and those growing in Hanzhong（汉中）are of good quality, and thus it is called Hanfangji（汉防己）. It grows everywhere in Jiangnan（江南）. There are different kinds of Fangji（fourstamen stephania root）under the same species. It is different in size, for it grows on different soil. Its lines inside are all like spokes. There is one kind called Mufangji（木防己）. Mufangji（木防己）got this name because its stem is similar to the wood, and people in Hanzhong（汉中）and other places all use this name. Mufangji（木防己）is actually Tongcao（通草）, which means that it is a hollow herb. It is not true that those growing in Hanzhong（汉中）are called Hanfangji（汉防己）, and those growing in other places are called Mufangji（木防己）. Various ancient formulas all mentioned Mufangji Tang [木防己汤, Cocculus Root Decoction], which proves that Mufangji（木防己）is actually the original name of Fangji（fourstamen stephania root）. Those growing in Hanzhong（汉中）are of good quality, and thus people later on called it Hanfangji（汉防己）. Its stem spreads like Ge [葛, pueraria, Puerariae Radix]. Blow air from one end into a cut stem, and the air can flow through the whole stem, just like Mutong（木通）. Its root is yellow inside and white outside, and it is covered with black lines when cut, thus it is called Jieli（解离）.

Pungent in taste and mild in property, it is white in color with black lines and receives the qi transformation from the mutual generation of metal and water. Its stem is like the wood which can restrict（防）earth. Ji（己）means earth. Thus, it is called Fangji（fourstamen stephania root）. It can mainly treat wind-cold diseases, warm malaria and the diseases caused by heat qi. The pathogen of wind cold is stored in the kidney, resulting in warm malaria featuring first fever and then chills. Warm malaria is the malaria with excessive heat qi. *Huang Di Nei Jing* [《黄帝内经》, *Huangdi's Inner Classic*] says, "Warm malaria is marked by fever followed by chills. It is caused by the attack of wind cold in winter, which is stored in the kidney." Fangji（fourstamen stephania root）activates water essence below and transports it outside, thus Fangji（fourstamen stephania root）can treat the above diseases. It can eliminate epilepsy and disperse pathogen. Pathogen invades the pericardium, resulting in epilepsy in cattle, horses, pigs, sheep and chickens. It can dredge the meridians inward and reach the collateral vessel outward through its hollow stems and spreading vines, thus it can eliminate epilepsy and disperse pathogen. It can purge defecation and disinhibit urination. Earth is promoted when meeting wood, and wood can control earth. Earth qi is disinhibited, thus defecation can be naturally purged, and urination can be naturally disinhibited.

Note by Zhang Zhicong (张志聪): Pungent in taste and mild in property, it has a hollow stem, spreading vines and root lines similar to spokes. It can activate water essence downward to flow upward and dredge the meridians inward to reach outward. Thus, *Jin Gui Yao Lüe* [《金匮要略》, *Synopsis of the Golden Chamber*] says, "The thoracic fluid retention is accompanied by symptoms, such as panting and fullness, epigastric mass, dark complexion and deep-tense pulse. The disease can continue for many days. Emetics and purgatives have been used, but with no signs of recovery. Mufangji Tang [木防己汤, Cocculus Root Decoction] can mainly treat it." *Jin Gui Yao Lüe* [《金匮要略》, *Synopsis of the Golden Chamber*] also says, "Fangji Huangqi Tang [防己黄芪汤, Stephania and Astragalus Decoction] can mainly treat wind edema with floating pulse and heavy body, sweating and aversion to wind. Skin edema is accompanied by symptoms, such as the edema in the limbs, the fluid retention in the skin and the slight twitching in the limbs. Fangji Fuling Tang [防己茯苓汤, Stephania and Poria Decoction] can mainly treat it." *Qian Jin Fang* [《千金方》, *Important Formulas Worth a Thousand Gold Pieces*] says that Sanwu Mufangji Tang [三物木防己汤, Three Ingredients and Cocculus Root Decoction] can mainly treat enuresis and difficult urination. Li Dongyuan (李东垣) said, "Fangji (fourstamen stephania root) is a herb which enters the low energizer and the blood aspect to treat diseases, thus it cannot be used to treat the diseases of the upper energizer and the qi aspect." Take a look at the diseases treated by various formulas in *Jin Gui Yao Lüe* [《金匮要略》, *Synopsis of the Golden Chamber*]. Do they really occur in the qi or blood aspect? Or in the upper or lower energizer? Fangji (fourstamen stephania root) is a herb which can move qi to disinhibit the upper part and has the similar actions as those of Wuyao［乌药, combined spicebush root, Radix Linderae］and Mutong［木通, ricepaperplant stempith, Medulla Tetrapanacis］. People later on regarded it as a herb for the lower part, which is actually groundless. Li Dongyuan（李东垣）also said, "Severely bitter in taste and cold in property, it can disinhibit the dampness heat in the blood. Comparing it to human beings, it is like an evil but healthy man who takes pleasure in other people's misfortune and whose ability can in turn be a curse. However, he can defend against danger and get away from disaster when used appropriately. Thus, it is a herb of strong reaction after taking it. For this reason, sages save it rather than abolishing it." Shennong（神农）used medium-grade herbs as minister medicinals mainly to disinhibit and regulate blood qi and expel pathogen to treat diseases. Doctors need to be sure whether the herb is toxic or non-toxic in property, consider its suitability of application and use it according to different diseases. As Fangji（fourstamen stephania root）is classified as a medium-grade herb and it is non-toxic in property, it can be used as medicinal to move qi and clear heat. The view that it is very effective but has a lot of side effects can not be found the record, while later generations abide by it as a motto and fear of it as much as poison. Aren't those who made the groundless statement the sinners to sages? Most of the statements from Li Dongyuan（李东垣）were groundless, because he was rich but greedy for fame, never studying the principles of things and valuing practice. Li Shizhen（李时珍）said that Li Dongyuan（李东垣）had been the greatest scholar studying medical classics since ancient times, which is totally wrong. How stupid he was! Is there any way to make Shennong（神农）govern the country again and repeatedly publicize the main principles of medical classics?

140. 木 通

木通 气味辛平,无毒。主除脾胃寒热,通利九窍血脉关节,令人不忘,去恶虫。

木通《本经》名通草,茎中有细孔,吹之两头皆通,故名通草。陈士良撰《食性本草》改为木通,今药中复有所谓通草,乃是古之通脱木也,与此不同。始出石城山谷及山阳,今泽潞、汉中、江淮、湖南州郡皆有,绕树藤生,伤之有白汁出，一枝五叶，茎色黄白，干有小大，伤水则黑，黑者勿用。

木通藤蔓空通，其色黄白，气味辛平，禀土金相生之气化，而通关利窍之药也。禀土气，故除脾胃之寒热。藤蔓空通，故通利九窍、血脉、关节。血脉通而关窍利，则令人不忘。禀金气，故去恶虫。

防己、木通皆属空通蔓草。防己取用在下之根，则其性自下而上，从内而外。木通取用在上之茎，则其性自上而下，自外而内，此根升梢降，一定不易之理。后人用之，主利小便，须知小便不利，亦必上而后下，外而后内也。

140. Mutong [木通, trifoliate akebia, Akebiae Trifoliatae Caulis]

It is pungent in taste, mild and non-toxic in property, and it is mainly used to eliminate the cold and heat in the spleen and stomach, disinhibit the nine orifices, blood vessels and joints, strengthen memory and expel pathogenic worms.

It is mentioned as Tongcao (通草) in *Shen Nong Ben Cao Jing* [《神农本草经》, *Shennong's Classic of Materia Medica*]. There are small holes in its stem, and the air blown into the stem from one end can come out from the other end, thus it is called Tongcao (通草). Chen Shiliang (陈士良) changed Tongcao (通草) into Mutong (trifoliate akebia) in his book *Shi Xing Ben Cao* [《食性本草》, *Materia Medica on Diet Habits*]. Tongcao (通草) can still be found in some formulas today, which is actually Tongtuomu [通脱木, rice-paper plant, Tetrapanax Papyriferum] of the ancient times and is different from Tongcao (通草) mentioned above. Firstly recorded to be growing in the valleys of Shicheng (石城) and Shanyang (山阳), now it grows everywhere in Zelu (泽潞), Hanzhong (汉中), Jianghuai (江淮) and Hunan (湖南). It creeps along the tree, and the white juice will flow out of the vein when it is cut. Its branch has five leaves, and its stem is yellow-white in color. Its sections are different in size, and they will blacken when processed in water for a long time and will not be suitable to be used as medicinal.

With hollow vines, it is yellow-white in color, pungent in taste, and mild in property. It can free the joints and can dredge the orifices by receiving qi transformation from the mutual generation of earth and metal. It receives earth qi, thus it can eliminate the cold and heat in the spleen and stomach. It has hollow vines, thus it can disinhibit the nine orifices, blood vessels and joints. Blood vessels, orifices and joints are disinhibited, and memory can then be strengthened. It receives metal qi, and thus it can expel pathogenic worms.

Both Fangji［防己, fourstamen stephania root, Radix Stephaniae Tetrandrae］ and Mutong（trifoliate akebia）are hollow creeping weeds. The below roots of Fangji（fourstamen stephania root）are used, thus it tends to move from the bottom to the top and from the inside to the outside. The above stem of Mutong（trifoliate akebia）is used, thus it tends to move from the top to the bottom and from the outside to the inside. The root of Mutong（trifoliate akebia）can ascend while its tip can descend, which is an unchangeable truth. People later on used it mainly to disinhibit urination. It should be known that treating dysuria should follow the up-to-down and outside-to-inside principle.

141. 葛 根

葛根 气味甘辛平,无毒。主治消渴,身大热,呕吐,诸痹,起阴气,解诸毒。

葛处处有之,江浙尤多,春生苗,延引藤蔓,其根大如手臂,外色紫黑,内色洁白,可作粉食,其花红紫,结实如黄豆荚,其仁如梅核,生嚼腥气。《本经》所谓葛谷者是也。

葛根延引藤蔓,则主经脉,甘辛粉白,则入阳明,皮黑花红,则合太阳,故葛根为宣达阳明中土之气,而外合于太阳经脉之药也。主治消渴身大热者,从胃府而宣达水谷之津,则消渴自止,从经脉而调和肌表之气,则大热自除。治呕吐者,和阳明之胃气也,治诸痹者,和太阳之经脉也。起阴气者,藤引蔓延,从下而上也,解诸毒者,气味甘辛,和于中而散于外也。

元人张元素曰:葛根为阳明仙药,若太阳初病,未入阳明,而头痛者,不可便用升麻、葛根,用之反引邪入阳明,为引贼破家也。愚按:仲祖《伤寒论》方有葛根汤,治太阳病,项背强几几,无汗,恶风。又治太阳与阳明合病。若阳明本病,只有白虎、承气诸汤,并无葛根汤证,况葛根主宣通经脉之正气以散邪,岂反引邪内入耶。前人学不明经,屡为异说。李时珍一概收录,不加辩证,学者看本草发明,当合经论参究,庶不为前人所误。

卢子由曰:《本经》痹字与风寒湿相合之痹不同,如消渴、身热、呕吐及阴气不起,与诸毒皆痹也,故云诸痹。

141. Gegen [葛根, kudzuvine root, Radix Puerariae]

It is sweet and pungent in taste, mild in property, and it is mainly used to relieve consumptive thirst, eliminate severe fever, treat vomiting and various impediments, invigorate yin qi and resolve various toxins.

　　Ge [葛, pueraria, Materia Medica Ge] grows everywhere, a large amount of which grows in Jiangsu (江苏) and Zhejiang (浙江). It sprouts in spring, its stem grows upright, and its vines grow sideways. Its root is as big as a human arm, with the outer color being purple-black and the inner being white, which can be ground into powder to make food. It has red-purple flowers. Its fruits are like soybean pods. Recorded as Gegu [葛谷, pueraria seed, Puerariae Semen] in *Shen Nong Ben Cao Jing* [《神农本草经》, *Shennong's Classic of Materia Medica*], its kernel is like a plum pit and tastes stinky when it is chewed raw.

Its stem grows upright, and its vines grow sideways, so it is related with the meridians. Sweet and pungent in taste, it is white when it is ground into powder, so it enters yang brightness. Its bark is black, and its flowers are red, so it is in accordance with greater yang. Thus, it is a medicinal which is externally in accordance with the meridians of greater yang to move the qi of center earth from yang brightness upward and outward. It can mainly treat consumptive thirst and severe fever by assisting the flow of fluids of water and grain from the stomach. Thus, consumptive thirst can be naturally relieved. It can harmonize the qi of the fleshy exterior from the meridians. Thus, severe fever can be naturally eliminated. It can treat vomiting by harmonizing stomach qi from yang brightness. It can treat various impediments by harmonizing the meridians of greater yang. It can invigorate yin qi, because its stem grows upright, and its vines grow sideways, moving from the bottom to the top. It can resolve various toxins, because it is sweet and pungent in taste and can harmonize the middle and dissipate to the exterior.

　　Zhang Yuansu (张元素) of the Yuan Dynasty said, "Gegen (kudzuvine root) is a magic herb featuring yang brightness. Greater yang has just suffered from the disease without invading yang brightness, which will result in headache, and then it is not allowed to use Shengma［升麻, largetrifoliolious bugbane rhizome, Rhizoma Cimicifugae］and Gegen（kudzuvine root）. Using them will in turn guide the pathogen into yang brightness, which is equal to leading the thief to mess the house." Note by Zhang Zhicong（张志聪）: Gegen Tang［葛根汤, Pueraria Decoction］recorded in *Shang Han Lun*［《伤寒论》, *Treatise on Cold Damage Diseases*］written by Zhang Zhongjing（张仲景）can treat greater yang diseases, including stiffness in the back and neck, no sweating and aversion to wind. The decoction can also treat the combination of greater yang diseases and yang brightness diseases. Baihu Chengqi Tang［白虎承气汤, White Tiger Purgative Decoction］can treat yang brightness principal diseases without using Gegen Tang［葛根汤, Pueraria Decoction］. In addition, Gegen（kudzuvine root）can mainly free the healthy qi of the meridians to dispel pathogenic qi. Then how can it in turn lead the pathogen inside? Predecessors did not have a thorough understanding of the classics, which has led to the rise of many fallacies. As to these fallacies, Li Shizhen（李时珍）included them all in his book instead of treating them in a dialectical way. Learners should examine the theory about materia medica together with the study of the classics in order not to be easily misled by predecessors.

Lu Ziyou（卢子由）said, "Bi［痹, impediment］recorded in *Shen Nong Ben Cao Jing*［《神农本草经》, *Shennong's Classic of Materia Medica*］means differently from that caused by the combination of wind, cold and dampness. Consumptive thirst, fever, vomiting, inactivated yin qi and various toxins all pertain to the category of impediment, and thus various impediments are used here."

142. 葛 谷

葛谷 气味甘平，无毒。主治下痢，十岁以上。

142. Gegu［葛谷, pueraria seed, Puerariae Semen］

It is sweet in taste, mild and non-toxic in property, and it is mainly used to treat dysentery continuing for over ten years.

143. 葛 花 附

葛花 附　气味甘平,无毒。主消酒《别录》,治肠风下血。《本草纲目》附。

143. Gehua [葛花, flowerof lobedkudzuvine, Flos Puerariae] *supplement*

It is sweet in taste, mild and non-toxic in property. It is mainly used to dispel the effects of alcohol. Recorded in *Ming Yi Bie Lu* [《名医别录》, *Miscellaneous Records of Famous Physicians*]. It can also treat bloody stool. Supplemented in *Ben Cao Gang Mu* [《本草纲目》, *Compendium of Materia Medica*].

144. 葛 叶 附

葛叶 附　主治金疮,止血,按傅之。《别录》附。

144. Geye [葛叶, pueraria leaf, Puerariae Folium] *supplement*

It can mainly treat incised wound and stop bleeding by rubbing and applying it to the affected area. Supplemented in *Ming Yi Bie Lu* [《名医别录》, *Miscellaneous Records of Famous Physicians*].

145. 葛 蔓 附

葛蔓 附　主治卒喉痹,烧研,水服方寸匕。《唐本草》附。

145. Geman [葛蔓, pueraria stem, Puerariae Caulis] *supplement*

It is mainly used to treat sudden pharyngitis by burning, grinding and taking one square-cun-spoon of it with water. Supplemented in *Tang Ben Cao* [《唐本草》, *Tang Materia Medica*].

146. 麻 黄

麻黄 气味苦温,无毒。主治中风伤寒头痛,温疟,发表出汗,去邪热气,止咳逆上气,除寒热,破症坚积聚。

麻黄始出晋地,今荥阳、中牟、汴州、彭城诸处皆有之。春生苗,纤细劲直,外黄内赤,中空有节,如竹形,宛似毛孔。

植麻黄之地,冬不积雪,能从至阴而达阳气于上。至阴者,盛水也,阳气者,太阳也。太阳之气,本膀胱寒水,而气行于头,周遍于通体之毛窍。主治中风伤寒头痛者,谓风寒之邪,病太阳高表之气,而麻黄能治之也。温疟发表出汗,去邪热气者,谓温疟病藏于肾,麻黄能起水气而周遍于皮毛,故主发表出汗,而去温疟邪热之气也。治咳逆上气者,谓风寒之邪,闭塞毛窍,则里气不疏而咳逆上气。麻黄空细如毛,开发毛窍,散其风寒,则里气外出于皮毛,而不咳逆上气矣。除寒热,破症坚积聚者,谓在外之寒热不除,致中土之气不能外达,而为症坚积聚。麻黄除身外之寒热,则太阳之气出入于中土,而症坚积聚自破矣。

146. Mahuang [麻黄, ephedra, Herba Ephedrae]

It is bitter in taste, warm and non-toxic in property, and it is mainly used to treat wind stroke, cold damage, headache and warm malaria, relieve exterior and induce sweating, eliminate pathogenic-heat qi, treat cough with dyspnea and descend adverse-rising qi, eliminate cold and heat and resolve abdominal mass.

Firstly recorded to be growing in the Jin (晋) area, now it grows everywhere in Xingyang (荥阳), Zhongmou (中牟), Bianzhou (汴州) and Pengcheng (彭城). It sprouts in spring, straight and thin. Red inside and yellow outside, it is hollow with bamboo-like nodes. Its hollow inside is as thin as a pore.

Mahuang (ephedra) grows in the area where there is no snow in winter, because it is able to move yang qi from the beginning of yin to the upper part. The beginning of yin can manage water, and yang qi is greater yang. The qi of greater yang, originating from the cold water of the bladder, moves through all the pores in the human body from the head. It can mainly treat wind stroke, cold damage and headache. The pathogen of wind cold can cause diseases in the qi of high exterior of greater yang, and Mahuang (ephedra) is able to treat it. It can treat malaria, relieve exterior and induce sweating as well as eliminate pathogenic-heat qi. Malaria is stored in the kidney. Mahuang (ephedra) can invigorate water qi to flow through the skin and the body hair. Thus, it can mainly release exterior and induce sweating, treat malaria and eliminate pathogenic-heat qi. It can treat cough with dyspnea and descend adverse-rising qi. The pathogen of the wind cold can block the pores, and interior qi is therefore obstructed, resulting in cough with dyspnea and adverse-rising qi. Its hollow inside is as thin as hair. It can open the pores and disperse wind cold, and interior qi can therefore be released through the skin and the body hair, resulting in the treatment of cough with dyspnea and the descending of adverse-rising qi. It can eliminate cold and heat and resolve abdominal mass. If external cold and heat is not eliminated, then the qi of center earth cannot spread out, resulting in abdominal mass. Mahuang (ephedra) is able to eliminate the cold and heat outside the body, and the qi of greater yang can therefore move in and out of center earth, resulting in the resolving of abdominal mass.

147. 白 芷

白芷　气味辛温,无毒。主治女人漏下赤白,血闭,阴肿,寒热头风侵目泪出,长肌肤,润泽颜色,可作面脂。

白芷处处有之,吴地尤多,根长尺余,粗细不等,色白气香。

白芷臭香色白,气味辛温,禀阳明金土之气化。主治妇人漏下赤白,血闭阴肿者,《经》云:阳明胃脉,其气下行而主阖。白芷辛温,禀阳明燥金之气下行,则漏下赤白,血闭阴肿可治也。治寒热头风侵目泪出者,白芷芳香,气胜于味,不但禀阳明燥金之气下行,且禀阳明中土之气上达,故寒热头风侵目泪出可治也。土主肌肉,金主皮肤,白芷得阳明金土之气,故长肌肤,面乃阳明之分部,阳气长,则其颜光,其色鲜,故润泽颜色。白芷色白,作粉如脂,故可作面脂。

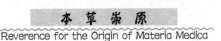
147. Baizhi〔白芷, dahurian angelica root, Radix Angelicae Dahuricae〕

It is pungent in taste, warm and non-toxic in property, and it is mainly used to treat metrostaxis with red and white leukorrhea, amenorrhea, the swelling of the vulva, cold-heat diseases, the headache due to the invasion of wind into the head and eyes with tearing, promote the muscle growth, moisten the skin and brighten the complexion. It can be used to make face lotion.

It grows everywhere and grows especially in bulk in the Wu (吴) area. Its root, white in color, fragrant in smell, is over one Chi deep and varies in thickness.

Fragrant in smell, white in color, pungent in taste and mild in property, it receives the qi transformation of metal and earth from yang brightness. It can mainly treat metrostaxis with red and white leukorrhea, amenorrhea and the swelling of the vulva. *Huang Di Nei Jing*〔《黄帝内经》, *Huangdi's Internal Classic*〕says that yang brightness is the meridian of the stomach, and its qi descends and is responsible for closing. Pungent in taste and mild in property, Baizhi (dahurian angelica root) receives the qi of dryness metal from yang brightness to descend, and thus it can treat the above diseases. It can treat cold-heat diseases, the headache due to the invasion of wind into the head and eyes with tearing. It has a fragrant smell, which is stronger than its taste. It descends by receiving the qi of dryness metal from yang brightness and ascends by receiving the qi of the center earth from yang brightness. Thus, it can treat the above diseases. Earth governs the muscles, and metal governs the skin. Baizhi (dahurian angelica root) obtains the qi of dryness metal from yang brightness, and thus it can promote the muscle growth. The face is the location where yang brightness lies. Exuberant yang qi can make the facial skin glowing and delicate, and thus Baizhi (dahurian angelica root) can moisten the skin and brighten the complexion. White in color, it looks like the grease when it is ground into powder, and thus it can be used to make face lotion.

148. 荆 芥

荆芥 气味辛温,无毒。主治寒热鼠瘘,瘰疬生疮,破结聚气,下瘀血,除湿疸。

荆芥《本经》名假苏,以其辛香如苏也,处处有之,本系野生,今多栽种,二月布子生苗,辛香可茹,方茎细叶,淡黄绿色,八月开小花,作穗成房,如紫苏。房内有细子黄赤色,今采者,凡茎叶穗子一概收用。

荆芥味辛,性温臭香,禀阳明金土之气,而肃清经脉之药也。寒热鼠瘘,乃水脏之毒,上出于脉,为寒为热也。本于水脏,故曰鼠,经脉空虚,故曰瘘,此内因之瘘也。瘰疬生疮,乃寒邪客于脉中,血气留滞,结核生疮,无有寒热,此外因之瘘也。荆芥味辛性温,肃清经脉,故内因之寒热鼠瘘,外因之瘰疬生疮,皆可治也。其臭芳香,故破结聚之气。破结聚,则瘀血自下矣。阳明之上,燥气主之,故除湿。

148. Jingjie [荆芥, fineleaf schizonepeta herb, Herba Schizonepetae]

It is pungent in taste, warm and non-toxic in property, and it is mainly used to treat cold-heat diseases, mouse fistula and the ulcer due to scrofula, disperse the stagnation of qi, relieve blood stasis and eliminate dampness jaundice.

It is mentioned as Jiasu (假苏) in *Shen Nong Ben Cao Jing* [《神农本草经》, *Shennong's Classic of Materia Medica*], for it has a pungent taste and a fragrant smell, similar to those of Su [苏, perilla, Perillae Folium]. It grows everywhere, but it used to grow in the wild. It is now planted in many places. Sow the seeds in the second lunar month, which will begin to sprout afterwards. Its seedling tastes spicy and delicious. It has a square stem and thin leaves, which are light yellow-green. It blossoms in the eighth lunar month with small flowers. It has spikes of flowers and will have corollas after the flowers fall, which are similar to those of Zisu [紫苏, perilla, Perillae Folium]. There are fine yellow-red seeds inside the corollas. Its stems, leaves, spikes and seeds are all collected today to be used as medicinal.

Pungent in taste, mild in property and fragrant in smell, it is a medicinal which receives the qi of metal earth from yang brightness to pure the meridians. The toxin of the water zang-organ flows upward and goes out of the meridians, resulting in cold-heat diseases and mouse fistula, which are manifested as cold and heat. The root cause of mouse fistula（鼠瘘）lies in the water zang-organ, thus mouse［鼠, mouse pertaining to water］is used. There is deficiency in the meridians, thus fistula［瘘, a hollow pipe］is used. Mouse fistula is the fistula of the internal cause. Cold pathogen invades the meridians, and blood qi retains and stagnates, resulting in subcutaneous node and ulcer with no cold or heat. Thus, the ulcer due to scrofula forms, which is the scrofula of the external cause. Pungent in taste and mild in property, Jingjie（fineleaf schizonepeta herb）can pure the meridians, and thus it can treat cold-heat diseases and the mouse fistula of the internal cause as well as the ulcer due to scrofula of the external cause. It is fragrant in smell, and thus it can disperse the stagnation of qi. The stagnation of qi is dispersed, and then blood stasis can be naturally relieved. When yang brightness governs the heaven, and dryness qi dominates the season, it can eliminate the dampness jaundice.

149. 贝 母

贝母 气味辛平,无毒。主治伤寒烦热,淋沥邪气,疝瘕,喉痹,乳难,金疮风痉。

贝母《尔雅》名莔,《国风》名䖵。河中、荆襄、江南皆有,唯川蜀出者为佳,其子在根下,内心外瓣,其色黄白,如聚贝子,故名贝母。

贝母川产者味甘淡,土产者味苦辛。《本经》气味辛平,合根苗而言也。根形象肺,色白味辛,生于西川,清补肺金之药也。主治伤寒烦热者,寒邪在胸,则为烦为热。贝母清肺,故胸中之烦热可治也。淋沥邪气者,邪入膀胱,不能随太阳而出于肤表。则小便淋沥。贝母通肺气于皮毛,故淋沥邪气可治也。疝瘕乃肝木受病。治疝瘕,金能平木也。喉痹乃肺窍内闭,治喉痹,通肺气也。乳难乃阳明津汁不通。金疮风痉,乃阳明经脉受伤,贝母色白味辛,禀阳明秋金之气,内开郁结,外达皮肤故皆治之。

149. Beimu [贝母, fritillaria, Fritillariae Bulbus]

It is pungent in taste, mild and non-toxic in property, and it is mainly used to treat cold damage with vexing fever, dribbling urination due to pathogenic qi, hernia and movable abdominal mass, pharyngitis, difficult lactation, incised wound and wind tetany.

It is mentioned as Meng (菌) in *Er Ya* [《尔雅》, *On Elegance*] and Meng (虻) in *Guo Feng* [《国风》, *Guofeng*]. It grows in Hezhong (河中), Jingxiang (荆襄) and Jiangnan (江南), but only those growing in Chuanshu (川蜀) are of good quality. Its bulb grows under the roots, with scale leaves outside and the heart inside, both of which are yellow-white in color. Its bulb is similar to a lot of Beizi [贝子, cowrie shell, Monetariae Concha] gathering together, thus it is called Beimu [贝母, mother of cowrie shells].

Beimu (fritillaria) growing in Sichuan (四川) tastes slightly sweet while the local one tastes bitter and pungent. *Shen Nong Ben Cao Jing* [《神农本草经》, *Shennong's Classic of Materia Medica*] says that it is pungent in taste and mild in property regarding its roots and seedlings. It grows in Xichuan (西川). It is white in color and pungent in taste, and its root is shaped like the lung, with the effects of clearing and tonifying lung metal. It can mainly treat cold damage with vexing fever. Cold pathogen invades the chest, resulting in vexing fever. It can clear the lung, and thus it can treat the vexing fever in the chest. The pathogen invades the bladder and cannot be excreted from the skin and the hair along with greater yang, resulting in dribbling urination. It can free lung qi through the skin and the body hair, and thus it can treat the dribbling urination due to pathogenic qi. Diseases invade liver wood, resulting in hernia and movable abdominal mass. Metal can calm wood, and thus it can treat hernia and movable abdominal mass. Pharyngitis is caused by the internal block of the lung orifice. Treating it requires freeing lung qi. Difficult lactation is caused by the obstruction of fluid from yang brightness. The yang brightness meridians are hurt, resulting in incised wound and wind tetany. Beimu (fritillaria) is white in color and pungent in taste, and receives the qi of autumn metal from yang brightness, and thus it can relieve depression inside and move outside to the skin, resulting in the treatment of the above diseases.

150. 苍耳子

苍耳子 气味甘温,有小毒。主治风头寒痛,风湿周痹,四肢拘挛痛,恶肉死肌,膝痛。久服益气。

《诗》名卷耳。《本经》名菓耳。处处有之,七八月开细白花,结实如妇女珥珰,外壳坚韧,刺毛密布,生青熟黄,中列两仁,其色黄白,嫩苗熟食可以救饥,其仁炒,去皮研为面,可作烧饼食。

苍耳《本经》名菓耳,该茎叶而言也。今时用实,名苍耳子,子内仁肉,气味甘温,外多毛刺,故有小毒,花白实黄,禀阳明燥金之气。金能制风,故主治风头寒痛,谓头受风邪,为寒为痛也。燥能胜湿,故主治风湿周痹,四肢拘挛痛,谓风湿之邪,伤周身血脉而为痹,淫于四肢而为拘挛疼痛也。夫周痹,则周身血脉不和,周痹可治,则恶肉死肌,亦可治也。四肢拘挛痛可治,则膝痛亦可治也。久服则风湿外散,经脉流通,故益气。

150. Cang'erzi [苍耳子, siberian cocklebur fruit, Fructus Xanthii]

It is sweet in taste, warm and slightly toxic in property, and it is mainly used to treat the cold and pain of the head caused by the attack of wind, wind dampness and general impediment, the spasm and pain of the limbs, malign muscles, the numbness of the muscles and the pain of the knees. Long-term taking of it can replenish qi.

It is mentioned as Juan'er (卷耳) in *Shi Jing* [《诗经》, *The Book of Songs*] and Xi'er (菓耳) in *Shen Nong Ben Cao Jing* [《神农本草经》, *Shennong's Classic of Materia Medica*]. It grows everywhere. It blossoms with fine white flowers in the seventh and eighth lunar months. It bears fruits similar to women's earrings with jewelry. Its fruit has a crust that is strong and densely covered with bristles. The fruit is blue-green when unripe and turns yellow when ripe. Inside the fruit, there are two kernels, which are yellow-white in color. Its seedlings can relieve hunger when cooked. Fry its kernels, peel them and grind them into powder, which can be used to make pancakes.

It is mentioned as Xi'er (菓耳) in *Shen Nong Ben Cao Jing* [《神农本草

经》, Shennong's Classic of Materia Medica] regarding its stems and leaves. It is called Cang'erzi（苍耳子）, because its fruits are used today. It has kernels inside its fruits, which are sweet in taste and warm in property. It has bristles on the crust, which make its fruits slightly toxic. It has white flowers and yellow fruits, and it receives the qi of dryness metal from yang brightness. It can mainly treat the cold and pain of the head caused by the attack of wind since metal can control wind. It is stated that wind pathogen invades the head, resulting in cold and pain. It can mainly treat wind-dampness, general impediment and the spasm of the limbs since dryness can restrict dampness. It is stated that wind-dampness pathogen damages the blood vessels all over the body, resulting in impediment. The pathogen is excessive in the limbs, resulting in spasm and pain. General impediment can cause the disharmony of the blood vessels all over the body. If general impediment can be treated, so can malign muscles and the numbness of the muscles. If the spasm and pain of the limbs can be treated, so can the pain of the knees. Long-term taking of it can dissipate wind dampness out of the body and dredge the meridians, which can therefore replenish qi.

151. 款冬花

款冬花　气味辛温,无毒。主治咳逆上气,善喘喉痹,诸惊痫,寒热邪气。

　　款冬花出关中、雍州、华州山谷溪涧间,花开红白,放紫萼于冰雪中。又名款冻。款,至也,谓至冻而花也。又名钻冻,谓钻冰取款冬也。十二月采蕊阴干,其色红白相兼,至灯节后,则毛萼大开,不堪入药。

　　款冬生于水中,花开红白,气味辛温,从阴出阳,盖禀水中之生阳,而上通肺金之药也。太阳寒水之气,不从皮毛外交于肺,则咳逆上气而善喘。款冬禀水气而通肺,故可治也。厥阴、少阳木火之气,结于喉中,则而喉痹。款冬得金水之气,金能平木,水能制火,故可治也。惊痫寒热邪气为病,不止一端,故曰:诸惊痫寒热邪气,款冬禀太阳寒水之气而上行外达,则阴阳水火之气,自相交会,故可治也。

　　愚按:款冬气味辛温,从阴出阳,主治肺气虚寒之咳喘,若肺火燔灼,肺气焦满者,不可用。《济生方》中,用百合、款冬二味为丸,名百花丸。治痰嗽带血,服之有愈有不愈者,寒嗽相宜,火嗽不宜也。卢子由曰:款冬《本经》主治咳逆上气,善喘喉痹,因形寒饮冷,秋伤于湿者,宜之。如火热刑金,或肺气焦满,恐益销烁矣。

151. Kuandonghua〔款冬花, common coltsfoot flower, Flos Farfarae〕

It is pungent in taste, warm and non-toxic in property, and it is mainly used to treat cough with dyspnea, descend adverse-rising qi and resolve frequent dyspnea, pharyngitis, fright epilepsy and the cold-heat diseases caused by pathogenic qi.

It originally grew in the valleys and streams of Guanzhong（关中）, Yongzhou（雍州）and Huazhou（华州）. It blossoms with red-white flowers, and its purple calyx grows in snow and ice. It is also called Kuandong（款冻）. Kuan（款）can mean to arrive, which demonstrates that it blossoms when frozen. It is also called Zuandong（钻冻）, which means that it can be obtained by breaking the ice. Collect its stamens or pistils in the twelfth lunar month and dry them in the shade, the color of which are red-white. Its hairy calyx grows bigger after the Lantern Festival, which cannot be used as medicinal.

Growing in water, pungent in taste, warm in property, it blossoms with red-white flowers. It passes out to yang from yin, because it is a medicinal receiving kidney yang from water and connecting lung metal upward. The qi of cold water from greater yang does not meet the lung outward through the skin and hair, resulting in cough with dyspnea, adverse-rising qi and frequent dyspnea. It receives water qi and connects the lung, and thus it can treat the above diseases. The qi of wood and fire from reverting yin and lesser yang stagnates in the throat, resulting in pharyngitis. Metal can calm wood, and water can control fire. Thus, it can treat the above disease by obtaining the qi of metal and water. Besides epilepsy and cold-heat diseases, there are other diseases caused by pathogenic qi. Thus, it is stated that it can move upward and flow outward to make the qi of yin, yang, water and fire interact with each other by receiving the qi of cold water from greater yang, and thus the above diseases can be treated.

Note by Zhang Zhicong（张志聪）: It can mainly treat the cough and dyspnea caused by deficiency cold of lung qi as it is pungent in taste and warm in property, and it passes out to yang from yin. It is not suitable for those having burning and scorching lung fire and parched and full lung qi. In *Ji Sheng Fang* [《济生方》, *Prescriptions to Aid the Living*], Baihua Pill [百花丸, Lily Bulb and Common Coltsfoot Flower Pill], made from Baihe [百合, lily bulb, Bulbus Lilii] and Kuandong (common coltsfoot flower), can treat phlegm cough containing blood. Some can be treated after taking the pill, but some cannot. It is suitable for treating cold cough, not fire cough. Lu Ziyou (卢子由) said that it can mainly treat cough with dyspnea, descend adverse-rising qi and cure frequent dyspnea and pharyngitis as recorded in *Shen Nong Ben Cao Jing* [《神农本草经》, *Shennong's Classic of Materia Medica*]. It is suitable for those being physically cold, consuming the cold food and drinks and suffering from the attack by dampness in autumn. Those suffering from fire heat tormenting metal or parched and full lung qi may be more emaciated because of fire heat after taking it.

152. 紫 菀

紫菀 气味苦温,无毒。主治咳逆上气,胸中寒热结气,去蛊毒,痿蹙,安五脏。

紫菀之根紫色,而其质柔宛,故名紫菀。近道处处有之,三四月布地生苗,本有白毛,其叶二四相连,五六月开黄白紫花,结黑子。其根细而白者,白菀,即女菀也。

紫,黑赤之间色也。黑赤,水火之色也。紫菀气味苦温,禀火气也。其质阴柔,禀水气也。主治咳逆上气者,启太阳寒水之气,从皮毛而合肺也。治胸中寒热结气者,助少阴火热之气,通利三焦而上达也。蛊毒在腹属土,火能生土,故去蛊毒。痿蹙在筋,属木,水能生木,故去痿蹙。水火者,阴阳之征兆也。水火交,则阴阳合,故安五脏。

152. Ziwan [紫菀, tatarian aster root, Radix Asteris]

It is bitter in taste, warm and non-toxic in property, and it is mainly used to treat cough with dyspnea, descend adverse-rising qi, cure the cold-heat diseases in the chest and the diseases caused by qi stagnation, eliminate parasitic toxin and atrophy-flaccidity and harmonize the five zang-organs.

It has purple and soft roots, and thus it is called Ziwan（紫菀）（紫，purple；菀，soft）. It grows everywhere in the places nearby. Sow the seeds in the third and fourth lunar months, which will then begin to sprout. There is white hair on its stem. Two or four leaves grow together. It blossoms with yellow, white or purple flowers and bears black seeds in the fifth and sixth lunar months. Those having thin and white roots are called Baiwan（白菀）, which is actually Nüwan（女菀）.

Purple is a color intermediate between black and red. Black and red pertain to water and fire. Bitter in taste and warm in property, Ziwan（tatarian aster root）receives fire qi. Soft in texture, it receives water qi. It can mainly treat cough with dyspnea and descend adverse-rising qi by activating the qi of cold water from greater yang and relating itself to the lung through the skin and body hair. It can treat the cold-heat diseases in the chest and the disease caused by qi stagnation by assisting the qi of fire heat from lesser yin and dredging the triple energizer to flow upward. Parasitic toxin occurs in the abdomen pertaining to earth. Fire can generate earth, and thus Ziwan（tatarian aster root）can eliminate parasitic toxin. Atrophy-flaccidity occurs in the sinews pertaining to wood. Water can generate wood, and thus it can eliminate atrophy-flaccidity. Water and fire are the symbols of yin and yang. The interaction of water and fire leads to the harmony of yin and yang, and thus it can harmonize the five zang-organs.

153. 知 母

知母 气味苦寒，无毒。主治消渴热中，除邪气，肢体浮肿，下水，补不足，益气。

知母《本经》名连母，又名蚳母，又名地参，又名水参。出频河、怀卫、彰德、解州、滁州、彭城诸处。形似菖蒲而柔润，其根皮黄，肉白，而外毛，以肥大质润者为佳。

知母质性滋润，得寒水之精，故气味苦寒，有地参、水参之名。又名连母、蚳母者，皮有毛而肉白色，禀秋金清肃之气，得寒水之精，而禀秋金之气，须知水之有母也。禀寒水之精，故主治消渴热中。皮外有毛，故除皮毛之邪气。肉厚皮

黄,兼得土气,故治肢体浮肿,下水。补不足者,补肾水之不足。益气者,益肺气
之内虚。夫金生其水,故补肾水之不足。土生其金,故益肺气也。

153. Zhimu〔知母, common anemarrhena rhizome, Rhizoma Anemarrhenae〕

It is bitter in taste, cold and non-toxic in property, and it is mainly used to treat consumptive thirst and heat strike, eliminate pathogenic qi, relieve the edema of the limbs, disinhibit urination, tonify insufficiency and replenish qi.

It is mentioned as Lianmu（连母）in *Shen Nong Ben Cao Jing*〔《神农本草经》, *Shennong's Classic of Materia Medica*〕. It is also called Chimu（蚔母）, Dishen（地参）and Shuishen（水参）. It grows in Pinhe（频河）, Huaiwei（怀卫）, Zhangde（彰德）, Xiezhou（解州）, Chuzhou（滁州）and Pengcheng（彭城）. It is shaped like Changpu〔菖蒲, acorus, Acori Tatarinowii Rhizoma〕, but it is softer and moister. Its root has yellow bark, with white flesh inside and hair outside. Those that are bigger and moister are of good quality.

It is moist in nature, and it receives the essence of cold water. Thus it is bitter in taste and cold in property, and it is also called Dishen（地参）and Shuishen（水参）. It is also named Lianmu（连母）and Chimu（蚔母）, because it has hair outside on the bark and white flesh inside, and it receives the pure qi of autumn metal and the essence of cold water. Zhimu（common anemarrhena rhizome）can receive the qi of autumn metal, so it knows that it pertains to water, which is generated by metal. It receives the essence of cold water, and thus it can mainly treat consumptive thirst and heat strike. It has hair outside on the bark, and thus it can eliminate the pathogenic qi of the skin and body hair. It has thick flesh and yellow bark, and it obtains earth qi. Thus it can relieve the edema of the limbs and disinhibit urination. Tonifying insufficiency is to tonify the insufficiency of kidney water. Replenishing qi is to replenish the internal deficiency of lung qi. Metal generates water, and thus Zhimu（common anemarrhena rhizome）can tonify the insufficiency of kidney water. Earth generates metal, and thus it can replenish lung qi.

154. 瓜蒌根

瓜蒌根 气味苦寒，无毒。主治消渴，身热，烦满大热，补虚，安中，续绝伤。

瓜蒌所在皆有之，三四月生苗，延引藤蔓，七月开花浅黄色，实在花下，大如拳，生青至九月熟黄，形如柿，内有扁子，壳色褐，仁色绿，其根直下，生年久者，长数尺，皮黄肉白，入土深者良。《本经》气味主治合根实而概言之。至陶弘景以根名天花粉，又名瑞雪。后人又分实名瓜蒌，子名瓜蒌仁，功用遂有异同。

瓜蒌根入土最深，外黄内白，气味苦寒，盖得地水之精气，而上达之药也，其实黄色，内如重楼，其仁色绿多脂，性能从上而下，主治消渴、身热者，谓启在下之水精上滋，此根之功能也。治烦满大热者，谓降在上之火热下泄，此实之功能也。补虚安中，续绝伤，合根实而言也。水火上下交济，则补虚而安中，藤蔓之药能资经脉，故续绝伤。

《乘雅》云：瓜蒌根实补虚安中者，热却则中安，亦即所以补液之虚耳。

154. Gualougen [瓜蒌根, root of snakegourd fruit, Trichosanthis Radix]

It is bitter in taste, cold and non-toxic in property, and it is mainly used to treat consumptive thirst, fever, vexation and fullness as well as severe heat, tonify deficiency, harmonize the middle and cure severe injury.

Gualou [瓜蒌, snakegourd fruit, Fructus Trichosanthis] grows everywhere. It sprouts in the third and fourth lunar months. Its main stem grows upward, and its vines grow sideways. It blossoms in the seventh lunar month with light yellow flowers. Its fruit, as big as a fist, grows under the flowers. The fruit is blue-green when unripe and turns yellow in the ninth lunar month when ripe, which is shaped like Shizi [柿子, persimmon, Kaki Fructus]. Inside the fruit, there are flat seeds. The crust is brown in color, and the kernel is green in color. Its root grows directly downward and can be as long as several Chi deep after some years, which is white inside and yellow outside. Those with the roots spreading deeply into the soil are of good quality. The property, taste and actions introduced in *Shen Nong Ben Cao Jing* [《神农本草经》, *Shennong's Classic of Materia Medica*] are actually those of its root and fruits. Tao Hongjing (陶弘景) named its root Tianhuafen (天花粉) and Ruixue (瑞雪). People later on named its fruits Gualou (snakegourd fruit) and its seeds Gualouren [瓜蒌仁, trichosanthes seed, Trichosanthis Semen]. Thus, their actions and uses began to have similarities and differences.

Yellow inside and white outside, bitter in taste and cold in property, Gualougen (root of snakegourd fruit) grows the deepest into the soil. It is a medicinal receiving the essential qi of earth water and going upward. The fruit of Gualougen (root of snakegourd fruit) is yellow in color, with its inside similar to that of Chonglou [重楼, paris root, Rhizoma Paridis]. The kernel of Gualougen (root of snakegourd fruit) is green in color and rich in fat, which tends to move from the upper part to the lower part. Gualougen (root of snakegourd fruit) can mainly treat consumptive thirst and fever, which is said to result from the effect of activating water essence in the lower part and guiding essence to nourish the upper part. The fruit of Gualougen (root of snakegourd fruit) can treat vexation and fullness as well as severe heat, which is said to result from the effect of descending and discharging the fire heat in the upper part. Both the root and the fruit can tonify deficiency, harmonize the middle and cure severe injury. The interaction of water and fire can tonify deficiency and harmonize the middle. Medicinals made from vines can be used for nourishing the meridians, and thus it can cure severe injury.

Bencao Chengya Banji [《本草乘雅半偈》, *Explanation on Materia Medica from Two Aspects*] says, "The root and fruit can tonify deficiency and harmonize the middle. If heat descends, the middle will be harmonized, which is why they can be used for tonifying the deficiency of fluids.

155. 瞿 麦

瞿麦 气味苦寒,无毒。主治关格诸癃结,小便不通,出刺,决痈肿,明目去翳,破胎堕子,下闭血。

瞿麦今处处有之,根紫黑色,其茎纤细有节,高尺余,开花有红紫粉兰数色,斑斓可爱,人家多栽莳,呼为洛阳花,结实如燕麦,内有小黑子,其茎叶穗实与麦相似,穗分两岐,故名瞿麦。雷敩曰:只用蕊壳,不用茎叶,若一时同用,令人气噎,小便不禁也。

瞿者,如道路通衢,有四通八达之意。麦者,肝之谷,有东方发生之意。瞿麦一本直上,花红根紫,禀厥阴少阳木火之气化。苦者,火之味。寒者,水之性。气味苦寒,乃水生木而木生火也。主治关格诸癃结,小便不通者,厥阴肝木主疏泄,少阳三焦主决渎也。出刺决痈肿者,津液随三焦出,气以温肌肉,则肌肉之刺可出,而肌肉之痈肿可决也。明目去翳者,肝通窍于目,肝气和而目明也。破胎堕子者,少阳属肾,肾气泄,则破胎堕子。下血闭者,厥阴主肝,肝气通,则月事时行而下血闭。

155. Qumai〔瞿麦, lilac pink herb, Herba Dianthi〕

It is bitter in taste, cold and non-toxic in property, and it is mainly used to treat anuria and vomiting, ischuria and the retention of urine, withdraw stabs, expel abscess and swelling, remove nebula to improve vision, induce abortion and relieve amenorrhea.

It grows everywhere now. Its roots are purple-black. Its stem is thin, which is about one Chi tall with nodes on it. It blossoms with the lovely flowers of several colors, such as red, purple, pink and blue. It is a widely cultivated herb, and it is popularly called Luoyanghua (洛阳花). It bears fruits similar to those of Yanmai〔燕麦, bromegrass, Bromi Caulis et Folium〕, with small black seeds inside. Its stems, leaves, ears and fruits are similar to those of Mai〔麦, wheat, Tritici Semen〕. Its ear is divided into two branches, and thus it is called Qumai (lilac pink herb). Leixiao (雷敩) said, "Its seed shells, rather than its stems and leaves, are used as medicinal. Using the seed shells together with stems and leaves will result in choking caused by qi and urinary incontinence."

Qu (瞿) in Chinese means that the road can reach everywhere. Mai (麦) in Chinese refers to the grain pertaining to the liver, which has the meaning of growing in the east. Its root is straight and purple, its flowers are red, and it receives the qi transformation of wood fire from reverting yin and lesser yang.

Bitterness is the taste of fire, and cold is the property of water. Being bitter in taste and cold in property are caused by the fact that water generates wood and wood generates fire. It can mainly treat anuria and vomiting, ischuria and retention of urine, for liver wood from reverting yin governs the free flow of qi, and the triple energizer from lesser yang governs the dredging of water pathway. It can withdraw stabs and expel abscess and swelling, for the body fluids come out from the triple energizer, and qi can warm the muscles. Thus, stabs can be withdrawn, and abscess and swelling can be expelled. It can remove nebula to improve vision, for the liver is connected to the upper eyes. Thus, liver qi is harmonized, and vision can be improved. It can induce abortion, for lesser yang pertains to the kidney. Kidney qi is leaked, resulting in induced abortion. It can relieve amenorrhea, for reverting yin governs the liver. Liver qi is unblocked, and thus menstruation can be induced, and amenorrhea can be relieved.

156. 苦 参

苦参　气味苦寒,无毒。主治心腹结气,症瘕积聚,黄疸,溺有余沥,逐水,除痈肿,补中,明目,止泪。

苦参《本经》名水槐,一名地槐,又名苦骨。近道处处有之。花开黄白,根色亦黄白,长五七寸许,叶形似槐,味苦性寒,故有水槐、地槐之名。苦以味名,参以功名,有补益上中下之功,故名曰参。参犹参也。

苦参气味苦寒,根花黄白,禀寒水之精,得中土之化,水精上与君火相参,故主治心腹结气,参伍于中土之中,故治症瘕积聚而清黄疸。禀水精,则能资肾,故治溺有余沥。苦主下泄,故逐水。苦能清热,故除痈肿。得中土之化,故补中。水之精,上通于火之神,故明目止泪。

156. Kushen〔苦参, lightyellow sophora root, Radix Sophorae Flavescentis〕

It is bitter in taste, cold and non-toxic in property, and it is mainly used to treat qi stagnation in the heart and abdomen, abdominal mass, jaundice and dribbling after urination, expel water, eliminate abscess and swelling, tonify the middle, improve vision and stop epiphora.

It is mentioned as Shuihuai (水槐) in *Shen Nong Ben Cao Jing* [《神农本草经》, *Shennong's Classic of Materia Medica*]. It is also called Dihuai (地槐) or Kugu (苦骨). It grows everywhere in the places nearby. Both its flowers and root are yellow-white in color. It is five to seven Cun tall. Its leaves are quite similar to Huaiye [槐叶, sophora leaf, Sophorae Folium]. It is bitter in taste and cold in property, which is why it is named Shuihuai (水槐) or Dihuai (地槐). Ku (苦) indicates its taste. Shen (参) indicates that the herb has similar actions to those of Renshen [人参, ginseng, Ginseng Radix], which demonstrates that it can tonify the triple energizer, and thus it is called Shen (参). Kushen (lightyellow sophora root) is just a kind of Shen (参, ginseng).

Bitter in taste and cold in property, it has yellow-white roots and flowers, receives the essence of cold water and obtains the transformation of center earth. Water essence flows upward to correlate with monarch fire, and thus it can mainly treat the qi stagnation in the heart and abdomen. It can treat abdominal mass and eliminate jaundice by the synthetic analysis of center earth. It receives water essence, which enables it to nourish the kidney, and thus it can treat dribbling after urination. Bitterness can mainly be used for purgation, and thus it can expel water. Bitterness can also clear heat, and thus it can eliminate abscess and swelling. It obtains the transformation of center earth, and thus it can tonify the middle. Water essence flows upward to interact with shen (spirit or mind) of fire, and thus it can improve vision and stop epiphora.

157. 青 蒿

青蒿 气味苦寒,无毒。主治疥瘙痂痒恶疮,杀虱,治留热在骨节间,明目。《纲目》误注下品,今改正。

青蒿处处有之,春生苗叶极细可食。至夏高四五尺,秋后开细淡黄花颇香,结实如麻子。凡蒿叶皆淡青,此蒿独深青,如松桧之色,深秋余蒿并黄,此蒿犹青,其气芬芳,其根白色,春夏用苗叶,秋冬用子根。寇氏曰:青蒿得春最早。

青蒿春生苗叶,色青根白,气味苦寒,盖受金水之精,而得春生之气。主治疥瘙痂痒恶疮者,气味苦寒,苦杀虫而寒清热也。又曰:杀虱者,言不但治疥瘙,而且杀虱也。又曰:治留热在骨节间者,主不但治痂痒恶疮,且治留热在骨节间也。禀金水之精,得春生之气,故明目。

157. Qinghao〔青蒿, sweet wormwood herb, Herba Artemisiae Annuae〕

It is bitter in taste, cold and non-toxic in property, and it is mainly used to treat scabies, pruritus, crust, itching and malign sore, kill louses, relieve bone steaming with heat in the joints and improve vision. It has been mislabeled as a low-grade herb in *Ben Cao Gang Mu*〔《本草纲目》, *Compendium of Materia Medica*〕, and thus it is corrected here.

It grows everywhere. In spring, it sprouts with very thin and edible leaves. In summer, it grows to four or five Chi tall. In autumn, it blossoms with small fragrant light yellow flowers and bears fruits as big as Damazi〔大麻子, cannabis fruit, Cannabis Fructus〕. The leaves of Hao(蒿) are all light green, except Qinghao(sweet wormwood herb), which has dark green leaves, the color of which is similar to those of pine and juniper. In late autumn, when the leaves of other kinds of Hao(蒿) turn yellow, its leaves remain green. It is fragrant, and it has white roots. Its seedlings and leaves are used in spring and summer, and its fruits and roots are used in autumn and winter. Kou Zongshi(寇宗奭) once said that Qinghao(sweet wormwood herb) sprouts earlier than other herbs in spring.

It sprouts in spring with green leaves and white roots, and it is bitter in taste and cold in property. It obtains the qi of spring resuscitation by receiving the essence of metal and water. It can mainly treat scabies, pruritus, crust, itching and malign sore through its bitterness and cold. Bitterness can kill louses, and cold can clear heat. It is stated that not only it can treat scabies and pruritus, but also it can kill louses. It is also stated that it can not only treat crust, itching and malign sore, but also relieve the bone steaming with heat in the joints. It receives the essence of metal and water and obtains the qi of spring resuscitation, thus it can improve vision.

158. 石苇

石苇 气味苦平,无毒。主治劳热邪气,五癃闭不通,利小便水道。

石苇始出华阴山谷,今晋绛、滁海、福州、江宁皆有,丛生石旁及阴崖险罅处。其叶长者近尺,阔寸余,背有黄毛,亦有成金星者,凌冬不凋,柔韧如皮,故《别录》名石皮,采处以不闻水声及人声者良。

水草、石草皆主在肾。石苇生于石上,凌冬不凋,盖禀少阴之精气,叶背有金星,有黄毛,乃金水相生。肾上连肺也,主治劳热邪气者,劳热在骨,邪气在皮,肺肾之所主也。五癃者,五液癃闭,小便不利也。石苇助肺肾之精气,上下相交,水津上濡,则上窍外窍皆通。肺气下化,则水道行而小便利矣。夫水声泄肾气,人声泄肺气,不闻水声、人声者,藏水天之精,以助人之肺肾也。

158. Shiwei〔石苇,pyrrosia,Pyrrosiae Folium〕

It is bitter in taste and mild and non-toxic in property, and it is mainly used to treat the overstrained heat caused by pathogenic qi, resolve five kinds of blocks caused by retention of urine and disinhibit urination and water passage.

Firstly recorded to be growing in the valleys of Huayin(华阴), now it grows in Jinjiang(晋绛), Chuhai(滁海), Fuzhou(福州)and Jiangning(江宁). Clumps of Shiwei(石苇)grow around rocks, in shady precipices and steep cracks. Its leaf can be as long as one Chi and as wide as one Cun, which has yellow hair in the back. There is one kind with golden stellate hair in the back of its leaves. It does not wither even in winter and it is as pliable as leather, and thus it is mentioned as Shipi〔石皮, rock leather〕in *Ming Yi Bie Lu*〔《名医别录》, *Miscellaneous Records of Famous Physicians*〕. Those collected in the place where water sounds and human voices cannot be heard are of better quality.

Both the aquatic weeds and the weeds growing around rocks are related with the kidney. Due to its receiving essence from lesser yin, Shiwei(pyrrosia)grows on rocks and does not wither even in winter. It has golden stellate hair or yellow hair in the back of its leaves, which results from its receiving the mutual generation of metal and water. The kidney connects upward to the lung, thus it can mainly treat the overstrained heat caused by pathogenic qi. Overstrained heat occurs in the bones, pathogenic qi occurs in the skin, and the bones and skin are governed respectively by the lung and the kidney. Five kinds of blocks caused by retention of urine are manifested as inhibited urination. Shiwei (pyrrosia) can assist the essential qi of the lung to interact with that of the kidney, and fluids can flow upward to moisten the lung, resulting in the unobstruction of the upper and lower orifices. The downward transformation of lung qi can disinhibit waterways as well as urination. Water sounds leak kidney qi, and human voices leak lung qi. Herbs can store the essence of water and heaven when growing in the places where water sounds and human voices cannot be heard, which allows them to be beneficial to the kidney and the lung.

159. 海 藻

海藻 气味苦咸寒,无毒。主治瘿瘤结气,散颈下硬核痛,痈肿,症瘕坚气,腹中上下雷鸣,治十二水肿。

　　海藻生东海岛中,今登莱诸处海中皆有,黑色如乱发,海人以绳系腰,没水取之。

咸能软坚,咸主润下,海藻生于海中,其味苦咸,其性寒洁,故主治经脉外内之坚结,瘿瘤结气,颈下硬核痛,痈肿,乃经脉不和而病结于外也。症瘕坚气,腹中上下雷鸣,乃经脉不和。而病结于内也。海藻形如乱发,主通经脉,故治十二经水肿,人身十二经脉流通,则水肿自愈矣。

159. Haizao〔海藻, seaweed, Sargassum〕

It is bitter and salty in taste, cold and non-toxic in property, and it is mainly used to treat goiter and tumor as well as qi stagnation, disperse the pain caused by hard node in the neck, resolve abscess and abdominal mass caused by qi stagnation, relieve thunderous rumbling in the upper and lower abdomen and treat twelve kinds of edema.

　　Originally growing on the islands in the East China Sea, now it grows everywhere in the waters of Dengzhou (登州) and Laizhou (莱州). It is black, and it looks like messy hair. Fishermen collect it by diving into the sea with strings fastened to their waists.

Saltiness can soften hardness and has the effects of moistening and descending. Haizao (seaweed), growing in the sea, is bitter and salty in taste and cold and clean in nature, and thus it can mainly treat the diseases caused by hard node in and out of the meridians. Goiter and tumor as well as qi stagnation, the pain caused by hard node in the neck and abscess are all externally accumulated diseases caused by the disharmony of meridians. Abdominal mass caused by qi stagnation and thunderous rumbling in the upper and lower abdomen are internally accumulated diseases caused by the disharmony of meridians. Haizao (seaweed), in the shape of messy hair, can mainly dredge the meridians, and thus it can treat twelve kinds of edema in the meridians. Edema can be naturally treated following the dredging of the twelve meridians in the body.

160. 水　萍

水萍　气味辛寒,无毒。主治暴热身痒,下水气,胜酒,长须发,止消渴。久服轻身。

水萍处处池泽止水中皆有。季春始生,而盛于夏。一叶过宿即生数叶,叶下有微须,即其根也。叶小而圆,面青背紫,其紫赤若血者,谓之紫背浮萍,入药为良。七月收采,置竹筛内,下以盆水映之晒日中,方易干也。

太阳之气,根于水中,而外浮于肤表。萍生水中,浮于水面,盖禀太阳之气化。其背紫赤,皆连于水,乃太阳之气,根于水中也。盛于暑夏,乃太阳之气,开浮而主夏也。气味辛寒者,辛属乾金,太阳如天而合乾。寒本太阳,太阳标阳而本寒也。主治暴热身痒者,风热之邪,暴客皮肤,一身苦痒。水萍禀寒水之气,外行肤表,故暴热身痒可治也。下水气者,太阳之气外达皮毛,则膀胱之水气自下也。胜酒者,酒性辛温而慓悍,先行皮肤。水萍辛寒而解热,亦先行皮肤,故能胜酒。长须发者,太阳为诸阳主气,而熏肤泽毛,须发长也。得寒水之精气,故止消渴。久服则阴精盛而阳气充,故轻身。

太阳之气出于水中,上与君火相合而主日。水萍下为水映,上为日晒方干,乃太阳之气,上下相通,此物理自然之妙用也。

160. Shuiping〔水萍, common duckweed, Spirodelae Herba〕

It is pungent in taste, cold and non-toxic in property, and it is mainly used to treat the itching caused by fulminant heat, disinhibit urination, dispel the effects of liquor, promote the hair growth and relieve consumptive thirst. Long-term taking of it can keep healthy.

It grows everywhere in ponds, lakes and the stagnant water. It starts to grow in the third month of spring and thrives in summer. One Shuiping (common duckweed) can grow several leaves after a night, with short branching roots under them, which are actually its roots. Its leaves are small and round, with the surface being blue-green and the back being purple. The one whose back of the leaf is as purplish red as blood is called Zibei Fuping (紫背浮萍), which is good to be used as medicinal. Collect it in the seventh lunar month, put it in a bamboo sieve, place a basin of water under the sieve to mirror it and dry it in the sun at noon, otherwise it will not be easily dried up.

The qi of greater yang is rooted in water and floats outside on the skin and hair. Shuiping (common duckweed) grows in water and floats on the water surface, because it receives the qi transformation of greater yang. The back of its leaf is purplish red, and all its leaves are connected to water, because the qi of greater yang is rooted in water. It thrives in summer, because the qi of greater yang can flow around and upward, which also governs summer. It is pungent in taste and cold in property. Pungency pertains to qian (乾) gold, because greater yang is like the heaven in accordance with qian (乾). The root of greater yang is cold, and the branch is yang. It can mainly treat the itching caused by fulminant heat. Wind-heat pathogen invades the skin fulminnatly, resulting in itching all over the skin. Shuiping (common duckweed) receives the qi from cold water and moves outside on the skin and hair, thus it can treat the itching caused by fulminant heat. It can disinhibit urination by moving the qi of greater yang outside to the skin and the body hair. It can dispel the effects of liquor. Pungent in taste, warm and strong in property, liquor moves firstly on the skin. Pungent in taste and warm in property, Shuiping (common duckweed) can clear heat and also moves firstly on the skin, and thus it can dispel the effects of liquor. It can promote the hair growth, because greater yang is the main qi of various yang with the actions of warming the skin and moistening the hair, which can therefore promote the hair growth. It obtains the essential qi of cold water, and thus it can relive consumptive thirst. Long-term taking of it can result in exuberant yin essence and sufficient yang qi, and thus it can keep healthy.

The qi of the greater yang originates from water and governs the sun by being in accordance with sovereign fire. Shuiping (common duckweed) will not be dried up in the sun unless placed in a basin of water to mirror it, because the upper and lower part of the qi of greater yang are connected, which shows the magical effect of the laws of nature.

161. 萆 薢

萆薢　气味苦平,无毒。主治腰脊痛强,骨节风寒湿周痹,恶疮不瘳,热气。

萆薢处处有之,出川蜀、怀庆者佳。苗引延蔓,茎叶俱青有刺,叶作三叉,花有红黄白数种,亦有无花结白子者,根黄白色,多枝节而硬,故《别录》一名赤节萆薢,犹卑解也。以其专精在根,性引延上,从下解上之义。

凡草木之根荄,坚硬而骨胜者,主肾。有刺而藤蔓者,走经脉。萆薢骨胜藤蔓,故主治腰脊痛强,骨节风寒而主肾。又,治湿痹、周痹,而主经脉。苦能清热,故治恶疮不瘳之热气。

161. Bixie [萆薢, fish poison yam, Dioscoreae Hypoglaucae seu Semptemlobae Rhizoma]

It is bitter in taste, mild and non-toxic in property, and it is mainly used to treat the pain and stiffness of the waist and spine, the wind-cold diseases in the joints, damp impediment, generalized impediment, the malign sore difficult to cure and the diseases caused by heat qi.

It grows everywhere, and those growing in Chuanshu (川蜀) and Huaiqing (怀庆) are of good quality. Its seedlings grow upward, and its vines grow sideways. Both its stems and leaves are blue-green with thorns. It has leaves with three lobes. It has red, yellow or white flowers. One kind of Bixie (萆薢) is flowerless and bears white seeds. It has strong red-yellow roots with many nodes, and thus it is also called Chijie Bixie (赤节草薢) in *Ming Yi Bie Lu* [《名医别录》, *Miscellaneous Records of Famous Physicians*], which has the effect of treating diseases with the lower part. It has the essence stored in the roots, and thus it can treat the diseases in the upper part of the human body through the lower part, resulting from its medicinal property of flowing from the lower to the upper.

Herb roots, which are strong with many nodes, are all related with the kidney. The effect of herb vines with thorns can penetrate the meridians. Bixie (fish poison yam), having roots with many nodes and vines growing sideways, can mainly treat the pain and stiffness of the waist and spine and the wind-cold diseases in the joints, both of which are related with the kidney. It can also treat damp impediment and generalized impediment, both of which are related with the meridians. Bitterness can clear heat, and thus it can treat the malign sore difficult to cure and the diseases caused by heat qi.

162. 白茅根

白茅根 气味甘寒,无毒。主治劳伤虚羸,补中益气,除瘀血血闭,寒热,利小便。

　　茅草处处由田野有之,春生芽,布地如针,俗谓之茅针。其叶如矛,边有锋棱,又名刀茅。茅有白茅、菅茅、黄茅、香茅、芭茅数种,叶皆相似白茅,根甚洁白,味甘如蔗,其根柔软如筋,故一名地筋,干之夜视有光,故腐则变为萤火茅,叶可以苫盖,及供祭祀苞苴之用。

白茅色白味甘,上刚下柔,根多津汁,禀土金水相生之气化。主治劳伤羸瘦者,烦劳内伤,则津液不荣于外,而身体羸瘦。茅根禀水精而多汁,故治劳伤羸瘦。补中益气者,中土内虚,则气不足。茅根禀土气而味甘,故能补中益气。除瘀血血闭者,肝气内虚,则血不荣经,而为瘀血血闭之证。茅根禀金气而色白,故除瘀血血闭。肺金之气外达皮毛,则寒热自愈。皮毛之气下输膀胱,则小便自利。

162. Baimaogen〔白茅根, lalang grass rhizome, Rhizoma Imperatae〕

It is sweet in taste, cold and non-toxic in property, and it is mainly used to treat overstrained damage and debility, tonify the middle and replenish qi, eliminate blood stasis and amenorrhea, treat cold-heat diseases and disinhibit urination.

Maocao〔茅草, curculigo, Curculiginis Rhizoma〕grows everywhere on the field. It sprouts in spring, and its buds spread all over the field like needles, which are popularly called Maozhen（茅针）. Its leaves with sharp edges are like spears, which are also called Daomao（刀茅）. There are several kinds of Maocao（curculigo）, such as Baimao（白茅）, Jianmao（菅茅）, Huangmao（黄茅）, Xiangmao（香茅）and Bamao（芭茅）, whose leaves are all similar to those of Baimao（白茅）. Baimaogen（lalang grass rhizome）is brilliant white and tastes as sweet as Ganzhe〔甘蔗, sugarcane, Sacchari Caulis〕. It is also as soft as tendon, which is why it is also called Dijin（地筋）. When dried, it gives off glimmer at night. Thus, it turns into Yinghuomao（萤火茅）when rotten. Its leaves can be used to cover things and wrap meat or fish for the sacrificial purpose.

Baimao（白茅）is white in color, sweet in taste, firm in the upper and soft in the lower part. Baimaogen（lalang grass rhizome）has abundant juice and receives the qi transformation of the mutual generation of earth, metal and water. It can mainly treat overstrained damage and debility. Vexing overstrain and internal damage can lead to the failure of body fluids to nourish the body, resulting in debility. Baimaogen（lalang grass rhizome）receives water essence and has abundant juice, and thus it can treat overstrained damage and debility. It can tonify the middle and replenish qi. The internal deficiency of center earth can cause qi deficiency. Baimaogen（lalang grass rhizome）receives earth qi and it is sweet in taste, and thus it can tonify the middle and replenish qi. It can eliminate blood stasis and amenorrhea. The internal deficiency of liver qi can lead to the failure of the blood to nourish the meridians, resulting in blood stasis and amenorrhea. Baimaogen（lalang grass rhizome）receives metal qi, and it is white in color, and thus it can eliminate blood stasis and amenorrhea. The qi of lung metal moves externally to the skin and body hair, and cold-heat diseases can therefore be naturally cured. The qi of the skin and hair transports downward to the bladder, and urination can therefore be naturally disinhibited.

163. 狗 脊

狗脊 气味苦平,无毒。主治腰背强,机关缓急,周痹,寒湿膝痛,颇利老人。

狗脊出常山川谷及太行山、淄青、眉州山野,处处有之。茎节如竹有刺,叶圆有赤脉,两两对生,边有锯齿,根形如狗之脊骨凸凹巃嵸,金毛密布。李时珍曰:狗脊有二种,一种根黑色如狗脊骨,一种有金黄毛如狗形,皆名狗脊。《本经》一名百枝,以形名也,《别录》一名强膂,一名扶筋,以功名也。

狗脊根坚似骨,叶有赤脉,主利骨节而通经脉之药也。治腰背强,机关缓急,利骨节也。血脉不和,则为周痹,或因于寒,或因于湿,皆能为痹。治周痹寒湿,通经脉也。又曰膝痛者,言机关缓急,则膝亦痛。老人精血虚而机关不利,故颇利老人。

163. Gouji〔狗脊, cibot rhizome, Rhizoma Cibotii〕

It is bitter in taste, mild and non-toxic in property, and it is mainly used to resolve the stiffness of the waist and back, relieve the spasm of the spine and treat the generalized impediment due to cold dampness and the pain of the knees. It is beneficial for the old people.

It grows everywhere in the valleys of Changshan Mountain (常山), in Taihang Mountain (太行山) and in the fields of Ziqing (淄青) and Meizhou (眉州). Its stem is similar to that of Zhu〔竹, bamboo, Bambusoideae〕with nodes on it. Its stem is also covered with thorns. Its leaves are round with red veins and serrated edges, growing in pairs in opposition. Its root is shaped like a dog's unsmooth spine and is covered with golden hair. Li Shizhen (李时珍) said, "There are two kinds of Gouji (cibot rhizome): One has a black root in the shape of a dog's spine while the other has a root in the shape of a dog covered with golden hair. Both of them are called Gouji (cibot rhizome)." It is mentioned as Baimei (百枚) because of its shape in *Shen Nong Ben Cao Jing* [《神农本草经》, *Shennong's Classic of Materia Medica*]. It is mentioned as Qianglü (强膂) and Fujin (扶筋) because of its actions recorded in *Ming Yi Bie Lu* [《名医别录》, *Miscellaneous Records of Famous Physicians*].

Its root is as strong as a bone, with red veins on its leaves. It is a medicinal which mainly has the actions of benefiting the joints and dredging the meridians. Thus, it can resolve the stiffness of the waist and back, relieve the spasm of the spine and benefit the joints. The disharmony of the blood and the vessels is manifested as generalized impediment, which is caused either by cold or dampness. Both cold and dampness can cause impediment. Thus, it can treat the generalized impediment due to cold dampness and dredge the meridians. It can also treat the pain of the knees, which results from the spasm of the spine. It is beneficial for the old people owing to the fact that they suffer from the dysfunction of the spine caused by the deficiency of essence and blood.

164. 淫羊藿

淫羊藿　气味辛寒,无毒。主治阴痿绝伤,茎中痛,利小便,益气力,强志。

　　淫羊藿出上郡阳山山谷,江东陕西、泰山、汉中、湖湘间皆有。茎高一二尺,一茎三桠,一桠三叶,叶似杏叶,上有刺,关中呼为三枝九叶草。枝茎细劲,经冬不凋,四月开白花,亦有紫花者,生处不闻水声者良。陶隐居云:西川北部有淫羊,一日百遍交合,盖食此藿所致,因以为名。《唐本草》名仙灵脾,有仙灵脾酒,益丈夫,兴阳,理腰膝冷。

　　羊为火畜,藿能淫羊,盖禀水中之天气,而得太阳阳热之气化也。禀水中之天气,故气味辛寒。得太阳之阳热,故主治阴痿绝伤。太阳合膀胱寒水之气,故治茎中痛,利小便。太阳之气,上合于肺,内通于肾,故益气力,强志。

　　淫羊藿禀太阳之气,而功能治下,与紫萍禀太阳之气,而浮越于肤表者,少有不同,故生处不闻水声者良。欲使太阳之气藏于水中,而不征现于外也。圣人体察物性,曲尽苦心,学者潜心玩索,庶几得之。

164. Yinyanghuo〔淫羊藿，epimedium herb，Herba Epimedii〕

It is pungent in taste, cold and non-toxic in property, and it is mainly used to treat impotence with flaccidity and the pain in the penis, disinhibit urination, replenish qi and energy, and strengthen memory.

Originally growing in the valleys of Yangshan Mountain（阳山）in Shangjun（上郡），now it grows in Jiangdong（江东），Shaanxi（陕西），Hanzhong（汉中），Hubei（湖北）and Hunan（湖南）as well as on Mount Tai. Its stem can be as tall as one or two Chi with three twigs. Each twig has three leaves, which are similar to Xingye〔杏叶，apricot leaf，Armeniacae Folium〕，with thorns on them. It is called Sanzhi Jiuye Cao（a herb with three twigs and nine leaves）by people in Guanzhong（关中）. Both its stem and twigs are thin but firm and do not wither even in winter. It blossoms in the fourth lunar month with white or purple flowers. Those growing in the place where there is no sound of running water are of good quality. Tao Yinju（陶隐居）said, "Some sheep growing in the north of Xichuan（西川）can mate one hundred times a day, because they have eaten Yinyanghuo（epimedium herb），thus Yinyanghuo（epimedium herb）is called such a name." It is mentioned as Xianlingpi（仙灵脾）in *Tang Ben Cao*〔《唐本草》，*Tang Materia Medica*〕. The liquor made from Xianlingpi（仙灵脾）can benefit men, invigorate yang and regulate the cold of the waist and knees.

Sheep pertain to fire. They can have strong sexual desire after eating Yinyanghuo（epimedium herb），which obtains the qi transformation of yang heat from greater yang by receiving heaven qi from water. It receives heaven qi from water, and thus it is pungent in taste and cold in property. It obtains yang heat from greater yang, and thus it can mainly treat impotence with flaccidity. Greater yang is in accordance with the qi of cold water from the bladder, and thus Yinyanghuo（epimedium herb）can treat the pain in the penis and disinhibit urination. The qi of greater yang is in accordance with the lung upward and flows inside to the kidney, and thus it can replenish qi and energy, and strengthen memory.

It can treat the diseases occurring in the lower part by receiving the qi of greater yang, which is slightly different from the property of Ziping〔紫萍, duckweed, Spirodela polyrrhiza（L.）Schleid〕. Ziping（duckweed）can float on the skin and muscles by receiving the qi of greater yang. Thus, Yinyanghuo（epimedium herb）growing in the place where there is no sound of running water is of good quality, intending to store the qi of greater yang in the water instead of displaying it outside. The sages have been at pains to understand the nature of things, and scholars may be able to know that if they devote themselves to pondering.

165. 紫 葳

紫葳 气味酸,微寒,无毒。主治妇人产乳余疾,崩中,症瘕血闭,寒热羸瘦,养胎。

紫葳处处皆有,多生山中,人家园圃亦或栽之。蔓延木上,高数丈,年久者藤大如杯,春初生枝,一枝数叶,尖长有齿,自夏至秋,花开五瓣,赭黄色,有细点,秋深更赤,今名凌霄花,谓其花之极高也,根花并用。

紫葳延引藤蔓,主通经脉,气味酸寒,主清血热,故《本经》主治如此。近时用此,为通经下胎之药。仲景鳖甲煎丸,亦用紫葳以消症瘕,必非安胎之品。《本经》养胎二字,当是堕胎之讹耳。

165. Ziwei〔紫葳, campsis flower, Campsis Flos〕

It is sour in taste, slightly cold and non-toxic in property, and it is mainly used to treat postpartum blood stasis, metrorrhagia, abdominal mass and amenorrhea, cold-heat diseases and debility, and nurture fetus.

It grows everywhere and can mostly be found in the mountains. It is sometimes cultivated in gardens. Its vines can grow to as tall as several Zhang along the tree. Years later, its vines can be as thick as a cup. In early spring, it begins to branch, with on one branch having several leaves. Its leaves are long and pointed with teeth on edges. It blossoms from summer to autumn, with ocher flowers having five petals and fine dots, which will turn red in late autumn. Its flower is now called Lingxiaohua（凌霄花）, which means that the flower can grow very high. Its flowers and roots can be used as medicinal.

It can mainly dredge the meridians because of its extending vines and can mainly clear blood heat because of its sour taste and cold property, thus it has such actions recorded in *Shen Nong Ben Cao Jing* [《神农本草经》, *Shennong's Classic of Materia Medica*]. It has recently been used as the herb to dredge the meridians and induce abortion. It is also used in Zhang Zhongjing's (张仲景) Biejia Jianwan [鳖甲煎丸, Decocted Turtle Shell Pill] to eliminate abdominal mass. Thus, it is not actually the one used for calming fetus. The words "nurture fetus" in *Shen Nong Ben Cao Jing* [《神农本草经》, *Shennong's Classic of Materia Medica*] must be an error of the words "induce abortion".

166. 薤 白

薤白 气味辛苦温滑,无毒。主治金疮疮败,轻身,不饥,耐老。

薤处处有之,正月发苗,叶状似韭,韭叶中实而扁,有剑脊,薤叶中空似细葱,而有棱,气亦如葱。二月开细花紫白色,一茎一根,根如小蒜,叶青根白,入药只用其根,故曰薤白、与韭白、葱白同一义也。根之色亦有微赤者,赤者苦而不辛,白者辛而不苦,入药以白者为佳。

薤用在下之根,气味辛温,其性从下而上,主助生阳之气上升者也。《金匮》胸痹证,有瓜蒌薤白白酒汤,瓜蒌薤白半夏汤,枳实薤白桂枝汤,皆取自下而上从阴出阳之义。金疮疮败,则皮肌经脉虚寒。薤白辛温,从内达外,故能治之,生阳上升,则轻身不饥耐老。

166. Xiebai [薤白, longstamen onion bulb, Bulbus Allii Macrostemonis]

It is pungent and bitter in taste, warm, slippery and non-toxic in property, and it is mainly used to treat incised wound and severe sore, keep healthy, tolerate hunger and prevent aging.

It grows everywhere. It sprouts in the first lunar month. Its leaves are similar to those of Jiu [韭, Chinese leek, Allii Tuberosi Folium]. The leaf of Jiu (Chinese leek) is flat and solid with a sword-like ridge in the middle. Xieye

[薤叶, Chinese chive leaf, Allii Folium] is hollow with edges, just like the leaf of Xicong [细葱, chive, Allii Schoenoprasi Herba seu Caput Radicis]. Xieye (Chinese chive leaf) also smells like scallion. It blossoms with fine purple-white flowers in the second lunar month. It has one stem and one root. Its root is white in color and is similar to that of Xiaosuan [小蒜, scorodoprasum, Allii Scorodoprasi Bulbus] while its leaves are green in color. Only its root can be used as medicinal, and thus it is called Xiebai (longstamen onion bulb). So Xiebai (longstamen onion bulb), Jiubai [韭白, Chinese leek root, Allii Tuberosi Radix] and Congbai [葱白, scallion white, Allii Fistulosi Bulbus] all have the same Chinese character "白" (Bai), which means the root. Some Xiebai (longstamen onion bulb) have light red roots, which are bitter but not pungent in taste. Xiebai (longstamen onion bulb) with a white root is pungent but not bitter in taste. It is better to use Xiebai (longstamen onion bulb) with a white root as medicinal.

Its roots are used, which are astringent in taste and warm in property. They tend to move from the lower to the upper, which can mainly help the rise of kidney-yang qi. According to *Jin Gui Yao Lüe* [《金匮要略》, *Synopsis of the Golden Chamber*], chest impediment can be cured by Gualou Xiebai Baijiu Tang [瓜蒌薤白白酒汤, Trichosanthes, Chinese Chive and White Liquor Decoction], Gualou Xiebai Banxia Tang [瓜蒌薤白半夏汤, Trichosanthes, Chinese Chive and Pinellia Decoction], or Zhishi Xiebai Guizhi Tang [枳实薤白桂枝汤, Unripe Bitter Orange, Chinese Chive and Cinnamon Twig Decoction], which all include Xiebai (longstamen onion bulb) because of its effects of moving from the lower to the upper and passing out to yang from yin. Incised wound and severe sore can cause the deficiency cold of the meridians in the cutaneous muscles. Xiebai (longstamen onion bulb), pungent in taste and warm in property, can reach the outside from the inside, and thus it can treat incised wound and severe sore. Kidney-yang rises, and thus it can keep healthy, tolerate hunger and prevent aging.

167. 龙 胆

龙胆 气味苦涩,大寒,无毒。主治骨间寒热,惊痫邪气,续绝伤,定五脏,杀蛊毒。

　　龙胆始出齐朐山谷及冤句，今处处有之，以吴兴者为胜，宿根生苗，一窠有根十余条，类牛膝而短，黄白色，其茎高尺余，纤细状如小竹枝，花开青碧色，冬后结子苗便枯，俗名草龙胆。又一种山龙胆，其叶经霜雪不凋，此同类而别种也。

龙胆草根味极苦，气兼涩，性大寒。茎如竹枝，花开青碧，禀东方木气，故有龙胆之名。龙乃东方之神。胆主少阳甲木，苦走骨，故主治骨间寒热。涩类酸，故除惊痫邪气。胆主骨，肝主筋，故续绝伤。五脏六腑皆取决于胆，故定五脏。山下有风曰虫，风气升而蛊毒自杀矣。

167. Longdan〔龙胆，Chinese gentian，Radix Gentianae〕

It is bitter and astringent in taste, severely cold and non-toxic in property, and it is mainly used to resolve the cold and heat in the bones and the fright epilepsy caused by pathogenic qi, treat severe injury, stabilize the five zang-organs and kill parasitic toxin.

　　Firstly recorded to be growing in the valleys of Qiqu（齐朐）and in Yuanju（冤句）, now it grows everywhere, and those growing in Wuxing（吴兴）are of better quality. Its perennial roots sprout. One Longdan（Chinese gentian）can have a dozen yellow-white roots, similar to those of Niuxi〔牛膝, achyranthes, Achyranthis Bidentatae Radix〕, but short in size. Its stem can grow to about one Chi tall, as thin as the small bamboo twig. It blossoms with blue-green flowers. It produces seeds after winter and withers afterwards, which is popularly called Caolongdan（草龙胆）. There is another herb called Shanlongdan（山龙胆）whose leaves do not wither even when exposed to frost and snow. They are different species under the same family.

Its root is astringent and severely bitter in taste and severely cold in property. Its stem is similar to the bamboo twig. Its flowers are blue-green. It receives wood qi in the east, which is why it is called Longdan（Chinese gentian）. Long〔龙, dragon〕is the god of the east; Dan〔胆, gallbladder〕governs the jia wood of lesser yang; the effect of bitterness can penetrate the bones, and thus Longdan〔龙胆, Chinese gentian〕can mainly resolve the cold and heat in the bones.

Astringency is quite like sourness, thus Longdan (Chinese gentian) can resolve the fright epilepsy caused by pathogenic qi. The gallbladder governs the bones, the liver governs the sinews, and thus it can treat severe injury. Both the five zang-organs and the six fu-organs depend on the gallbladder, and thus it can stabilize the five zang-organs. Parasites are caused by the wind arising from the foot of the hill. Wind qi rises, and parasitic toxin will naturally dissipate.

168. 黄 芩

黄芩 气味苦寒,无毒。主治诸热,黄疸,肠澼,泄痢,逐水,下血闭,恶疮,疽蚀,火疡。

黄芩《本经》名腐肠,又名空肠,又名妒妇,谓外皮肉,而内空腐,妒妇心黯,黄芩心黑同也。出川蜀及陕西河东,近道皆有。芩者黔也,黑色也。其根黑而黄,故曰黄芩。

黄芩色黄内空,能清肠胃之热,外肌皮而性寒,能清肌表之热,乃手足阳明兼手太阴之药也。主治诸热黄疸,肠澼泄痢者,言诸经之热,归于胃土而为黄疸,归于大肠而为泄痢。黄芩中空,主清肠胃之热,故能治之。肠胃受浊,得肺气通调,则水津四布,血气运行,逐水下血闭者,黄芩外肌皮而清肌表。肌表清,则肺气和,而留水可逐,血闭自下矣。火热之气留于肌肉皮肤,则为恶疮疽蚀。恶疮疽蚀名曰火疡。黄芩治之,清肌表也。

168. Huangqin〔黄芩, baical skullcap root, Radix Scutellariae〕

It is bitter in taste, cold and non-toxic in property, and it is mainly used to treat various diseases caused by heat, jaundice, dysentery and diarrhea, expel water, relieve amenorrhea and cure severe sore, the deep-rooted carbuncle and swollen sore caused by fire toxin.

It is mentioned as Fuchang (腐肠), Kongchang (空肠) and Dufu (妒妇) in *Shen Nong Ben Cao Jing*〔《神农本草经》, *Shennong's Classic of Materia Medica*〕. It has yellow bark and flesh, but it is loose and rotten-like inside. It is called Dufu〔妒妇, jealous women〕, because it is black inside. It is generally believed that jealous women are usually black-hearted. Originally growing in

Chuanshu（川蜀）, Shaanxi（陕西）and Hedong（河东）, now it grows everywhere in the places nearby. Qin（芩）means Qian（黔）, which indicates that the color is black. Its root is black and yellow, and thus it is called Huangqin［黄芩, baical skullcap root］.

It is yellow in color, loose inside and can clear the heat of the intestines and the stomach. Its bark and flesh outside are cold in property and can clear the heat from the fleshy exterior. Thus, it is a medicinal for hand yang brightness, foot yang brightness and hand greater yin. It can mainly treat various diseases caused by the heat, jaundice, dysentery and diarrhea. It is said that jaundice is caused by the heat of various meridians flowing to the stomach earth, and diarrhea is caused by the heat of various meridians flowing to the large intestine. It is loose inside and can mainly clear the heat of the intestines and the stomach, and thus it can treat the above diseases. Lung qi can free and regulate the turbidity water of the intestines and the stomach, the water fluid can then distribute all through the body, and blood and qi can flow smoothly. It can expel water and relieve amenorrhea, because its bark and flesh outside can clear the heat from the fleshy exterior. The heat of the fleshy exterior is cleared, and then lung qi can be harmonized, water can be expelled, and amenorrhea can be naturally relieved. Heat qi rested in the skin and muscles can cause severe sore and deep-rooted carbuncle, both of which can be called swollen sore caused by fire toxin. Huangqin（baical skullcap root）can treat these diseases by clearing the heat from the fleshy exterior.

169. 藁 本

藁本 气味辛温,无毒。主治妇人疝瘕,阴中寒肿痛,腹中急,除风头痛,长肌肤,悦颜色。

藁本始出崇山山谷,今西川河东、兖州、杭州山中皆有。根似芎䓖而轻虚,味麻不堪作饮,正月、二月采根,曝干三十日成。

藁,高也。藁本始生崇山,得天地崇高之气,禀太阳标本之精。故下治妇人疝瘕,阴中寒肿痛,中治腹中拘急,上除头风痛。盖太阳之脉本于下,而上额交巅,出入于中上也。太阳阳气有余,则长肌肤,悦颜色。

169. Gaoben〔藁本, Chinese lovage, Rhizoma Ligustici〕

It is pungent in taste, warm and non-toxic in property, and it is mainly used to treat hernia and movable abdominal mass of women, cold, the swelling and pain of the vulva and spasmodic pain in the abdomen, eliminate the headache caused by the invasion of wind into the head, promote the growth of the muscles and luster complexion.

Firstly recorded to be growing in the valleys of Chongshan Mountain (崇山), now it grows in the mountains of Xichuan (西川), Hedong (河东), Yanzhou (兖州) and Hangzhou (杭州). Its root is similar to that of Xiongqiong〔芎藭, Szechwan Lovage Rhizome, Chuanxiong Rhizoma〕, but light and loose. The root is tongue-numbing, which makes it not suitable for drinking. The root collected in the first and second lunar months should be dried for thirty days before preparation for use.

Gao (藁) means being high. Originally growing in Chongshan Mountain (崇山), it has obtained the lofty qi of the heaven and the earth, and received the essence of branches and rootes from greater yang. Thus, it can treat hernia and movable abdominal mass of women and cold, the swelling and pain of the vulva occurring in the lower part of the human body; treat spasmodic pain in the abdomen occurring in the middle; treat the headache caused by the invasion of wind into the head occurring in the upper. This is because the greater yang meridian starts from the lower part, runs along the forehead, reaches the vertex and comes in and out of the middle and upper energizer. It can promote the growth of muscles and luster complexion when the yang qi of greater yang is abundant.

170. 百 合

百合　气味甘平,无毒。主治邪气腹胀心痛,利大小便,补中益气。

百合近道山谷处处有之。三月生苗,高二三尺,一茎直上,叶如竹叶,又似柳叶,四向而生,五月茎端开白花,芬芳六出,四垂向下,昼开夜合,故名夜合花。其根如蒜,细白而长,重叠生二三十瓣。煮食甘美,取瓣分种,如种蒜法,一种花红不四垂者,山丹也。一种花红带黄而四垂,上有黑斑点,其子黑色,结在枝叶间者,卷丹也。其根皆同百合,皆可煮食,而味不美。盖一类三种,唯白花者入药,余不可用。

百合色白属金,味甘属土,昼开夜合,应天道之昼行于阳,夜行于阴,四向六合,应土气之达于四旁。主治邪气腹胀心痛者,邪气下乘于脾,则地气不升而腹胀。邪气上乘于肺,则天气不降而心痛。盖腹者脾之部,肺者心之盖也。利大小便者,脾气上升,肺气下降,则水津四布,糟粕运行矣。补中者,补脾。益气者,益肺也。

170. Baihe〔百合, lily bulb, Bulbus Lilii〕

It is sweet in taste, mild and non-toxic in property, and it is mainly used to treat abdominal distension and the heart pain due to pathogenic qi, purge defecation, disinhibit urination, tonify the middle and replenish qi.

It grows everywhere in the nearby valleys. It sprouts in the third lunar month, with its seedlings growing up to two or three Chi tall. It has one stem growing straight upward with leaves similar to Zhuye〔竹叶, bamboo leaf, Lophatheri Folium〕or Liuye〔柳叶, willow leaf, Salicis Folium〕. Its leaves spread to four directions. It blossoms with fragrant white flowers growing at the end of the stem in the fifth lunar month. The flower has six petals hanging to four directions. It blooms during the day and closes at night, which is why it is called Yehehua〔夜合花, dwarf magnolia, Magnoliae Coco Flos〕. Its bulb is long, thin and white, similar to that of Suan〔蒜, garlic, Allii Sativi Bulbus〕, with twenty or thirty overlapping scale leaves, which tastes delicious when cooked. The method of planting it is similar to that of planting garlic which is to split the bulb and plant the leaves separately. The one whose flowers are red in color but do not hang down is called Shandan〔山丹, morningstar lily bulb, Lilii Concoloris Bulbus〕. The one, which has hanging red-yellow flowers with black spots and fruits growing between leaves and branches, is called Juandan (卷丹). Their bulbs are the same as Baihe (lily bulb), both of which can be cooked and eaten, but not delicious. They are the three different species under the same family. All three cannot be used as medicinal, except the one with white flowers.

Its color is white, which pertains to metal. Its taste is sweet, which pertains to earth. It blooms during the day and closes at night, which corresponds to the principle of the heaven that defense qi flows in the yang channel during the day and in the yin channel at night. The flowers hanging to four directions correspond to the fact that earth qi reaches its surroundings. It can mainly treat the abdominal distension and the heart pain, which are caused by the fact that pathogenic qi attacks the spleen downward, and earth qi can not ascend, resulting in abdominal distention. Pathogenic qi attacks the lung upward, and heaven qi cannot descend, resulting in heart pain. The above phenomena result separately from the abdomen being the location where yang brightness lies and the lung being the canopy of the heart. It can purge defecation and disinhibit urination, because spleen qi ascends, and lung qi descends, resulting in the distributing of water fluid all over the body and the moving of waste. Tonifying the middle is to tonify the spleen, and replenishing qi is to benefit the lung.

171. 干 姜

干姜 气味辛温,无毒。主治胸满咳逆上气,温中,止血,出汗,逐风湿痹,肠澼下痢,生者尤良。

干姜用母姜晒干,以肉厚而白净,结实明亮如天麻者为良,故又名白姜。临海、章安、汉温、池州诸处皆能作之,今江西、浙江皆有,而三衢开化者佳。

太阴为阴中之至阴,足太阴主湿土,手太阴主清金。干姜气味辛温,其色黄白,乃手足太阴之温品也。胸满者,肺居胸上,肺寒则满也。咳逆上气者,手足太阴之气不相通贯,致肺气上逆也。温中者,言干姜主治胸满咳逆上气,以其能温中也。脾络虚寒,则血外溢。干姜性温,故止血也。出汗者,辛以润之,开腠理,致津液通气也。逐风湿痹者,辛能发散也。肠澼下痢,乃脾脏虚寒。《伤寒论》云:脾气孤弱,五液注下,下焦不合,状如豚肝。干姜能温脾土,故治肠澼下痢。生者尤良,谓生姜能宣达胃气,用之尤良。

按:桂枝、葛根、柴胡诸汤,并胃逆呕吐,表寒诸证,多用生姜。夫生姜乃老姜所生之子姜,主宣达阳明胃土之气,阳明为太阴之府,故干姜治脾,生姜治胃,脏腑者,子母之谓也。

按:《神农本经》只有干姜、生姜,而无炮姜,后人以干姜炮黑,谓之炮姜。《金匮要略》治肺痿,用甘草干姜汤,其干姜亦炮,是炮姜之用,仲祖其先之矣。姜味本辛,炮过则辛味稍减,主治产后血虚身热,及里寒吐血,衄血,便血之证。若炮制太过,本质不存,谓之姜炭,其味微苦不辛,其质轻浮不实,又不及炮姜之功能矣。即用炮姜,亦必须三衢开化之母姜,始为有力。今药肆中多以伤水变味之生姜,晒干炮用,未免有名无实。

171. Ganjiang [干姜, dried ginger, Rhizoma Zingiberis]

It is pungent in taste, warm and non-toxic in property, and it is mainly used to relieve chest fullness, treat cough with dyspnea, descend adverse-rising qi, warm the middle, staunch bleeding, promote sweating, expel the impediment caused by wind and dampness, and treat dysentery and diarrhea. The raw one is especially effective.

Ganjiang (dried ginger) is actually dried Mujiang (母姜). As solid and clear as Tianma [天麻, tall gastrodia tuber, Rhizoma Gastrodiae], those having thick and white flesh are of good quality and are therefore also called Baijiang [白姜, dried ginger, Zingiberis Rhizoma]. It can be processed in Linhai (临海), Zhang'an (章安), Hanwen (汉温) and Chizhou (池州) and now grows everywhere in Jiangxi (江西) and Zhejiang (浙江). Those growing in Kaihua (开化) of Sanqu (三衢) are of better quality.

Greater yin is beginning of the yin of all yin, foot greater yin governs damp earth, and hand greater yin governs clear metal. Pungent in taste, mild in property, yellow-white in color, Ganjiang (dried ginger) is the one used for warming foot and hand greater yin. The lung is placed above the chest. Cold enters the lung, resulting in chest fullness. Cough with dyspnea will occur when the qi of hand great yin and foot great yin does not connect with each other, resulting in adverse-rising lung qi. Ganjiang (dried ginger) can mainly relieve chest fullness, treat cough with dyspnea and descend adverse-rising qi, for it can warm the middle. The deficiency cold of the spleen collateral can cause the external bleeding. It is warm in property, and thus it can staunch bleeding. It can promote sweating since its pungency can help achieve its nourishing effect, and thus it can open the striae and interstice, which will result in the free flow of liquid and qi. It can expel the impediment caused by wind and dampness, for pungency has the dissipating effect. Dysentery and diarrhea are caused by the deficiency cold of the spleen. *Shang Han Lun* [《伤寒论》, *Treatise on Cold Damage*] says, "Weak spleen qi can cause the uncontrolled flow of five kinds of fluid and the disharmony of the lower energizer. Blood condenses downward into the shape of a pig's liver." Ganjiang (dried ginger) can warm spleen earth, and thus it can treat dysentery and diarrhea. The raw one is especially effective. It is stated that Shengjiang [生姜, fresh ginger, Zingiberis Rhizoma Recens] can disinhibit lung qi, which is especially effective to be used as medicinal.

Note by Zhang Zhicong (张志聪): Shengjiang (fresh ginger) is mostly used in Guizhi Tang [桂枝汤, Cinnamon Twig Decoction], Gegen Tang [葛根汤, Pueraria Decoction] and Chaihu Tang [柴胡汤, Bupleurum Decoction] and in treating stomach qi ascending counterflow, vomiting and exterior cold. Shengjiang (fresh ginger) is the rhizome grown from Laojiang [老姜, old ginger, Zingiberis Rhizoma Vetum], which can mainly disinhibit the stomach earth qi of yang brightness. Yang brightness is the house of greater yin, thus Ganjiang (dried ginger) can treat the diseases of the spleen, and Shengjiang (fresh ginger) can treat those of the stomach. The relationship between the stomach and the spleen is like that between the mother and the son.

Note by Zhang Zhicong (张志聪): Ganjiang (dried ginger) and Shengjiang (fresh ginger), not Paojiang [炮姜, blast-fried ginger, Rhizoma Zingiberis Preparata], can be found in *Shen Nong Ben Cao Jing* [《神农本草经》, *Shennong's Classic of Materia Medica*]. People later on blast-fried Ganjiang (dried ginger) to make Paojiang (blast-fried ginger). It is recorded in *Jin Gui Yao Lüe* [《金匮要略》, *Synopsis of the Golden Chamber*] that Gancao Ganjiang Tang [甘草干姜汤, Licorice and Dried Ginger Decoction] can treat lung atrophy. Ganjiang (dried ginger) used in the decoction is blast-fried to make it have the same action as that of Paojiang (blast-fried ginger). Thus, Zhang Zhongjing (张仲景) has been the first man to record this use. Ginger is pungent in taste, and the blast-fried one will be less pungent. It can mainly treat postpartum blood-deficiency fever, interior cold, hematemesis, epistaxis and bloody stool. Ginger's essence will be lost when excessively blast-fried, and it will become Jiangtan（姜炭）later. Slightly bitter and not pungent in taste, Jiangtan（姜炭）is floating and light in nature, and its actions are inferior to those of Paojiang（blast-fried ginger）. It is necessary to use Mujiang（母姜）growing in Kaihua（开化）of Sanqu（三衢）to make Paojiang（blast-fried ginger）to guarantee its effect. Currently, businessmen running drug stores usually dry and blast-fry Shengjiang（fresh ginger）whose taste has been changed when processed in water, which has made Paojiang（blast-fried ginger）produced there exist in name only.

172. 赤小豆

赤小豆　气味甘酸平,无毒。主下水肿,排痈肿脓血。

赤豆出江淮间,今关西、河北、汴洛皆有,夏至后下种,苗科高尺许,枝叶似豇豆,至秋开花淡银褐色,有腐气,结荚长二三寸,皮色微白带红,豆如绿豆而色赤,可作粥饭,煮熟署黯,可作香豉入药,以紧小而赤黯者为良。豆谷类也,赤小豆乃赤豆之小者,今药肆中不知以何物,草子赤黑相间者,伪充赤小豆,其谬已甚。夫既名为豆,岂可于谷外求之耶。

赤豆煮熟,其味则甘,生时其气微酸,故曰甘酸平。豆者,水之谷也,其性下沉,是主从上而下,由外而内,色赤属火,又主从下而上,由内而外。《本经》主下水肿,乃从上而下,由外而内也。排痈肿脓血,乃从下而上,由内而外矣。

172. Chixiaodou〔赤小豆, rice bean, Phaseoli Semen〕

It is sweet and sour in taste, mild and non-toxic in property, and it is mainly used to resolve edema, and eliminate abscess and purulent blood.

Originally growing in Jianghuai（江淮）Region, now Chidou（rice bean）grows everywhere in Guanxi（关西）, Hebei（河北）, Bian and Luo（汴洛）area. Its seeds are sown after the Summer Solstice（夏至）, and its seedlings can be as tall as one Chi. Its branches and leaves are similar to those of Jiangdou〔豇豆, cowpea, Vignae Sinensis Semen〕. It blossoms in autumn with light silver-brown flowers, giving off rotten smells. Its pod, slightly white in color with a touch of red, can be as long as two or three Cun. Its bean, like Lüdou [绿豆, mung bean, Phaseoli Radiati Semen], is red in color, which can be used for cooking porridge and rice. Cover its beans until they turn all black while cooking them. They can be made into Xiangchi [香豉, fermented soybean, Sojae Semen Fermentatum] so as to be used as medicinal. It will be more effective to choose the small one which is dark red in color. Beans pertain to the grain, and Chixiaodu (rice bean) is the small kind of Chidou (rice bean). Businessmen running drug stores nowadays are using something unknown, a kind of red and black herb fruit, to fake Chixiaodou (rice bean). This kind of mistake has already been very severe. Since it is named Dou (bean), how can they use something even not pertaining to the grain to fake it?

The taste of Chidou (rice bean) is sweet when cooked, but it is slightly sour when raw, which is why it is said to be sweet and sour in taste and mild in property. The bean is the grain pertaining to water, which has a descending property, and thus it can mainly move from the upper to the lower and from the outside to the inside. It is red in color, and the red color pertains to fire, and thus it can also move from the lower to the upper and from the inside to the outside. *Shen Nong Ben Cao Jing* [《神农本草经》, *Shennong's Classic of Materia Medica*] says that it can mainly resolve edema, because it moves from the upper to the lower and from the outside to the inside. It can eliminate abscess and purulent blood, because it moves from the lower to the upper and from the inside to the outside.

173. 大豆黄卷

大豆黄卷 气味甘平,无毒。主治湿痹、筋挛、膝痛,不可屈伸。

黑大豆水浸出芽,约五寸长,使干之,名为黄卷。李时珍曰:一法壬癸日以井华水浸大豆,候生芽,取皮阴干用。

《金匮》薯蓣丸治虚劳不足,风气百疾,内用大豆黄卷,义可知矣。

173. Dadou Huangjuan [大豆黄卷, soybean sprout, Semen Glycines Siccus]

It is sweet in taste, mild and non-toxic in property, and it is mainly used to treat damp impediment, muscular spasm, the pain of the knees and the inability to bend and stretch.

Heidadou［黑大豆, black soybean, Sojae Semen Atrum］ will sprout when soaked in water. Dry the sprout when it grows to five Cun tall. The dried sprout is called Huangjuan（黄卷）. Li Shizhen（李时珍）said, "Another method of preparation：Soak Dadou［大豆, soybean, Sojae Semen］ in the first bucket of water fetched from the well in the morning on the Rengui （壬癸）Day until it sprouts. Dry its peel in the shade for medical use."

As recorded in *Jin Gui Yao Lüe*［《金匮要略》, *Synopsis of the Golden Chamber*］, consumptive diseases with insufficiency and all kinds of diseases caused by wind qi can be treated by Shuyu Wan［薯蓣丸, Dioscorea Pill］, with Dadou Huangjuan（soybean sprout）as its raw material. People can know the actions of Dadou Huangjuan（soybean sprout）from what has been mentioned above.

174. 白 薇

白薇 气味苦咸平,无毒。主治暴中风,身热肢满,忽忽不知人,狂惑邪气,寒热酸疼,温疟洗洗,发作有时。

白薇《本经》名春生,出陕西及舒、滁、润、辽诸处。其根黄白色,类牛膝,而短小柔软可曲者,白薇也。坚直易断者,白前也。《乘雅》云:根似牛膝而细长尺许,色黄微白,芳香袭人者,白薇也。色白微黄,折之易断者,白前也。

凡草木皆感春气而生,唯《本经》号白薇为春生。谓其能启水天之精气,随春气而生升也。其味苦咸,咸者水也。苦者火也。禀太阳寒水之气在下,标阳之气在上也。根色黄白,又得阳明秋金之气,而秋金之气,合肺气于皮毛,亦太阳之所主也。太阳标阳之气,行于肌表,故主治暴中风。太阳寒水之气,周于一身,故主治身热。肢满,风邪淫于四末也。忽忽,眩晕貌。忽忽不知人,风邪行于头目也。夫风者,百病之长,善行数变。狂惑邪气,风淫血分而涉于心包矣。寒热酸痛,风淫肌腠而涉于经脉矣。白薇禀秋金之气,故治诸风之变证。先热后寒,名曰温疟。温疟洗洗,如水洒身之寒也。温疟发作有时,白薇禀寒水之气,上行外达,故治温疟。又得太阳之标阳,故治温疟之洗洗。

174. Baiwei［白薇，blackend swallowwort root，
Radix Cynanchi Atrati］

It is bitter and salty in taste, mild and non-toxic in property, and it is mainly used to treat sudden wind stroke, fever and the distension of the limbs, unconsciousness, the mania due to pathogenic qi, cold-heat diseases and aching muscles as well as warm malaria with shivering occurring at set times.

It is mentioned as Chunsheng（春生）in *Shen Nong Ben Cao Jing*［《神农本草经》, *Shennong's Classic of Materia Medica*］. It originally grew in Shaanxi（陕西）, Shuzhou（舒州）, Chuzhou（滁州）, Runzhou（润州）and Liaozhou（辽州）. It has yellow-white roots similar to those of Niuxi［牛膝, achyranthes, Achyranthis Bidentatae Radix］. The root of Baiwei（blackend swallowwort root）is short, soft and bendable, and the root of Baiqian［白前, willowleaf rhizome, Rhizoma Cynanchi Stauntonii］is straight and easy to break. *Bencao Chengya Banji*［《本草乘雅半偈》, *Explanation on Materia Medica from Two Aspects*］says, "Its root is as thin as that of Niuxi（牛膝）, which is about one Chi long. Its root is yellow with a touch of white and fragrant, and the root of Baiqian（willowleaf rhizome）is white with a touch of yellow and easy to break when bended."

Plants all grow by sensing spring qi, but Baiwei（blackend swallowwort root）is the only one called Chunsheng（春生）in *Shen Nong Ben Cao Jing*［《神农本草经》, *Shennong's Classic of the Materia Medica*］, which demonstrates that it can not only activate the essential qi of water and heaven, but also grow and move upward along with spring qi. It is salty and bitter in taste. Saltiness pertains to water, and bitterness pertains to fire. It receives the qi of cold water from greater yang downward and the qi of branch yang upward. Its root is yellow-white in color and obtains the qi of autumn metal from yang brightness. The qi of autumn metal is in accordance with lung qi in the skin and the body hair, which are also governed by greater yang. The qi of branch yang from greater yang flows on the fleshy exterior, thus Baiwei（blackend swallowwort root）can mainly treat sudden wind stroke. The qi of cold water from greater yang flows through the whole body, thus it can mainly treat fever. The wind pathogen is excessive in the limbs, resulting in the distention of the limbs. Unconsciousness is actually vertigo. The wind pathogen flows in the head and eyes, resulting in unconsciousness. Wind is a primary factor responsible for all diseases and tends to move and change. The wind pathogen is excessive in the blood aspect, which involves the pericardium, resulting in mania. The pathogen is excessive in the skin, which involves the meridians, resulting in cold-heat diseases and aching muscles. Baiwei (blackend swallowwort root), having received the qi of autumn metal, can treat various complications caused by wind. Warm malaria is named like this because it is marked by fever followed by chills. People who suffer from warm malaria with shivering feel as cold as being spilled on by water. It occurs at set times. Baiwei (blackend swallowwort root) can treat warm malaria by receiving the qi of cold water, going upward and reaching outside. It can also treat the shivering due to warm malaria by receiving branch yang from greater yang.

175. 败 酱

败酱 气味苦平,无毒。主治暴热火疮赤气,疥瘙,疽痔,马鞍热气。

败酱俗名苦菜,处处原野皆有。春初生苗,深冬始凋,野人多食之。

败酱味苦性寒,故主治暴热火疮赤气,而疥瘙疽痔,马鞍热气,皆为火热之病。马者,火之畜也。《金匮》方有薏苡附子败酱散,亦主肠痈而消热毒。

175. Baijiang [败酱, patrinia, Patriniae Herba]

It is bitter in taste, mild and non-toxic in property, and it is mainly used to treat fulminant heat, burn with heat qi, scabies and itching, carbuncle and hemorrhoids, and the heat qi in the skin due to riding horse.

It is popularly called Kucai (苦菜) and grows everywhere on plains. It sprouts in early spring and begins to wither in late winter. People living in the wild tend to eat it.

It is bitter in taste and cold in property, and thus it can mainly treat fulminant heat and burn with heat qi. Scabies and itching, carbuncle and hemorrhoids, and the heat qi in the skin due to riding horses are all fire-heat diseases. Horses are the livestock pertaining to fire. As recorded in *Jin Gui Yao Lüe*〔《金匮要略》, *Synopsis of the Golden Chamber*〕, Yiyi Fuzi Baijiang San〔薏苡附子败酱散, Coix, Aconite and Patrinia Powder〕can be used to treat intestinal abscess and eliminate heat toxin.

176. 白藓根皮

白藓根皮　气味苦寒,无毒。主治头风,黄疸,咳逆,淋沥,女子阴中肿痛,湿痹死肌,不可屈伸起止行步。

白藓出河中江宁、滁洲、润州皆有之,以川蜀者为胜。苗高尺余,茎青叶稍白,四月开花紫白色,根皮白色,根心内实,其气腥膻。

白藓臭腥色白,气味苦寒,禀金水之精,而治风热之证。主治头风,金能制风也。治黄疸,水能清热也。禀金气而益肺,故治咳逆。禀水气而益膀胱,故治男子淋沥,女子之阴中肿痛。燥气属金,故治湿痹之死肌。水气主骨,故治骨属不可屈伸,及不可起止行步也。

176. Baixian Genpi〔白藓根皮, dictamnus root bark, Cortex Dictamni〕

It is bitter in taste, cold and non-toxic in property, and it is mainly used to treat head wind, jaundice, cough with dyspnea, stranguria, the swelling and pain of the vulva, damp impediment, the numbness of the muscles and the inability to bend, stretch and walk.

Baixian〔白藓, dictamnus, Dictamnus dasycarpus Turcz〕grows in Hezhong（河中）, Jiangning（江宁）, Chuzhong（滁洲）and Runzhou（润州）, and those growing in Chuanshu（川蜀）are of better quality. It has seedlings which are about one Chi tall, a blue-green stem and slightly white leaves. It blossoms in the fourth lunar month with purple-white flowers. Its root bark is white in color, and its root is solid. It root smells stinky and has the smell of mutton.

Stinky in smell and white in color, bitter in taste and cold in property,

Baixian Genpi (dictamnus root bark) receives the essence of metal and water, and thus it can treat wind-heat diseases. It can mainly treat head wind, for metal can control wind. It can treat jaundice, for water can clear heat. It receives metal qi to benefit the lung, and thus it can treat cough with dyspnea. It receives water qi to benefit the bladder, so it can treat male stranguria and the swelling and pain of the vulva. Dryness qi pertains to metal, and thus it can treat damp impediment and the numbness of the muscles. Water qi governs the bones, and thus it can treat the inability to bend, stretch and walk, which are all bone diseases.

177. 蓼 实

蓼实 气味辛温,无毒。主治明目,温中,耐风寒,下水气,面浮肿,痈疡。

蓼近水滨及下湿处皆有,其类甚多,有青蓼、香蓼、水蓼、马蓼、紫蓼、赤蓼、木蓼七种。又一种味极辛辣,谓之辣蓼。今时浸水和面,暑面是为神曲,又取燥末拌糯米饭一团,作酵造酒,而诸蓼与实用之者鲜矣。

177. Liaoshi〔蓼实, water pepper fruit, Polygoni Hydropiperis Fructus〕

It is pungent in taste, warm and non-toxic in property, and it is mainly used to improve vision, warm the middle, resist wind cold, purge the retention of water, relieve facial edema and resolve abscess and ulcer.

It grows everywhere near the shore and in the wet low-lying places. It has many kinds, seven of which are Qingliao (青蓼), Xiangliao (香蓼), Shuiliao (水蓼), Maliao (马蓼), Ziliao (紫蓼), Chiliao (赤蓼) and Muliao (木蓼). Another extremely pungent kind is called Laliao (辣蓼). Currently, soak it in water, knead the dough with it, cover the dough, and then Shenqu〔神曲, medicated leaven, Massa Medicata Fermentata〕is made. Or dry it, grind it into powder, mix the powder with sticky rice, knead the mixture into a ball and ferment the ball to make liquor. However, there are fewer and fewer Liaoshi (water pepper fruit) along with its practical applications.

178. 薇 衔

薇衔 气味苦平,无毒。主治风湿痹,历节痛,惊痫,吐舌,悸气,贼风,鼠瘘,痈肿。薇音眉。

薇衔生汉中川泽及冤句,邯郸。丛生,叶似芃蔚。有毛赤茎,《本经》名麋衔,一名鹿衔,言麋鹿有疾,衔此草即瘥也。又名吴风草。李时珍曰:按郦道元《水经注》云:魏兴、锡山多生薇衔草,有风不偃,无风独摇,则吴风当作无风乃通。

按:月令五月鹿角解,十一月麋角解,是麋鹿有阴阳之分矣。此草禀少阴水火之气,是以麋鹿咸宜,犹乌药之治猫狗也。《素问》黄帝问曰:有病身热懈惰,汗出如浴,恶风少气,此为何病? 岐伯曰:病名酒风,治之以泽泻、术各三分,麋衔五分,合以三指撮,为后饭后饭,先服药也。此圣方也。而后世不知用之,诚缺典矣。

178. Meixian [薇衔, Pyrola, Pyrolae Herba]

It is bitter in taste, mild and non-toxic in property, and it is mainly used to treat wind-dampness impediment, agonizing multiple arthralgia, fright epilepsy, protruding tongue, palpitation, the diseases caused by the abnormal weather, scrofula, and abscesses and swelling. 薇 should be pronounced as Mei (眉).

Meixian (Pyrola) grows in mountains and near waters in Hanzhong (汉中), and in Yuanju (冤句) and Handan (邯郸). It grows in dense tufts. Its leaves look like those of Chongwei [芃蔚, leonurus fruit, Leonuri Fructus], and its stem is red and hairy. It is called Mixian (麋衔) and Luxian [鹿衔, Pyrola, Pyrolae Herba] in *Shen Nong Ben Cao Jing* [《神农本草经》, *Shennong's Classic of Materia Medica*], which says that holding the herb in the mouth could help elks recover from illness. It is also known as Wufengcao (吴风草). Li Shizhen (李时珍) said, "According to *Shui Jing Zhu* [《水经注》, *Commentary to the River Classic*] by Li Daoyuan (郦道元), it grows mainly in Weixing (魏兴) and Xishan (锡山). It does not fall in wind but sways without wind. Then, Wufeng (吴风) is regarded as no wind."

Note by Gao Shishi（高世栻）: *Yue Ling*［《月令》, *The Phenology of Lunar Month*］says that deer shed their antlers in the fifth lunar month and elks in the eleventh lunar month. Hence, elks and deer pertain to yin and yang respectively. It receives the qi of water and fire from lesser yin, and it is suitable for both elks and deer, just as Wuyao［乌药, lindera, Linderae］for both cats and dogs. In *Huang Di Nei Jing: Su Wen*［《黄帝内经·素问》, *Huangdi's Internal Classic: Plain Questions*］, Huangdi asked, "What is the disease marked by body fever, the lassitude of limbs, profuse sweating, aversion to wind and shortness of breath?" Qibo answered, "It is called Jiufeng［酒风, Alcohol-Wind］. It can be treated by Zexie［泽泻, water plantain rhizome, Rhizoma Alismatis］（three Fen）, Baizhu［白术, white atractylodes rhizome, Rhizoma Atractylodis Macrocephalae］（three Fen）and Mixian（麋衔）（five Fen）, which are ground into powder to be taken three pinches before each meal." It is a very effective formula, but unfortunately it was seldom used by later generations due to lack of recordation.

179. 土瓜根

土瓜根 气味苦寒,无毒。主治消渴、内痹、瘀血、月闭、寒热酸疼,益气,愈聋。

> 土瓜《本经》名王瓜,俗名野甜瓜。月令云:四月王瓜生,即此瓜也。始生鲁地平泽田野及人家墙垣篱落间,四月生苗延蔓。其蔓多须叶,如瓜蒌叶,但无叉缺,有毛刺。五月开黄花,花下结子,熟时赤如弹丸,根如瓜蒌,根之小者,须掘深二三尺,乃得正根。三月采根,阴干候用。

> 愚按:土瓜非世俗所食之王瓜,又非世俗所食之甜瓜。《本经》虽有其名,今人未之识也。因仲景《伤寒论》有土瓜根为导之法,故存之。

> 按:月令所谓王瓜者,蔓延而生,茎叶上皆有细毛,其叶圆而上尖,一叶之下辄有一须,遇草木茎叶即能缠绕。六七月开花色黄五瓣,花下蒂长,即其实也。吾杭甚多,凡旷野隙地遍处有之,民间往往认作瓜蒌,高氏以为今人未之识者,盖以此故耳。

179. Tuguagen［土瓜根, cucumber gourd root, Trichosanthis Cucumeroidis Radix］

It is bitter in taste, cold and non-toxic in property, and it is mainly used to treat consumptive thirst, internal impediment, blood stasis, amenorrhea, cold and heat and the ache of the limbs, replenish qi and cure deafness.

Tugua (cucumber gourd) is called Wanggua (王瓜) in *Shen Nong Ben Cao Jing* [《神农本草经》, *Shennong's Classic of Materia Medica*], also popularly known as wild melon. *Yueling* [《月令》, *The Phenology of Lunar Month*] says that Wanggua (王瓜) grows in the fourth lunar month, which is actually Tugua (cucumber gourd). It originally grows in the wild and the plain wetland in Lu area (鲁地), and among courtyards and fences of houses. It sprouts seedlings and vines in the fourth lunar month. Its vine has lots of hairs and its leaves are like those of Gualuo [瓜蒌, snakegourd fruit, Trichosanthes kirilowii Maxim]. It has burrs but no branches. It blossoms yellow in the fifth lunar month. It bears fruits after the withering of flowers, which are as red as shooting balls when ripening. Its root is like that of Gualuo (snakegourd fruit), and it's so tiny that the taproot can only be dug out two or three Chi underground. Its root will be collected in the third lunar month and dried in the shade for future use.

Note by Zhang Zhicong (张志聪): Tugua (cucumber gourd) is neither Wanggua (王瓜) nor melon, both of which are commonly eaten. Few recognize it nowadays although it is recorded in *Shen Nong Ben Cao Jing* [《神农本草经》, *Shennong's Classic of Materia Medica*]. It has been passed down due to *Shang Han Lun* [《伤寒论》, *Treatise on Exogenous Febrile Diseases*] by Zhang Zhongjing (张仲景) in which its root is used as efficacy enhancer added to medicine.

Note by Gao Shishi (高世栻): Wanggua (王瓜) recorded in *Yue Ling* [《月令》, *The Phenology of Lunar Month*] grows with its vines spreading outwards and fine hairs in both stems and leaves, and its leaves are round and pointed in the upper part. A fibrous root is always under each leaf and intertwines with whatever plant it meets. It blossoms yellow with five-petal flowers in the sixth and seventh lunar months, and the fruits grow after the withering of flowers. It is very common in Hangzhou（杭州）and grows everywhere in the wild and open field. It is usually mistaken for Gualuo（snakegourd fruit）, which, according to Gao's（高氏）, may be the reason why nobody recognizes it nowadays.

180. 厚 朴

厚朴 气味苦温,无毒。主治中风,伤寒,头痛寒热,惊悸,气血痹,死肌,去三虫。

厚朴取其木质朴而皮厚以命名,一名烈朴,又名赤朴,谓其性辛烈而色紫赤也。洛阳、陕西、江淮、河南、川蜀山谷中,往往有之,近以建平、宜都及梓州、龙州者为上。木高三四丈,径一二尺,肉皮极厚,以色紫油湿润者为佳,春生叶如槲叶,四季不凋,五六月开红花,结实如冬青子,生青熟赤,实中有核,其味甘美。厚朴之实,别名逐折。《别录》云:主疗鼠瘘,明目,益气。

厚朴气味苦温,色赤性烈,花实咸红,冬不落叶,肉厚色紫,盖禀少阳木火之精,而通会于肌腠者也。主治中风伤寒头痛寒热者,谓能解肌而发散也。助木火之精气,故能定肝心之惊悸也。气血痹者,津液随三焦出气以温肌肉,肝主冲任之血,充肤热肉,痹则气血不和于肌腠。厚朴气温色紫,能解气血之痹而活死肌也。去三虫者,三焦火气内虚,则生虫。厚朴得少阳之火化,而三虫自去矣。

愚按:厚朴色赤性烈,生用则解肌而达表,禀木火之气也。炙香则运土而助脾,木生火而火生土也。《金匮》方中厚朴大黄汤,用厚朴一尺,取象乎脾也。

180. Houpo〔厚朴, magnolia bark, Cortex Magnoliae Officinalis〕

It is bitter in taste, warm and non-toxic in property, and it is mainly used to treat wind stroke, cold damage, headache, chills and fever, fright palpitation, qi and blood impediment and necrotic muscles, and eliminate three worms.

Houpo（magnolia bark）is named for its plain wood and thick bark, also known as Liepo（烈朴）and Chipo（赤朴）for it is acrid and drying in property and purplish red in color. It grows in the mountain valleys of Luoyang

（洛阳）, Shaanxi（陕西）, Jianghuai（江淮）, Henan（河南）, and Sichuan（四川）. In recent years, those growing in Jianping（建平）, Yidu（宜都）, Zizhou（梓州）and Longzhou（龙州）are of the best quality. It is three or four Zhang in height and one or two Chi in diameter. Its bark and flesh are extremely thick, and the oil-infused one in purple color is the best in quality. Its leaves sprout out in spring like oak leaves and stay green all the year round. It blossoms red in the fifth and sixth lunar months. Its fruits, like Dongqingzi［冬青子, Chinese ilex, Ilicis Chinensis Semen］, are green at first and turn red when ripening, which have kernels inside and taste sweet. Its fruit is also called Zhuzhe（逐折）. *Ming Yi Bie Lu*［《名医别录》, *Miscellaneous Records of Famous Physicians*］says that it is mainly used to treat scrofula, improve vision, and replenish qi.

Houpo（magnolia bark）is bitter in taste, warm and drying in property, and red in color. Both its flowers and fruits are red, its leaves stay green in winter, and its flesh is thick and purple in color. It receives the essence of wood and fire from lesser yang and can reach the interstices of the flesh. It can mainly treat the syndromes of wind stroke, cold damage, headache and chills and fever, because it can release the flesh and has the effect of dispersing. It can relieve liver and heart fright palpitation, because it assists the essence of wood and fire. Body fluids warm the muscles with the triple energizer discharging qi, the liver governs Chongren blood to fill the skin and warm the flesh, so qi and blood impediment leads to qi and blood disharmony in the interstices of the flesh. Warm in property and purple in color, it can resolve the qi and blood impediment, and invigorate necrotic muscles. When the triple energizer is deficient in fire qi, worms appear. It gets fire transformation from lesser yang, so it can eliminate three worms.

Note by Zhang Zhicong（张志聪）: Houpo（magnolia bark）, drying in property and red in color, can release the flesh and expel the pathogen from the exterior when the raw one is used, for it receives the qi of wood and fire. After stir-fried with liquid adjuvant, it can transport earth to assist the spleen, for wood generates fire and fire generates earth. Houbo Dahuagn Tang［厚朴大黄汤, Magnolia Bark Rhubarb Decoction］in *Jin Gui Yao Lue*［《金匮要略》, *Synopsisof Golden Chamber*］uses Houpo（magnolia bark）of one Chi in length, as it has the same image as the spleen.

181. 黄 檗

黄檗 气味苦寒,无毒。主治五脏肠胃结热,黄疸,肠痔,止泄痢,女子漏下赤白,阴伤蚀疮。檗,音百,俗作黄柏,省笔之讹。

　　黄檗木出汉中山谷及永昌、邵陵、房商、山东诸处皆有。今以蜀中出者,皮厚色深为佳,树高数丈,叶似紫椿,经冬不凋,皮外白里深黄色,入药用其根结块,如松下茯苓。

　　黄檗气味苦寒,冬不落叶,禀太阳寒水之精。皮厚色黄,质润稠粘,得太阴中土之化。盖水在地之下,水由地中行,故主治五脏肠胃中之结热,黄疸,肠痔。治结热者,寒能清热也。治黄疸、肠痔者,苦能胜湿也。止泄痢者,先热泄而后下痢,黄柏苦寒,能止之也。女子漏下赤白,阴伤蚀疮,皆湿热下注之病。苦胜湿而寒清热,故黄檗皆能治之也。以上主治,皆正气无亏,热毒内盛,所谓下者举之,结者散之,热者寒之,强者泻之,各安其气,必清必静,则病气衰气,归其所宗,此黄檗之治皆有余之病也。如正气稍虚,饮食不强,便当禁用。

　　愚按:黄檗禀寒水之精,得中土之化,有交济阴阳,调和水火之功,所治至广。而《真珠囊药性》云:黄檗疮用,一言蔽之。后人从事歌括者,信为疮药而已。其曰真珠,殆以鱼目欺世尔。

181. Huangbo [黄檗, root of Chinese mahonia, Radix Mahoniae]

It is bitter in taste, cold and non-toxic in property, and it is mainly used to treat the heat binding in the five zang-organs and in the stomach and intestines, jaundice, intestinal hemorrhoids, diarrhea and dysentery, the metrostaxis with red and white vaginal liquid, and the eroding sore due to genital ulceration. 檗 should be pronounced as bo (百). The herb is also popularly and mistakenly called Huangbo (黄柏) for the sake of convenience.

Huangbo (root of Chinese mahonia) grows in the mountain valleys of Hanzhong (汉中) and in Yongchang (永昌), Shaoling (邵陵), Fangshang (房商) and Shandong (山东). Those growing in Shuzhou (蜀中) is of the best quality with thick bark and dark color. The tree is several Zhang tall; its leaves are like those of Zichun (紫椿) and stay green in winter; its bark is white externally and dark-yellow internally; its rhizome is used as medicinal, like Fuling

［伏苓, poria sclerotium, Wolfiporia Cocos］growing under pine trees.

It is bitter in taste and cold in property, its leaves never fall in winter, and it receives the essence of cold water from greater yang. Its bark being thick, its color being yellow and its property being smooth and viscous, it gets the transformation of center earth from greater yin. It can mainly treat the heat binding in the five zang-organs and the stomach and intestines, jaundice and intestinal hemorrhoids because water is under the ground and runs through the ground. It treats heat binding because cold can clear heat. It treats jaundice and intestinal hemorrhoids because bitterness can predominate dampness. It checks diarrhea and dysentery, because being bitter and cold, it can discharge heat first and then purge dysentery. Both the metrostaxis with red and white vaginal liquid and the eroding sore due to genital ulceration are caused by damp-heat pouring down. Bitterness can predominate dampness and cold can clear heat, so it can treat these diseases. For the above diseases, healthy qi is sufficient and heat toxin is exuberant inside. It is said that diseases should be treated based on the following methods: treating fallen by raising, treating the pathogenic accumulation with dissipation, treating the heat with cold, treating the excess with purgation. Each method is responsible for tranquilizing healthy qi, making it undisturbed, thus Bingqi and Shuaiqi will decline and return to the due positions. Thus, the diseases treated by Huangbo (root of Chinese mahonia) all belong to the repletion pattern. If health qi is a little deficient and appetite is poor, it is forbidden to be used.

Note by Zhang Zhicong (张志聪): Huangbo (root of Chinese mahonia) receives the essence of cold water and gets the transformation of center earth. It can coordinate yin and yang, and harmonize water and fire, so it can treat wide varieties of diseases. Nevertheless, *Zhen Zhu Nang Yao Xing* [《真珠囊药性》, *Pouch of Pearls*] says that it could only be used to treat sores. The later generations engaged in putting formulas into verses just took it for granted. Thus, the book which calls itself as valuable as a pearl actually misleads the public.

182. 卮 子

卮子　气味苦寒,无毒。主治五内邪气,胃中热气,面赤,酒疱皶鼻,白癞,赤癞,疮疡。

　　卮,酒器也,卮子象之,故名,俗作栀。《本经》谓之木丹,《别录》谓之越桃,今南方及西蜀州郡皆有之。木高七八尺,叶如李,厚而深绿,春荣夏茂,凌冬不凋,五月花开,花皆六出,洁白芬芳,交秋结实,如诃子状,生青,熟则黄赤,其中仁穰亦红赤,入药宜用山卮子,皮薄而圆小,刻房七棱至九棱者为佳。李时珍曰:蜀中有红栀子,花烂红色,其实染物亦赭红色。

栀子气味苦寒,其色黄赤,春荣夏茂,凌冬不凋,盖禀少阴之气化。少阴寒水在下,而君火在上也。花多五瓣,而栀花六出。六者水之成数也。稍秒结实,味苦色赤,房刻七棱九棱,是下禀寒水之精,而上结君火之实。主治五内邪气,胃中热气者,禀寒水之精,而治热之在内也。面赤,酒疱鼻,白癞,赤癞,疮疡者,结君火之实,而治热之在外也。栀子能启寒水之精,清在上之火热,复能导火热之气以下降者,如此。

　　栀子生用能起水阴之气上滋,复导火热以下行,若炒黑则但从上而下,不能起水阴以上滋,故仲祖栀子豉汤生用不炒,有交姤水火,调和心肾之功。而后人委言栀子生用则吐,炒黑则不吐,且以栀子豉汤为吐剂。愚每用生栀及栀子豉汤,并未曾吐。夫不参经旨,而以讹传讹者,不独一栀子为然矣。

182. Zhizi [卮子, fruit of cape jasmine, Fructus Gardeniae]

It is bitter in taste, cold and non-toxic in property, and it is mainly used to treat the diseases in the five zang-organs caused by pathogenic qi, the severe heat in the stomach, red face, rosacea, white leprosy, red leprosy, sore and ulcer.

　　The Chinese character "卮" (zhi) means a liquor vessel. Zhizi (fruit of cape jasmine) gets its name because it is like a wine vessel, also popularly known as Zhi (栀). It is called Mudan (木丹) in *Shen Nong Ben Cao Jing* [《神农本草经》, *Shennong's Classic of Materia Medica*] and Yuetao (越桃) in *Ming Yi Bie Lu* [《名医别录》, *Miscellaneous Records of Famous Physicians*], which grows in the south and the areas in Xishu (西蜀). Its tree is seven or eight Chi in height. Its leaves, like those of the plum tree, are thick and dark green, which grow in spring, flourish in summer and stay green in winter. It blossoms in May, its flowers having six petals, white and fragrant. As autumn sets in, it bears fruits in the same shape as Hezi [诃子, medicine terminalia fruit,

Fructus Chebulae], which are green at first and turn yellow-red when ripening. Both of its fruit meat and seeds inside are red. Shan Zhizi [山栀子, gardenia, Gardeniae Fructus] which are round, small and thin-skinned should be used as medicinal. Those with seven-edge or nine-edge porocalyx are of the best quality. Li Shenzhen (李时珍) said, "Hong Zhizi (红栀子) grows in Sichuan (四川). It has red and brilliant flowers, and its fruits can be used as crimson dye."

Bitter in taste, cold in property and yellow-red in color, Zhizi (fruit of cape jasmine) grows in spring, flourishes in summer and stays green in winter. It receives the qi transformation from lesser yin. The cold water from lesser yin is in the lower while the sovereign fire is in the upper. In contrast to most flowers with five petals, its flowers have six petals and six is the figure constituting water. It bears fruits shortly after the flowers. Its fruits are bitter in taste, red in color, and have seven-edge or nine-edge porocalyx. Thus, it receives the essence of cold water in the lower and produces fruits of the sovereign fire in the upper. It can mainly treat the diseases in the five zang-organs caused by pathogenic qi, the severe heat in the stomach, because it receives the essence of cold water to clear the internal heat. It can treat red face, rosacea, white leprosy, red leprosy, sore and ulcer, because it bears fruits of the sovereign fire to clear the external heat. Therefore, it can clear the fire-heat in the upper by taking advantage of the essence of cold water and also the guide qi of fire-heat downward.

When the raw one is used, Zhizi (fruit of cape jasmine) can guide the qi of Shuiyin upward to nourish the body and also guide fire-heat downward. When stir-fried black, it can only act from upward to downward and fails to guide the qi of Shuiyin upward to nourish the body. Hence, Zhongzu (仲祖) used the raw one in Zhizi Chi Tang [栀子豉汤, Gardenia and Fermented Soybean Decoction], which has the effects of coordinating water and fire, and harmonizing the heart and the kidney. The later generations have said that the raw one makes people vomit while the stir-fired one does not and regarded Zhizi Chi Tang [栀子豉汤, Gardenia and Fermented Soybean Decoction] as an emetic formula. However, when I use them, I never vomit. They didn't understand what the medical canon really meant and spread false information. Zhizi (fruit of cape jasmine) is not the only medicinal that suffers this fate.

183. 杏 仁

杏仁 气味甘苦温,冷利,有小毒。主治咳逆上气,雷鸣,喉痹,下气,产乳,金疮,寒心奔豚。

杏叶似梅,二月开淡红花,五月实熟有数种,赭色而圆者,名金杏。甘而有沙者,名沙杏,黄而带酢者,名梅杏。青而带黄者,名柰杏,入药用苦杏。

杏仁气味甘苦,其实苦重于甘,其性带温,其质冷利。冷利者,滋润之意,主治咳逆上气者,利肺气也。肺气利而咳逆上气自平矣。雷鸣者,邪在大肠。喉痹者,肺窍不利。下气者,谓杏仁质润下行,主能下气。气下则雷鸣,喉痹皆愈矣。产乳者,产妇之乳汁也。生产无乳,杏仁能通之。金疮者,金刃伤而成疮也。金伤成疮,杏仁能敛之。寒心奔豚者,肾脏水气凌心而寒,如豚上奔。杏仁治肺,肺者金也,金为水之母,母能训子逆。又,肺气下行,而水逆自散矣。

183. Xingren [杏仁, apricot seed, Semen Armeniacae Amarum]

It is sweet and bitter in taste, warm, cold-purgation and slightly toxic in property, and it is mainly used to treat the cough with dyspnea, the thunderous sound in the throat and throat impediment, descend qi, promote lactation, and treat the sores caused by the incised wound, the pathogenic cold that damages the heart like running pig.

With its leaves like those of the plum, it blossoms light red in the second lunar month. Its fruits get ripe in the fifth lunar month and are of several types: those round and red-brown are called Jinxing (金杏), those sweet and with sand-like meat Shaxing (沙杏), those yellow and sour Meixing (梅杏), those yellow-green Naixing (柰杏). Kuxing (苦杏) is used as medicinal.

Xingren (apricot seed) tastes sweet and bitter, and apricot tastes more bitter than sweet. Xingren (apricot seed) is warm in property and cold-purgation in nature. Cold-purgation means moistening. It can mainly treat the cough with dyspnea, because it can promote the function of lung qi. The thunderous sound in the throat is caused by the pathogen in the large intestine, and throat impediment is caused by the dysfunction of the lung orifice. Being moistening in nature and having the effect of descending, it can descend qi, which in turn cures the thunderous sound in the throat and throat impediment. In addition, it can help women who have just given birth to promote lactation. Incised wound is the injury caused by metal. It can heal up the sores caused by incised wound. As for pathogenic cold that damages the heart like running pig, fluid retention in kidney attacks and damages the heart, just like the pig running upward. Xingren (apricot seed) governs the lung which is metal in nature. Metal is the mother of water and mother can discipline son. Thus, when lung qi is descending, water counterflow will dissipate naturally.

184. 桃 仁

桃仁 气味苦甘平,无毒。主治瘀血血闭,症瘕邪气,杀小虫。

　　桃种类颇多,唯山中野毛桃即《尔雅》所谓榹桃者,小而多毛,核粘味恶,其仁充满多脂,可入药用。

　　桃仁、杏仁味俱甘苦,杏仁苦胜,故曰甘苦,桃仁甘胜,故曰苦甘。桃色先青后紫,其味甘酸,禀木气也,其仁亦主疏肝,主治瘀血血闭,疏肝气也。症瘕邪气乃血与寒汁沫,留聚於肠胃之外,凝结而为症瘕,肝气和平,则症瘕邪气自散矣。杀小虫者,厥阴风胜则生虫,肝气疏通而虫自杀矣。

　　《素问》五果所属,以桃属金,为肺之果,后人有桃为肺果,其仁治肝之说。

　　愚按:桃味酸甘,其色生青熟紫,并无金体,窃疑《素问》之桃,乃胡桃也,俗名核桃,外壳内白,庶几似之。若谓桃,则唯毛桃仁之桃,皮色白有毛,余俱无矣。生时肉青白,熟则紫矣。若以外核内仁当之,则杏梅未始不如是,献疑于此,俟后贤正之。

184. Taoren〔桃仁, peach seed, Semen Persicae〕

It is bitter and sweet in taste, mild and non-toxic in property, and it is mainly used to treat static blood, blood block, the abdominal mass caused by pathogenic qi, and kill small worms.

　　Peaches are of wide varieties. However, only the wild peaches growing in mountains, also called Zitao (榹桃) in Er Ya [《尔雅》, On Elegance], can be used as medicinal. They are small, hairy and awful in taste, having sticky nuclei and plump, fatty seeds.

Xingren [杏仁, apricot seed, Semen Armeniacae Amarum] and Taoren (peach seed) are both sweet and bitter in taste. However, bitterness predominates in the former, so it is sweet-bitter while sweetness predominates in the latter, so it is bitter-sweet. Green at first then turning purple in color, and sweet and sour in taste, it receives wood qi. Taoren (peach seed) is effective in soothing the liver so it can mainly treat static blood and blood block to soothe liver qi. The blood and cold body fluid gathering outside the stomach and intestines causes pathogenic qi which congeals into abdominal mass. If liver qi is in harmony, then pathogenic qi will dissipate naturally. Worms will appear when reverting yin wind predominates and they will be killed when liver qi is freed.

According to Huang Di Nei Jing: Su Wen [《黄帝内经·素问》, Huangdi's Internal Classic: Plain Questions], among the five fruits, peach pertains to metal and it is the fruit of lung. Therefore, the later generations have held the view that peach is the fruit of the lung, and its seeds can be used to treat the diseases of the liver.

Note by Zhang Zhicong (张志聪): Peach, sour and sweet in taste, green at first and turning purple when ripening, is not like metal. I guess the peach mentioned in Huang Di Nei Jing: Su Wen [《黄帝内经·素问》, Huangdi's Internal Classic: Plain Questions] is Hutao [胡桃, walnut, Juglandis], popularly known as Hetao [核桃, walnut, Juglandis Semen], which has hard shell outside and white seeds inside, almost like metal. As for peach, the only metal-like peach is the one called Maotaoren (毛桃仁) with white skin and hair. It is green-white at first and turns purple when ripening. If the shell outside and the kernel inside decided the nature of a fruit, then apricot and plum would also pertain to metal. Actually, they don't. Here, I raise my doubts in hope that the virtuous people can correct it in the future.

185. 桃 胶 附

桃胶 附　气味苦平,无毒。炼服保中不饥,忍风寒。《别录》附。

桃茂盛时,以刀割树皮,久则胶溢出,采收以桑灰汤浸过晒干用。

185. Taojiao〔桃胶, peach resin, Persicae Resina〕 *supplement*

It is is bitter in taste, mild and non-toxic in property. Taking refined Taojiao (peach resin) can preserve central qi and enable people to tolerate hunger and cold wind. Supplemented in *Ming Yi Bie Lu*〔《名医别录》, *Miscellaneous Records of Famous Physicians*〕.

When the peach is flourishing, cut the bark with a knife and Taojiao (peach resin) will flow out after some time. After collected, it will be steeped in the mulberry ash decoction and dried in the sun for future use.

186. 乌　梅

乌梅　气味酸温平涩,无毒。主治下气,除热,烦满,安心,止肢体痛,偏枯不仁,死肌,去青黑志,蚀恶肉。志痣同。

梅实将熟时,采微黄者,篮盛于突上熏黑,若以稻灰淋汁,润湿蒸过,则肥泽不蛀。

梅花放于冬,而实熟于夏,独得先春之气,故其味酸,其气温平而涩,涩附于酸也。主下气者,得春生肝木之味,生气上升,则逆气自下矣。除热烦满者,禀冬令水阴之精,水精上滋,则烦热除而胸膈不满矣。安心者,谓烦热除而胸膈不满,则心气亦安。肢体痛,偏枯不仁,死肌,皆阳气虚微,不能熏肤充身泽毛,若雾露之溉。梅实结于春而熟于夏,主敷布阳气于肌腠,故止肢体痛,及偏枯不仁之死肌。阳气充达,则其颜光,其色鲜,故去面上之青黑痣,及身体虫蚀之恶肉。

愚按:乌梅味酸,得东方之木味,放花于冬,成熟于夏,是禀冬令之水精而得春生之上达也。后人不体经义,不穷物理,但以乌梅为酸敛收涩之药,而春生上达之义未之讲也,惜哉。

186. Wumei〔乌梅, mume, Mume Fructus〕

It is sour in taste, warm, mild, astringent and non-toxic in property, and it is mainly used to descend qi, relieve fever, vexation and fullness, tranquilize the heart, treat the pain of the limbs, hemiplegia and necrotic muscles, and remove bluish black spots and malign flesh. 志 means 痣 (Zhi).

When plums are about to ripen, pick the yellowish ones in the basket and hang it above the chimney to blacken them. If drizzled with rice ash liquid, moistened and steamed, plums will become plump and moist, without being damaged by worms.

The plum blossoms in winter and ripens in summer. It exclusively obtains the qi of early spring, so its taste is sour and its property is warm, mild and astringent, astringency attached to sourness. Wumei (mume) can mainly descend qi because it obtains the liver-wood flavor of spring resuscitation. When vital qi goes upward, conterflow qi will descend naturally. It can relieve fever, vexation and fullness because it receives the essence of water yin in winter. When water essence goes upward and nourishes the body, fever and vexation will be eliminated, and the chest and diaphragm will not feel full any longer. It can tranquilize the heart because when fever, vexation and fullness are relieved, heart qi will also be quieted. The pain of the limbs, hemiplegia and necrotic muscles are all caused by the debilitation of yang qi which, just like the fog and dew to moisturize the earth, is too weak to fumigate the skin, fill the body and moisturize the hair. Plums, growing in spring and ripening in summer, apply yang qi to the interstices of the flesh, thus it can treat the pain of the limbs, hemiplegia, and necrotic muscles. If yang qi is sufficient, the face will become shiny and bright, so it can remove bluish black spots and malign flesh that worms have eaten into.

Note by Zhang Zhicong (张志聪): Wumei (mume) is sour in taste for it obtains the liver-wood flavor. It blossoms in winter and ripens in summer for it receives the water essence of winter and obtains the vital qi of spring which moves upward. The later generations who don't understand the true meaning of medical canons and can't find out the nature of things only regard it as a sour and astringent medicinal, ignoring its obtaining the vital qi of spring which moves upward. It is really a pity.

187. 枳 实

枳实 气味苦寒,无毒。主治大风在皮肤中,如麻豆苦痒,除寒热结,止痢,长肌肉,利五脏,益气,轻身。

本 草 崇 原

Reverence for the Origin of Materia Medica

枳实出河内洛西及江湖州郡皆有。近时出于江西者为多,其木如橘而小,高五七尺,叶如橙,多刺,春开白花结实,至秋始成。《周礼》云:橘逾淮而北为枳,今江南枳橘皆有,江北有枳无橘,此是种类各别,非逾淮而变也。七八月采者为枳实,九十月采者为枳壳。愚按:实者乃果实之通称,言实壳亦在其中矣。

枳实气味苦寒,冬不落叶,禀少阴标本之气化,臭香形圆,花白多刺,穰肉黄白。又得阳明金土之气化,主治大风在皮肤中。如麻豆苦痒者,得阳明金气而制风,禀少阴水气而清热也。除寒热结者,禀少阴本热之气而除寒,标阴之气而除热也。止痢,长肌肉者,得阳明中土之气也。五脏发原于先天之少阴,生长于后天之阳明,故主利五脏,得少阴之阴,故益气,得阳明之气,故轻身。

仲祖本论,有大承气汤,用炙厚朴,炙枳实。小承气汤,用生厚朴,生枳实,生熟之间,有意存焉。学人不可不参。

187. Zhishi [枳实, processed unripe bitter orange, Fructus Aurantii Immaturus]

It is bitter in taste, cold and non-toxic in property, and it is mainly used to treat the diseases caused by the invasion of severe wind into the skin, the pain and itching like sesames and soybeans in the skin, eliminate cold and heat accumulation, check dysentery, promote the growth of muscles, harmonize the five zang-organs, replenish qi and keep people healthy.

Zhishi (processed unripe bitter orange) grows in Luoxi (洛西), Henei (河内) and many areas of Jianghu (江湖). In recent years, most of it grows in Jiangxi (江西). Its wood, like that of Ju [橘, tangerine, Citri Reticulatae Fructus], is thin, with five or seven Chi in height; its leaves, like those of oranges, are thorny. In spring, it blossoms white and bears fruits which are not ripe until the autumn. Zhouli [《周礼》, Rituals of the Zhou Dynasty] says that Ju (tangerine) changes into Zhi [枳, bitter orange, Poncirus trifoliate] when planted to the north of Huai River. Now both Zhi (bitter orange) and Ju (tangerine) grow in Jiangnan (江南) while only Zhi (bitter orange) grows in Jiangbei (江北), which shows that they belong to different types, and cannot be differentiated by the area where they grow. Those collected in the seventh and eighth lunar months are called Zhishi（processed unripe bitter orange）, and those collected in the ninth and tenth lunar months Zhiqiao［枳壳, bitter orange, Aurantii Fructus］. Note by Zhang Zhicong（张志聪）：Shi（实）is the general name of fruits, which also includes Qiao（壳）.

Bitter in taste, cold in property, with leaves staying green in winter, Zhishi（processed unripe bitter orange）receives the qi transformation of branches and roots from lesser yin; it is fragrant, thorny, and round in shape, with white flowers and yellow-white flesh. It obtains the qi transformation of metal and earth from yang brightness, so it can mainly treat the diseases caused by invasion of severe wind into the skin. It can treat the pain and itching like sesames and soybeans in the skin because it obtains metal qi from yang brightness to control wind and receives water qi from lesser yin to clear heat. It can eliminate cold and heat accumulation because it receives branch-heat qi from lesser yin to eliminate cold and root-yin qi to eliminate heat. It can check dysentery and promote the growth of muscles because it obtains the qi of center earth from yang brightness. The five zang-organs originate from the lesser yin of earlier heaven and grow in the yang brightness of later heaven, so it can harmonize the five zang-organs. It obtains yin from lesser yin, so it can replenish qi; it obtains qi from yang brightness, so it can keep people healthy.

In the books written by Zhang Zhongjing（张仲景）, there are Da Chengqi Tang［大承气汤, Major Purgative Decoction］using Zhihoupo［炙厚朴, mix-fried officinal magnolia bar, Magnoliae Officinalis Cortex cum Liquido Frictus］and Zhizhishi［炙枳实, mix-fried processed unripe bitter orange, Fructus Aurantii Immaturus］, and Xiao Chengqi Tang［小承气汤, Minor Purgative Decoction］using raw Houpu（magnolia bark）and raw Zhishi（processed unripe bitter orange）. Zhang Zhongjing（张仲景）deliberately used mix-fried medicinals in the former and raw ones in the latter. Scholars should pay attention to the different choices of the medicinals.

188. 枳 壳 附

枳壳 附　气味苦酸,微寒,无毒。主治风痹、淋痹,通利关节,劳气咳嗽,背膊闷倦,散留结胸膈痰滞,逐水,消胀满,大胁风,安胃,止风痛。《开宝本草》附。

上世本草只有枳实,至宋《开宝本草》,始分枳之小者为枳实,大者为枳壳。愚谓:小者其性藏密而气全,大者其性宣发而气散,或云:大者气足而力虚,小者气不足而力薄。不知气之足也,在于旺时,若过其时,则反薄矣。又,李东垣云:枳壳缓而枳实速。王好古云:枳壳主高,枳实主下,高者主气,下者主血,未免臆说不经。后学遵而信之,宁无黄乎。须知实与壳,其种未始有殊也。种既无殊,则缓速气血之说,何可分乎。

188. Zhiqiao〔枳壳, bitter orange, Aurantii Fructus〕*supplement*

It is bitter and sour in taste, slightly cold and non-toxic in property, and it is mainly used to treat wind impediment and strangury impediment, free joints, relieve overstrain cough and oppression and the fatigue of the back and arms, dissipate the phlegm stagnation bound in the chest and diaphragm, expel water, disperse distention and fullness, treat the diseases caused by the invasion of severe wind into the hypochondrium, harmonize the stomach and relieve wind pain. Supplemented in *Kai Bao Ben Cao*〔《开宝本草》, *Materia Medica of the Kaibao Era*〕

Only Zhishi〔枳实, processed unripe bitter orange, Fructus Aurantii Immaturus〕was recorded in *Shen Nong Beng Cao Jing*〔《神农本草经》, *Shennong's Classic of Materia Medica*〕. Up until the Song Dynasty, *Kai Bao Ben Cao*〔《开宝本草》, *Materia Medica of the Kaibao Era*〕began to classify small ones as Zhishi (processed unripe bitter orange) and big ones as Zhiqiao (bitter orange). In my humble opinion, for the small one, its property is storing and compact, so its qi is complete; for the big one, its property is ascent and dispersion, so its qi is dispersed. It is said that for the big one, qi is sufficient and weak, while for the small one, qi is insufficient and mild. However, those who hold this view don't know that it is at prosperous time that qi is sufficient; if the time is passed, qi will become mild. Besides, Li Dongyuan (李东垣) said, "As to treating disease, Zhiqiao (bitter orange) works slowly but Zhishi (processed unripe bitter orange) works quickly." Wang Haogu (王好古) said, "Zhiqiao (bitter orange) governs the upper while Zhishi (processed unripe bitter orange) governs the lower, so the former governs qi while the latter governs blood." These views are just their subjective speculations and may not be true. However, later scholars believed what they said and obeyed it. Did they not do this to flatter them? It must be known that Zhiqiao (bitter orange) and Zhishi (processed unripe bitter orange) grow from the same seeds. Since they have the same seeds, how can the above theories of Li Dongyuan (李东垣) and Wang Haogu (王好古) differentiate them?

189. 山茱萸

山茱萸　气味酸平,无毒。主治心下邪气寒热,温中,逐寒湿痹,去三虫,久服轻身。

　　山茱萸今海州、兖州,江浙近道诸山中皆有。木高丈余,叶似榆有刺,二月开花白色,四月结实如酸枣,色紫赤,九月十日采实,阴干去核用肉。

　　山茱萸色紫赤而味酸平,禀厥阴少阳木火之气化。手厥阴属心包,故主治心下之邪气寒热。心下乃厥阴心包之部也。手少阳属三焦,故温中。中,中焦也。中焦取汁,奉心化赤而为血,血生于心,藏于肝。足厥阴肝主之血,充肤热肉,故逐周身之寒湿痹。木火气盛,则三焦通畅,故去三虫。血充肌腠,故久服轻身。

　　愚按:仲祖八味丸用山茱萸,后人去桂附,改为六味丸,以山茱萸为固精补肾之药。此外并无他用,皆因安于苟简,不深探讨故也。今详观《本经》山茱萸之功能主治如此,学者能于《本经》之内会悟,而广其用,庶无拘隘之弊。

189. Shanzhuyu〔山茱萸, cornus, Fructus Corni〕

It is sour in taste, mild and non-toxic in property, and it is mainly used to treat the cold and heat caused by the pathogenic qi in the region below the heart, warm the middle, eliminate cold-dampness impediment and kill three worms. Long-term taking of it will keep people healthy.

Shanzhuyu (cornus) grows in Haizhou (海州), Yanzhou (兖州) and the mountains nearby in Jiangzhe (江浙). It is more than one Zhang in height, and its leaves are like those of elms and thorny. It blossoms white in the second lunar month, and bears fruits like the wild jujube and purple-red in color in the fourth lunar month, which will be collected in the ninth and tenth lunar months, and dried in the shade. Its flesh will be used as medicinal with the kernel being removed.

Purple-red in color, sour in taste and mild in property, Shanzhuyu (cornus) receives the qi transformation of wood and fire from reverting yin and lesser yang. The hand reverting yin pertains to the pericardium, so it can mainly treat the cold and heat caused by the pathogenic qi in the region below the heart which is home to the reverting yin pericardium. The hand lesser yang pertains to the triple energizer, so it can warm the middle which refers to the middle energizer. The middle energizer takes the liquid and supplies it to the heart where it is transformed into the red blood, and thus the blood is generated in the heart and stored in the liver. The blood governed by the foot reverting yin liver fills the skin and heats the flesh, so it can eliminate the cold-dampness impediment in the whole body. When wood fire qi is exuberant, the triple energizer will be free and uninhibited, so it can kill three worms. When the blood fills the interstices of the flesh, long-term taking of it will keep people healthy.

Note by Zhang Zhicong (张志聪): Shanzhuyu (cornus) is used in Bawei Dihuang Wan [八味地黄丸, Eight-Ingredient Rehmannia Pill] created by Zhang Zhongjing (张仲景). The later generations removed Guifu [桂附, Cinnamon Bark and Aconit] and changed it into Liuwei Dihuang Wan [六味地黄丸, Six-Ingredient Rehmannia Pill]. They believed that Shanzhuyu (cornus) was a medicinal to secure essence and tonify the kidney and had no other uses, which was all because they were content with their superficial knowledge about it and didn't make in-depth study. Nowadays, after reading *Shen Nong Ben Cao Jing* [《神农本草经》, *Shennong's Classic of Materia Medica*] carefully, we learn that it has different effects and accordingly can be used to treat different diseases. If scholars had really understood it from the book and wildly used it, maybe they would not have made such a mistake.

190. 吴茱萸

吴茱萸 气味辛温,有小毒。主治温中下气,止痛,除湿血痹,逐风邪,开腠理,咳逆寒热。

吴茱萸所在有之，江浙、蜀汉尤多。木高丈余，叶似椿而阔厚，紫色，三月开红紫细花，七八月结实累累成簇，似椒子而无核，嫩时微黄，熟则深紫，多生吴地，故名吴茱萸。九月九日采，阴干，陈久者良，滚水泡一二次，去其毒气用之。

山茱萸、吴茱萸咸禀木火之气。禀火气，故主温中。禀木气，故主下气。中焦温而逆气下，则痛自止矣。湿血痹者，湿伤肌腠，致充肤热肉之血凝泣为痹。少阳炎热之气，行于肌腠，肝主冲任之血，淡渗皮肤，则湿血痹可除矣。又曰：逐风邪者，言湿痹可除，而风邪亦可逐也。气味辛温，故开腠理。腠理开，则肺病之咳逆，皮肤之寒热皆治矣。

190. Wuzhuyu〔吴茱萸, evodia, Fructus Evodiae〕

It is pungent in taste, warm and slightly toxic in property, and it is mainly used to warm the middle, descend qi, relieve pain, eliminate damp and blood impediment, expel wind pathogen, open the striae and interstice, and treat the cough with dyspnea as well as cold and heat.

Wuzhuyu (evodia) grows in many areas, especially in Jiangzhe (江浙) and Shuhan (蜀汉). It is more than one Zhang (丈) in height; its leaves, like those of toona, are broad, thick and purple in color; its thin red-purple blossoms come out in the third lunar month; it bears clusters of fruits in the seventh and eighth lunar months, which are like peppers but have no kernels. The fruits are yellowish and turn deep purple when ripening. It mainly grows in Wudi (吴地), thus called Wuzhuyu (evodia). It will be collected on the ninth day of the ninth lunar month and dried in the shade. The one stored for a long time is of better quality. Before it is used as medicinal, it should be soaked in the boiling water once or twice to remove toxin.

Shanzhuyu〔山茱萸, cornus, Fructus Corni〕and Wuzhuyu (evodia) both receive wood and fire qi. Wuzhuyu (evodia) receives fire qi, so it can mainly warm the middle. It receives wood qi, so it can mainly descend qi. When the middle energizer is warmed and countflow qi is descended, the pain naturally will be relieved. When dampness damages the interstices of the flesh, the blood which can fill the skin and heat the flesh will congeal, thus causing damp and blood impediment. When the hot qi from lesser yang moves in the interstices of the flesh and the Chongren blood governed by the liver percolates blandly into the skin, damp and blood impediment will be eliminated. What's more, since it can eliminate damp and blood impediment, it also can expel wind pathogen. It is pungent in taste and warm in property, so it can open the striae and interstice. If the striae and interstice are open, then the cough with dyspnea caused by the lung disease and cold and heat will be treated, too.

191. 猪 苓

猪苓 气味甘平,无毒。主治痎疟,解毒蛊疰不祥,利水道。久服轻身耐老。

猪苓始出衡山山谷及济阴、冤句,今蜀州、习州亦有之。乃枫树之苓也,其皮黑,其肉白,而坚实者佳。任昉《异述记》云:南中有枫子鬼木之老者,为人形,亦呼为灵枫,盖瘿瘤也。至今越巫有得者,以之雕刻鬼神,可致灵异。《尔雅正义》云:枫子鬼乃枫木上寄生,枝高二三尺,天旱以泥涂之即雨。荀伯子《临川记》云:岭南枫木岁久生瘿,如人形,遇暴雷大雨,则暗长三五尺,谓之枫人,则枫为灵异之木,可知矣。

按:陶弘景曰:猪苓是枫树苓。苏颂曰:生土底不必枫根下始有。李时珍曰:猪苓是木之余气所结,如松之余气结茯苓之理。他木皆有,枫树为多。卢子由曰:木之有余于气与脂者,唯松与枫,松则兼气与脂而咸有余,枫则余气为苓,不复余脂为香。余脂为香,不复余气为苓,苓与香各禀气与脂之体与用也。合诸说,观之苓虽他木皆有,唯枫树下者,入药为良。犹寄生、螵蛸二物他树亦有,而唯取桑上者入药,亦此理耳。谓之猪苓者,以其形似猪矢命名。

枫树之瘿,遇雷雨则暗长,以泥涂之,即天雨,是禀水精所主之木也。猪苓新出土时,其味带甘,苓主淡渗,故曰甘平。痎疟,阴疟也。主治痎疟者,禀水精之气以奉春生,则阴疟之邪,随生气而升散矣。解毒蛊疰不详者,苓禀枫树之精华,结于中土,得土气则解毒,禀精华则解蛊疰不祥也。味甘平而淡渗,故利水道。久服则水精四布,故轻身耐老。

191. Zhuling〔猪苓, polyporus, Polyporus Umbellatus〕

It is sweet in taste, mild and non-toxic in property, and it is mainly used to treat malaria, remove toxin and parasitic toxin, treat pulmonary tuberculosis and the diseases caused by monsters, and promote the water passage in the body. Long-term taking of it will keep people healthy and prevent aging.

Firstly recorded to be growing in the valleys of Hengshan Mountain (衡山) and in Jiyin (济阴) and Yuanju (冤句), now Zhuling (polyporus) also grows in Shuzhou (蜀州) and Xizhou (习州). It is the polyporus of maple trees with black skin and white flesh. The one that is hard outside and plump inside is of the best quality. *Yi Shu Ji* [《异述记》, *Stories about Ghost*] by Ren Fang (任昉) records that in Nanzhong (南中), there are some old Fengzigui wood [枫子鬼木, ghost-like maple wood] which are like a human in shape, thus also called Lingfeng [灵枫, spiritual maple tree]; probably it's the tree tumor that makes it human-like. Nowadays, people in Yuewu (越巫) got it and carved it into ghosts and gods which are thought to be supernatural. *Er Ya Zheng Yi* [《尔雅正义》, *The Orthodox Interpretation of Erya*] says that Fengzigui [枫子鬼, ghost-like maple wood] is parasitic to the maple tree; its branches are two or three Chi in height; in drought, smear it with mud and it will rain. *Lin Chuan Ji* [《临川记》, *Travel Notes in Lin Chuan*] by Xun Bozi (荀伯子) records that the maple trees in Lingnan (岭南) will have the tree tumor when getting older, making it human-like; in thunderstorm and heavy rain, it can grow three or five Chi, called Fengren [枫人, human-like maple tree]; thus, it can be known that the maple tree is supernatural.

Note by Gao Shishi (高世栻): Tao Hongjing (陶弘景) said, "Zhuling (polyporus) is the polyporus of maple trees." Su Song (苏颂) said, "Polyporus does not necessarily grow under maple trees." Li Shizhen (李时珍) said, "Zhuling (polyporus) is transformed from the excessive qi of wood, just like Fuling [茯苓, poria, *Poria*] from the excessive qi of pine trees. It grows under many trees, but mainly under maple trees. Lu Ziyou (卢子由) said, "Among all trees, only pine trees and maple trees are excessive in qi and resin. For pine trees, both qi and resin are excessive; for maple trees, if qi is excessive which can be transformed into polyporus, resin will not be excessive which can be transformed into fragrance. Conversely, when resin is in excess, qi will not. Polyporus and fragrance have the same property and function as qi and resin. In one word, although it can also grow under other trees, only the one under maple trees can be used as medicinal, just as Jisheng [寄生, mistletoe, Taxilli Herba] and Piaoxiao [螵蛸, mantis egg-case, Mantidis Ootheca] can also grow on other trees, but only the one on mulberry can be used as medicinal. It is like a pig shit in shape, hence called Zhuling (polyporus).

The tree tumor of maple trees grows very quickly in thunderstorms; smear it with mud and it will rain; it receives water essence and is governed by the latter. When it springs out of the earth, it is sweet. Besides, polyporus is a bland medicinal. Therefore, it is sweet in taste and mild in property. Malaria is the yin malaria. It can mainly treat malaria because it receives the qi of water essence to supply spring resuscitation and the pathogen of yin malaria will ascend and dissipate with vital qi. It can remove toxin and parasitic toxin, and treat pulmonary tuberculosis and the diseases caused by monsters because it receives the essence of maple trees and grows in center earth. It obtains earth qi to remove toxin and parasitic toxin, and receives essence to treat pulmonary tuberculosis and the diseases caused by monsters. It is sweet in taste, mild in property and bland, so it can promote the water passage in the body. Long-term taking of it will spread water essence throughout the whole body, so it will keep people healthy and prevent aging.

192. 芜荑

芜荑 气味辛平，无毒。主治五内邪气，散皮肤骨节中淫淫温行毒，去三虫，化食。

芜荑生晋山川谷，今河东、河西近道处处皆有，而太原、延州、同州者良。其木名楩，《说文》曰：楩，山枌榆也，有刺，实为芜荑。叶圆而厚，其实早成，亦如榆荚，但气臭如犯，土人作酱食之，则味香美。性能杀虫，置物中亦能辟蛀。

芜荑，山榆仁也，榆受东方甲乙之精，得先春发陈之气，禀木气也。其味辛，其臭腥，其色黄白，其本有刺，禀金气也。木能平土，故主治五内之邪气。五内者，中土也。金能制风，故散皮肤骨节中淫淫温行毒。淫淫温行者，风动之邪也。风胜则生虫，去三虫，亦金能制木也。火衰则食不化，化食，乃木能生火也。

192. Wuyi [芜荑, great elm seed, Semen Ulmus Macrocarpa]

It is pungent in taste, mild and non-toxic in property, and it is mainly used to treat the diseases in the five zang-organs caused by pathogenic qi, disperse the retention of the pathogenic factors in the skin, remove pathogenic wind, febrile and toxic elements in the joints, expel three worms and digest food.

Wuyi (great elm seed) grows in the valleys of Jinshan Mountain (晋山). Nowadays, it is everywhere nearby in Hedong (河东) and Hexi (河西). Those growing in Taiyuan (太原), Yanzhou (延州) and Tongzhou (同州) are of better quality. Its wood is called Pian (楩). *Shuo Wen* Jie Zi [《说文解字》, *Explain Words*] says that Pian (楩), referring to the mountain-elm, is thorny, and its seeds are Wuyi (great elm seed). Its leaves are round and thick; its seeds mature early which are like ordinary elm seeds but as smelly as Xin [犿, pronounced as Xin, the name of an animal, beaver genus, like a cat but smaller, smelly]; the locals make it into paste, which tastes delicious. It can kill worms, so it is put in things to expel worms.

Wuyi (great elm seed) is the seed of the mountain-elm. The elm obtains the essence of Jia (甲) and Yi (乙) governed by the East and sprouting and growing the qi of early spring, so it receives wood qi. Pungent in taste, stinky in smell, yellow-white in color, its wood being thorny, it receives metal qi. Wood can pacify earth, so it can mainly treat the diseases in the five zang-organs caused by pathogenic qi. The five zang-organs belong to center earth. Metal can control wind, so it can disperse the retention of pathogenic factors in the skin and remove pathogenic wind and the febrile and toxic elements in the joints. These diseases are caused by the pathogen of wind stirring. When wind prevails, worms appear. It can expel three worms because metal can control wood. When fire debilitates, food will not be digested. It can digest food because wood can generate fire.

193. 皂荚

皂荚 气味辛咸温,有小毒。主治风痹死肌,邪气风头泪出,利九窍,杀精物。

皂荚处处有之，其树高大，叶如槐叶，枝间有刺，即皂角刺也。夏开细黄花，结实有三种，一种小如猪牙，一种大而肥厚，多脂而粘，一种长而瘦薄，枯燥不粘，皆可入药。《本经》用如猪牙者，其树多刺，难上采荚，以蔑箍其树，一夜自落，有不结实者，树凿一孔入生铁三五斤，泥封之即结荚。人以铁砧捶皂荚，即自损，铁碾碾之，久则成孔，铁锅爨之多爆片落。

愚按：纳生铁而即结荚者，铁乃金类，色黑属水，得金水之气，则木茂而结荚也。铁遇之而剥损者，荚色紫赤，具太阳火热之气，火能克金也。蔑箍其皮，荚即落者，太阳之气自下而上行于肤表，箍其皮则阳气不能上升，太阳气殒而荚落矣。

皂荚枝有刺而味辛，禀金气也。色紫赤而味兼咸，禀水气也。太阳之气合金气而出于肤表，合水气而下挟膀胱，故味辛咸而气温热，辛咸温热，则有小毒矣。风邪薄于周身，则为风痹死肌之证。风邪上薄于头，则为风头泪出之证。皂荚禀金气而制风，故能治也。九窍为水注之气，皂荚禀水气，故利九窍。太阳阳热之气，若天与日，天日光明，则杀精物，精物，犹百精老物也。

193. Zaojia［皂荚，gleditsia，Radix Gleditsiae］

It is pungent and salty in taste, warm and slightly toxic in property, and it is mainly used to treat wind impediment, necrotic muscles and the headache due to the invasion of pathogenic wind and pathogenic qi into the head with tearing, disinhibit the nine orifices and kill the strange pathogenic factors like ghosts.

Zaojia (gleditsia) exists everywhere, its tree is very tall and its leaves is like those of Huaiye［槐叶, sophora leaf, Sophorae Folium］. There are thorns among branches, which is Zaojiaoci［皂角刺, gleditsia thorn, Gleditsiae Spina］. In summer, its fine yellow blossoms come out. It has three kinds of fruits: one is as small as the pit tooth, another big, plump, fatty and sticky, and the third one long, thin, dry and non-sticky. All of them can be used as medicinal. The one like the pit tooth is used in *Shen Nong Ben Cao Jing*［《神农本草经》, *Shennong's Classic of Materia Medica*］. Its thorny tree makes it difficult to collect the fruit. However, when the tree is hooped with a thin bamboo, the fruit will fall by itself next day. For the tree which is not fruitful, cut a hole in the tree, put three or five Jin of pig iron into it and seal it with mud, and the tree will bear fruits. Zaojia (gleditsia) is so hard that if beaten with an anvil, it will destroy the anvil; if ground with an iron mill, it will make holes in the iron mill over time; if it is fried with an iron pot, it may explode the iron pot into pieces.

Note by Zhang Zhicong (张志聪): The pig iron helps the tree bear fruits, because iron, as a kind of metal, is black in color and pertains to water. It receives metal and water qi, which makes it grow thickly and bear fruits. Zaojia (gleditsia) can destroy iron, because it is purple-red and has the fire-heat qi from greater yang, and fire can restrict metal. When the tree is hooped with a thin bamboo, it will fall by itself, because the qi from greater yang, which moves along the bark of the tree from bottom to top, cannot rise if the tree is hooped with a bamboo. When the qi from greater yang perishes, it will fall down.

Pungent in taste and its branches being thorny, Zaojia (gleditsia) receives metal qi. Purple-red in color and salty in taste, it receives water qi. The qi from greater yang combines with metal qi to come out of the skin and combines with water qi to confine the bladder, so it is pungent and salty in taste and warm-heat and slightly toxic in property. Wind impediment and necrotic muscles are caused by pathogenic wind invading the whole body; headache and tearing are caused by pathogenic wind invading the head. Zaojia (gleditsia) receives metal qi to control wind, so it can treat these diseases. The nine orifices are where the body fluid flows and stays. Zaojia (gleditsia) receives water qi, so it can promote the nine orifices. The yang heat qi from greater yang is like the sky and the sun which are bright, so it can kill the strange pathogenic factors which are like ghosts.

194. 皂角刺 附

皂角刺 附 一名天丁,气味辛温,无毒。米醋熬嫩刺作煎,涂疮癣,有奇效。《图经本草》治痈肿,妒乳,风疠恶疮,胎衣不下,杀虫。《本草纲目》小儿重舌,小便淋闭,肠风痢血,大风疠痒,痈疽不溃,疮肿无头。诸方。去风,化痰,败毒攻毒,定小儿惊风发搐,攻痘疮起发,化毒成浆。隐庵增附。

194. Zaojiaoci [皂角刺, gleditsia thorn, Gleditsiae Spina] *supplement*

It is also called Tianding [天丁, gleditsia thorn, Gleditsiae Spina], pungent in taste, warm and non-toxic in property. The decoction boiled with tender thorns and rice vinegar is very effective in treating sores and tinea. *Tu Jing Ben Cao* [《图经本草》, *Illustrated Classic of Materia Medica*] It is used to treat abscesses and swelling, galactostasis, the malign sore caused by pestilential wind and the retention of the placenta, and kill worms. *Ben Cao Gang Mu* [《本草纲目》, *Compendium of Materia Medica*] It is used to treat the double tongue in children, dribbling urination, the blood dysentery caused by intestinal wind, the pestilential itching of great wind, unruptured abscesses and carbuncles, and headless swollen sores. *Zhu Fang* [《诸方》, *Various Prescriptions*]. It is effective in eliminating wind, dissolving phlegm, vanquishing toxin and attacking toxin, relieving child infantile convulsion, attacking the eruption of pox and sore and transforming toxin into thick fluid. Supplemented by Zhang Zhicong (张志聪).

195. 皂荚子 附

皂荚子 附　气味辛温,无毒。炒舂去赤皮,以水浸软,煮熟糖渍食之,疏道五脏风热壅。《本草衍义》核中白肉,入治肺药,核中黄心嚼食,治膈痰吞酸。《图经本草》仁和血,润肠,《用药法象》治风热,大肠虚秘,瘰疬肿毒,疮癣。《本草纲目》治疔肿便痈,风虫牙疼,妇人难产,里急后重,肠风下血,腰脚风痛。《诸方》治疝气,并睾丸肿痛。隐庵增附。

195. Zaojiazi [皂荚子, gleditsia seed, Gleditsiae Semen] *supplement*

It is pungent in taste, warm and non-toxic in property. It can be processed in this way: first stir-fried and pounded to remove the red skin, soaked soft in water, and finally cooked and sugared. Eating it can relieve the wind-heat congestion of the five-zang organs. *Ben Cao Yan Yi* [《本草衍义》, *Extention of Materia Medica*] The white flesh in the seed is used together with other medicinals to treat the lung diseases;

the yellow kernel can be chewed to treat diaphragm phlegm and acid swallowing. *Tu Jing Ben Cao* [《图经本草》, *Illustrated Classic of Materia Medica*] The seed can harmonize the blood and moisten the intestines. *Yong Yao Fa Xiang* [《用药法象》, *Method of Medication*] It is used to treat wind heat, the large intestinal constipation of deficiency type, scrofula, swelling, toxin, sores and tinea. *Ben Cao Gang Mu* [《本草纲目》, *Compendium of Materia Medica*] It is used to treat furuncle swelling, stool abscesses, wind-worm toothache, female difficult delivery, tenesmus, bloody defecation and the wind pain of lumbar and foot. *Zhu Fang* [《诸方》, *Various Prescriptions*] It is used to treat hernia and swelling and the pain of testicles. Supplemented by Zhang Zhicong (张志聪).

196. 肥皂荚 附

肥皂荚 附 气味辛温,微毒。主治去风湿,下痢便血,疮癣肿毒。《本草纲目》附。

肥皂荚种类与皂荚相同,以其厚而多肉,故名肥皂荚,内有黑子数颗,大如指头而不甚圆,色如黑漆而甚坚,中有白仁如栗,煨熟可食,外科用之消肿毒、瘰疬。《相感志》云:肥皂荚水能死金鱼,辟蚂蚁,麸见之则不就。

近时疡医用肥皂肉,捣罯无名肿毒。用核仁,治鼠瘘疽痔。方上游医,用为吐药,治症瘕痞积。内科用者,盖鲜焉。

196. Feizaojia [肥皂荚, gymnocladus fruit, Gymnocladi Fructus] *supplement*

It is pungent in taste, warm and slightly toxic in property, and it is mainly used to treat rheumatism, diarrhea with blood, swelling and toxin of sores and tinea. Supplemented in *Ben Cao Gang Mu* [《本草纲目》, *Compendium of Materia Medica*].

Of the same type as Zaojia [皂荚, gleditsia, Radix Gleditsiae], it is thick and fleshy, thus called Feizaojia (gymnocladus fruit). Inside there are several black seeds, which are as big as fingers and not very round. The seeds are like the black paint in color and very hard. In the middle there are white nucleoli like chestnuts, which can be eaten after it is roasted. In surgery, it is used to eliminate swelling, toxin and scrofula. *Xiang Gan Zhi* [《相感志》, *Encyclopedia of Life*] says that the water used to soak it can kill goldfish and drive ants away from bran.

Nowadays, the sore and wound doctors pound its flesh into pieces and apply it to the wound to treat the unknown swelling and toxin. Besides, its nucleolus is used to treat scrofula, carbuncle and hemorrhoid. Only some very good doctors use it as an emetic drug to treat abdominal mass, stuffiness and accumulation. It is seldom used in the internal medicine.

197. 秦 皮

秦皮　气味苦,微寒,无毒。主治风寒湿痹,洗洗寒气,除热,目中青翳白膜。久服头不白,轻身。

　　秦皮本名梣皮,出陕西州郡,河阳亦有之,其木似檀枝干,皆青绿色,叶细无花实,皮上有白点而不粗错,取皮渍水,色便青碧,书纸上视之亦青色者,为真。

　　秦木生于水旁,其皮气味苦寒,其色青碧,受水泽之精,具青碧之色,乃禀水木相生之气化。禀木气而春生,则风寒湿邪之痹证,及肤皮洗洗然之寒气,皆可治也。禀水气而清热,故主除热。目者肝之窍,木气盛,则肝气益,故治目中青翳白膜。发者,血之余,水精足,则血亦充,故久服头不白而轻身。

197. Qinpi〔秦皮, ash, Cortex Fraxini〕

It is bitter in taste, slightly cold and non-toxic in property, and it is mainly used to treat the impediment due to wind, cold and dampness, the chilliness and shivering due to cold qi, relieve fever, and relieve nebula and the white membrane in eyes. Long-term taking of it will prevent white hair and keep people healthy.

　　Qinpi (ash), originally called Cenpi (梣皮), grows in the areas of Shaanxi (陕西), which also can be seen in Heyang (河阳). Its wood, similar to that of Tan〔檀, sandal, Santali〕, is green in color. It has fine leaves but no flowers and fruits. On the bark there are neatly arranged white spots which turn green when it is soaked in water. The one that is green when placed on the paper is real.

　　The ash tree grows by water; its bark is bitter in taste, cold in property and green in color. It gets water essence, and it is green in color, because it receives the qi transformation of mutual generation between water and wood. It receives wood qi to promote spring resuscitation, so it can treat the impediment due to wind, cold and dampness and skin chilliness and shivering due to cold qi. It receives water qi to clear heat, so it can mainly relieve fever. The eye is the orifice of the liver. Exuberant wood qi replenishes liver qi, so it can relieve the nebula and white membrane in the eyes. The hair is transformed from the blood in excess. If water essence is sufficient, the blood is also sufficient, so long-term taking of it will prevent white hair and keep people healthy.

198. 箽竹叶

箽竹叶 气味苦寒,无毒。主治咳逆上气,溢筋急,消恶疡,杀小虫。

竹产处唯江河之南甚多,故戴凯之《竹谱》曰:九河鲜有,五岭实繁,茎直中通,四时青翠,茎有节,节有枝,枝有节,节有叶,叶必三之,枝必两之,六十年一花,其花结实,其竹则枯。竹之种类最多,《本经》用箽竹,后人兼用淡竹,苦竹。一种薄壳者,名甘竹,亦佳。竹禀冬令之水精,其根硬,喜行东南,是气禀西北,而体尚向东南也。冬时孕笋,春时抽箽,夏时解箨,秋日成竿,得天地四时之气。

竹叶凌冬不落,四季常青。凌冬不落者,禀太阳标阳之气也。太阳标阳本寒,故气味苦寒。四季常青者,禀厥阴风木之气也,木主春生,上行外达,故主治咳逆上气。溢筋急者,肝主筋,竹叶禀风木之精,能滋肝脏之虚急也。消恶疡者,恶疡主热,竹叶禀水寒之气,能清心脏之火热也。虫为阴类,竹叶得太阳之标阳,而小虫自杀矣。

198. Jinzhuye [箽竹叶, leaf of henon bamboo, Folium Phyllostachydis Henonis]

It is bitter in taste, cold and non-toxic in property, and it is mainly used to treat the cough with dyspnea, the spasm of the sinews and malign sores, and kill small worms.

The bamboo grows in many areas in the south of Jianghe (江河). Hence,

Zhu Pu [《竹谱》, *Bamboo Spectrum*] says that the bamboo is rare in Jiuhe (九河) but flourishes in Wuling (五岭); with its stems straight and hollow in the middle, it stays green all the year round; its stems have knots, knots have branches, branches have knots, and knots have leaves. For every branch knot, there must be three leaves; for every stem knot, there must be two branches. It blossoms every sixty years; when the flower bears fruits, the bamboo will wither. The bamboo has the most types. Jinzhu [菫竹, henon bamboo, Folium Phyllostachydis] is used in *Shen Nong Ben Cao Jing* [《神农本草经》, *Shennong's Classic of Materia Medica*]. The later generations used both Danzhu [淡竹, bamboo, Bambusae] and Kuzhu [苦竹, bitter bamboo, Pleioblasti]. Ganzhu (甘竹), a kind of bamboo with thin skin, is also of the best quality. The bamboo receives the water essence of winter. Its roots are hard and tend to grow in the southeastern direction. Thus, it receives northwestern qi, but stands in the southeastern direction. Bamboo shoots are bred underground in winter, break out of ground in spring, get rid of its shell in summer and grow into bamboo in autumn. Therefore, it obtains the qi of four seasons in the heaven and the earth.

Jinzhuye (leaf of henon bamboo) doesn't fall in winter and stays green all the year round. It doesn't fall in winter because it receives the qi of branch yang from greater yang. The branch yang from greater yang is cold itself, so it is bitter in taste and cold in property. It stays green all the year round because it receives the wind and wood qi from reverting yin. Wood governs the spring resuscitation featured by moving upward and flowing outward, so it can mainly treat the cough with dyspnea. It can treat the spasm of the sinews because the liver governs the sinews, and it receives wind and wood essence to nourish liver deficiency. It can treat malign sores because malign sores govern heat, and it receives water-cold qi to clear the fire-heat in the heart. Worms pertain to yin, and obtain the branch yang from greater yang, so naturally it can kill small worms.

199. 竹 沥 附

竹沥 附　气味甘大寒,无毒。主治暴中风,风痹,胸中大热,止烦闷,消渴,劳复。《别录》附。

　　簟竹、淡竹、苦竹皆可取沥，将竹截取二尺许劈开，以砖两片对立架竹于上，两头各出五七寸，以火炙出其沥，以盘承取。

朱震亨曰：竹沥滑痰，非助以姜汁不能行。

199. Zhuli [竹沥, bamboo sap, Bambusae Succus] *supplement*

It is sweet in taste, severely cold and non-toxic in property, and it is mainly used to treat sudden stroke, wind impediment, the great heat in the chest, relieve vexation and oppression, and treat consumptive thirst and overfatigue relapse. Supplemented in *Ming Yi Bie Lu* [《名医别录》, *Miscellaneous Records of Famous Physicians*].

　　Zhuli (bamboo sap) can be extracted from Jinzhu [簟竹, henon bamboo, Folium Phyllostachydis], Danzhu [淡竹, bamboo, Bambusae] and Kuzhu [苦竹, bitter bamboo, Pleioblasti]. Cut a two-Chi long bamboo and open it, place it onto two opposite bricks with both sides five or seven Cun out; stir-fry it to extract Zhuli (bamboo sap) out and collect it with dish.

　　Zhu Zhengheng (朱震亨) said, "Zhuli (bamboo sap) is effective in lubricating phlegm only with Jiangzhi [姜汁, ginger juice, Zingiberis Rhizomatis Succus]".

200. 竹 茹 附

竹茹 附　气味甘，微寒，无毒。主治呕哕温气，寒热，吐血，崩中。《别录》附。

　　用刀轻轻刮去竹皮上粉青，取青内之皮，谓之竹茹。今人用竹沥、竹茹，皆取大竹，不知淡竹、苦竹、簟竹皆细小不大，俱系野生，非家种也。

　　呕哕，吐逆也。温气，热气也。竹茹，竹之脉络也。人身脉络不和，则吐逆而为热矣。脉络不和，则或寒或热矣。充肤热肉，淡渗皮毛之血，不循行于脉络，则上吐血而下崩中矣。凡此诸病，竹茹皆能治之，乃以竹之脉络而通人之脉络也。

200. Zhuru [竹茹, bamboo shavings, Bumbusae Caulis in Taenia] *supplement*

It is sweet in taste, slightly cold and non-toxic in property, and it is mainly used to treat the vomiting of warm qi, cold and heat, hematemesis and metrorrhagia. Supplemented in *Ming Yi Bie Lu* [《名医别录》, *Miscellaneous Records of Famous Physicians*].

Zhuru (bamboo shavings) is the skin inside the green powder of the bamboo which can be scraped off by a knife. Both Zhuli [竹沥, bamboo sap, Bambusae Succus] and Zhuru (bamboo shavings) used nowadays are taken from big bamboos. Few know that Danzhu [淡竹, bamboo, Bambusae], Kuzhu [苦竹, bitter bamboo, Pleioblasti] and Jinzhu [箽竹, henon bamboo, Folium Phyllostachydis] are all thin and small, which are wild and not grown at home.

Vomiting refers to retching couterflow; warm qi refers to heat qi. Zhuru (bamboo shavings) is the vessels and networks of bamboos. The disharmony of human vessels and networks causes the retching counterflow of warm qi and cold and heat. If the blood which can fill the skin, heat the flesh and percolate the skin and hair blandly doesn't circulate in the vessels and networks, it will cause hematemesis and metrorrhagia. It can treat all of these diseases because the vessels and networks of bamboos can dredge the vessels and networks of the human body.

201. 石 膏

石膏 气味辛,微寒,无毒。主治中风寒热,心下逆气惊喘,口干舌焦,不能息,腹中坚痛,除邪鬼,产乳,金疮。

石膏出齐庐山及鲁蒙山,荆州、彭城、钱塘亦有。有软硬二种,软石膏生于石中,大块作层,如压扁米糕,细纹短密,宛若束针,洁白如膏,松软易碎,烧之白烂如粉。硬石膏作块而生,直理起棱,如马齿坚白,击之则段段横解,光亮如云母、白石英,有墙壁。烧之亦易散,仍硬不作粉,今用以软者为佳。

石膏质坚色白,气辛味淡,纹理如肌腠,坚白若精金,禀阳明金土之精,而为阳明胃府之凉剂,宣剂也。中风寒热者,风乃阳邪,感阳邪而为寒为热也。金能制风,故主治中风之寒热。心下逆气惊喘者,阳明胃络上通于心,逆则不能上通,致有惊喘之象矣。口干舌焦,不能息,腹中坚痛者,阳明之上,燥气治之,口干舌焦,燥之极也。不能息,燥极而阳明之气不和于上也。腹中坚痛,燥极而阳明之气不和于下也。石膏质重性寒,清肃阳明之热气,故皆治之。禀金气则有肃杀之能,故除邪鬼。生产乳汁,乃阳明胃府所生。刀伤金疮,乃阳明肌肉所主。石膏清阳明而和中胃,故皆治之。

《灵枢经》云:两阳合明,是为阳明。又云:雨火并合,故为阳明,是阳明上有燥热之主气,复有前后之火热,故伤寒有白虎汤,用石膏、知母、甘草、粳米,主资胃府之津,以清阳明之热。又,阳明主合而居中土,故伤寒有越脾汤。石膏配麻黄,发越在内之邪,从中土以出肌表,盖石膏质重则能入里,味辛则能发散,性寒则能清热。其为阳明之宣剂、凉剂者,如此。

201. Shigao [石膏, gypsum, Gypsum Fibrosum]

It is pungent in taste, slightly cold and non-toxic in property, and it is mainly used to treat the cold and heat due to pathogenic wind, the fright and dyspnea due to the qi counterflow from below the heart, the dryness of the mouth with a scorched tongue, the inability to breathe, and the stiffness and pain of the abdomen, eliminate the pathogenic factors like ghosts, promote lactation and treat incised wound.

Shigao (gypsum) is produced in Lushan Mountain (庐山) of Qi (齐) and Mengshan Mountain (蒙山) of Lu (鲁), which also exists in Shanzhou (荆州), Pengcheng (彭城) and Qiantang (钱塘). It has two types: soft and hard. The soft one exists in the stone in the form of large layers, like a flattened rice cake. With short and dense fine lines like bunches of needles, it is as white as the cream, soft and fragile. When burned, it changes into white powder. The hard one exists in blocks with straight texture and edges, and it is as hard and white as the horse teeth. When hit, it is broken horizontally into segments, as shiny as Yunmu [云母, muscovite, Muscovitum] and Baishiying [白石英, white quartz, Quartz Album] and having walls. When burned, it also tends to become loose but it is too hard to become powder. Nowadays, the soft one is of better quality as medicinal.

Bland and pungent in taste, hard and white like first-class gold, its texture like the interstices of the flesh, Shigao (gypsum) receives the essence of metal and earth from yang brightness, and it is the cool formula of yang brightness stomach which is a dispersing formula. Wind is the yang pathogen which will cause cold and heat. Metal can control wind, so it can mainly treat the cold and heat caused by pathogenic wind. The yang brightness stomach collateral is connected upward with the heart but qi counterflow prevents such connection, thus causing fright and dyspnea. The celestial qi above yang brightness is controlled by dryness qi. The dryness of the mouth with a scorched tongue is caused by extreme dryness, which also leads to the disharmony of qi from yang brightness with the upper body, thus causing the inability to breathe, and the disharmony of qi from yang brightness with the lower body, thus causing the stiffness and pain of the abdomen. Shigao (gypsum), heavy and cold in property, is effective in clearing the heat qi from yang brightness, so it can treat all the above diseases. It receives the metal qi and is able to kill, so it can eliminate the pathogenic factors like ghosts. Lactation is produced in the yang brightness stomach, and incised wound is governed by the yang brightness muscle. Shigao (gypsum), which clears yang brightness and harmonizes the stomach, is effective in promoting lactation and treating incised wound.

Huang Di Nei Jing: Ling Shu [《黄帝内经·灵枢》, *Huangdi's Internal Classic: Miraculous Pivot*] says that double yang combines with each other into brightness, thus called yang brightness. It also says that rain and fire combine with each other, thus becoming yang brightness. Yang brightness has the dominant qi of dryness-heat above and the fire-heat in the front and at the back. Therefore, Baihutang [白虎汤, white tiger decoction] is used to treat cold damage, which includes Shigao [石膏, gypsum, Gypsum Fibrosum], Zhimu [知母, anemarrhena, Anemarrhenae Rhizoma], Gancao [甘草, licorice, Glycyrrhizae Radix], and Jingmi [粳米, rice, Oryzae]. It can enrich the fluid of the stomach to clear the heat of yang brightness. In addition, yang brightness governs combination and dwells in center earth. Thus, Yuepitang [越脾汤, Spleen-Effusing Decoction] is used to treat cold damage, in which Shigao (gypsum) combines with Mahuang [麻黄, ephedra, Ephedrae Herba] to expel the internal pathogen from center earth to the exterior. Probably Shigao (gypsum) is heavy so it can enter the interior, pungent in taste so it can disperse, and cold in property so it can clear heat. That's why it is called the dispersing formula and the cool formula of yang brightness.

202. 慈 石

慈石　气味辛寒,无毒。主治周痹,风湿,肢节中痛,不可持物,洗洗酸消,除大热烦满,及耳聋。

慈石出太山山谷及慈山山阴。今慈州、徐州及南海旁山中皆有之。《南州异物志》云:涨海崎头水浅而多慈石,大舟以铁叶固之者,至此皆不得过。以此言之,南海所出尤多也。慈州者,岁贡最佳,能吸铁,虚连数十铁,或一二斤刀器,回转不落者,尤良。其石中有孔,孔中有黄赤色,其上有细毛,功用更胜。土宿真君曰:铁受太阳之气,始生之初,卤石产焉,百五十年而成慈石,二百年孕而成铁,是慈石乃铁之母精也。

慈石色黑味辛性寒,盖禀金水之精气所生。周痹者,在于血脉之中,真气不能周也。慈石能启金水之精,通调血脉,故能治之。风湿肢节中痛,不可持物,洗洗酸消者。风湿之邪伤于肢节而痛,致手不能持物,足洗洗酸消不能行。酸消,犹痿削也。慈石禀阳明、太阳金水之气,散其风湿,故能治之。除大热烦满及耳聋者,乃水济其火,阴交于阳,亦慈石引针,下而升上之义。

202. Cishi〔慈石, **magnetite ore**, **Magnetitum**〕

It is pungent in taste, cold and non-toxic in property, and it is mainly used to treat generalized impediment, wind-dampness, the pain of limbs that makes it difficult to hold anything and the chilliness with ache, eliminate severe heat, vexation and fullness, and treat deafness.

Originally produced in the valleys of Taishan Mountain（太山）and the shade of Cishan Mountain（慈山）, Cishi（magnetite ore）also exists in the mountains of Cizhou（慈州）, Xuzhou（徐州）and the mountains by South China Sea nowadays. *Nan Zhou Yi Wu Zhi*〔《南州异物志》, *Products and Customs in Nanzhou*〕says that the water in Qitou（崎头）of South China Sea is shallow and there are a lot of Cishi（magnetite ores）, so large ships fixed with ore cannot pass there. Accordingly, the South China Sea is abundant in it. In Cizhou（慈州）, the one given to the court every year is of the best quality, which can absorb ore. The one which can absorb dozens of interconnected ores or one or two Jin of ore instruments that turn around and don't fall is especially good. The one with yellow-red holes inside and fine hairs outside are more effective. Tusu Zhenjun（土宿真君）said, "Ore gets qi from greater yang. At the beginning of its birth, it is polyhalite which grows into Cishi（magnetite ore）after fifty or one hundred years and into iron after two hundred years. Thus, Cishi（magnetite ore）is the mother essence of iron."

Black in color, pungent in taste and cold in property, Cishi（magnetite ore）is born by receiving the essential qi of metal and water. Generalized impediment is caused by genuine qi failing to circulate with the blood to the whole body. It can treat it because it can arouse the essence of metal and water, dredge and regulate the blood and the vessels. As for the pain of the limbs that are difficult to hold anything and the chilliness with ache, wind-damp pathogen damages the limbs to make them painful so that it is difficult for hands to hold anything; feet are so cold and painful that they cannot walk. "酸消"（suanxiao）is also written as "痠削"（suanxiao）. Cishi（magnetite ore）which receives metal and water qi from yang brightness and greater yang can dissipate wind dampness, so it can treat these diseases. It can eliminate severe heat, vexation, fullness and treat deafness because water coordinate with fire and yin interacts with yang. It is also because Cishi（magnetite ore）can absorb needles, which connotes the meaning of "rising up".

203. 石硫黄

石硫黄 气味酸温，有毒。主治妇人阴蚀，疽痔恶血，坚筋骨，除头秃，能化金银铜铁奇物。奇，疑作等。

石硫黄出东海牧羊山谷及太行河西山中。今南海诸番岭外州郡皆有，然不及昆仑、雅州舶上来者良。此火石之精所结，所产之处必有温泉，泉水亦作硫黄气。以颗块莹净光腻，色黄，嚼之无声者，弥佳。夹土与石者，不堪入药。

硫黄色黄，其形如石。黄者，土之色。石者土之骨。遇火即焰，其性温热，是禀火土相生之气化。火生于木，故气味酸温，禀火气而温经脉，故主治妇人之阴蚀，及疽痔恶血。禀土石之精，故坚筋骨。阳气长则毛发生，故主头秃。遇火而焰，故能化金银铜铁奇物。

203. Shiliuhuang［石硫黄，sulphur，Sulfur］

It is sour in taste, warm and toxic in property, and it is mainly used to treat woman genital erosion, carbuncle, hemorrhoids and malign blood, strengthen the sinews and bones, treat baldness, and melt gold, silver, copper, iron and so on. "奇" (qi) maybe means "and so on" (等).

Shiliuhuang (sulphur) exists in the mountain valleys of the East China Sea which serve as pastures and the mountains in Hexi (河西), Taihang (太行). Nowadays, it exits in the areas outside the mountains of South China Sea, which, however, is inferior to the one from Kunlun (昆仑) and Yazhou (雅州). It is the product of essence of flint. Where it is produced, there must be hot springs, and the spring water also transforms into sulphur gas. The one with its blocks crystal clear, shiny, exquisite and yellow in color are of the best quality, which doesn't make any sound when being chewed. The one mixed with soil and stones cannot be used as medicinal.

Shiliuhuang (sulphur) is yellow in color and like a stone in shape. Yellow is the color of earth, and the stone is its bone. Flammable when meeting fire and warm-heat in property, it receives the qi transformation of mutual generation between fire and earth. Fire is generated by wood, so it is sour in taste and warm in property; it receives fire qi to warm the channel, so it can mainly treat woman genital erosion, carbuncle, hemorrhoids and malign blood. It receives the essence of flint, so it can strengthen the sinews and bones. The waxing of yang qi promotes the growth of hair, so it can treat baldness. It is flammable when meeting fire, so it can melt gold, silver, copper, iron and so on.

204. 阳起石

阳起石　气味咸，微温，无毒。主治崩中漏下，破子脏中血，症瘕结气，寒热腹痛无子，阴痿不起，补不足。

阳起石乃云母根也。出齐州之齐山，庐山及太山、云山、沂州、琅琊诸山谷。今唯齐州采取，他处不复识之矣。齐州仅一土山，石出其中，彼人谓之阳起山。其山常有暖气,虽盛冬大雪遍境,独此山无积白。盖石气薰蒸使然也。山唯一穴,官司常禁闭,每发冬初,州发丁夫,遣人监取上供,岁月积久,其穴益深,镵凿他石得之甚难。以白色明莹,云头雨脚轻松,如狼牙者为上。黄色者亦重,其上犹带云母者,绝品也。拣择供上,剩余者,州人方货之,不尔,无由得也。置雪中倏然没跡者为真。画纸上于日下扬之飞举者,乃真佳也。

阳起石者,此山之石,乃阳气之所起也,故大雪遍境,而山无积白。有形之石,阳气所钟,故置之雪中,倏然没跡,扬之日下,自能飞举。主治崩中漏下者,崩漏为阴,今随阳气而上升也。破子脏中血,及症瘕结气者,阳长阴消,阳气透发,则症结破散矣。妇人月事不以时下,则寒热腹痛而无子。阳起石贞下启元,阴中有阳,阴阳和而寒热除,月事调而生息繁矣。男子精虚,则阴痿不起。阳起石助阴中之阳,故治阴痿不起,而补肾精之不足。

204. Yangqishi〔阳起石,actinolite,Actinolitum〕

It is salty in taste, slightly warm and non-toxic in property, and it is mainly used to treat metrorrhagia and metrostaxis, the vaginal bleeding due to the uterine injury, the abdominal mass due to qi stagnation, cold and heat, the infertility due to abdominal pain and impotence, and tonify kidney essence deficiency.

Yangqishi (actinolite) is the root of Yunmu〔云母, muscovite, Muscotitum〕existing in Qishan Mountain (齐山) of Qizhou (齐州), Lushan Mountain (庐山), Taishan Mountain (太山), Yunshan Mountain (云山) and the mountain valleys of Yizhou (沂州) and Langya (琅琊). At present, it is only produced in Qizhou (齐州) and cannot be recognized in other places. It only exists in an earth piled hill of Qizhou (齐州), which is called Yangqi Mountain (阳起山) by the locals. Warm air often circles around the hill, and in freezing winter when heavy snow is everywhere else, this hill is not covered by snow. Probably it is due to the fumigation of stone gas. There is only one cave in the hill which is often closed by the local authority. In every early winter, laborers are dispatched and supervised by the local authority to mine for Yangqishi (actinolite), which is offered to the court. With time passing by, the cave is getting deeper and deeper and mining for it is becoming harder and harder. The one that are white, crystal clear, like the cloud in the upper and like the rain running down on the ground in the lower is of the best quality, which is light, loose and like the wolf tooth. The yellow one is also heavier, which is peerless if mixed with Yunmu [云母, muscovite, Muscotitum]. The high-quality Yangqishi (actinolite) is chosen to offer to the court, and the rest is sold as goods by the locals. It cannot be got otherwise. The one soon disappearing in the snow is real. The one that can fly in the wind when put on the drawing paper and thrown up under the sun is really excellent.

Yangqishi (actinolite) is the stone from which yang qi is rising, so when heavy snow is everywhere else, only the mountain where it exists has no snow. Yang qi accumulates in this tangible stone, so when put in the snow it soon disappears, and when thrown up under the sun it can fly in the wind by itself. It can mainly treat metrorrhagia and metrostaxis because they pertain to yin and will rise up with yang qi. It can treat the vaginal bleeding due to uterine injury, the abdominal mass due to qi stagnation, because as yang waxes and yin wanes, yang qi will disperse, so it can break and dissipate the abdominal mass due to qi stagnation. The irregularity of women's menstruation leads to cold and heat and the infertility due to the abdominal pain. It promotes the circulation of yin and yang and makes yang within yin, so the harmony of yin and yang can eliminate cold and heat and regulate the menstruation which in turn promotes fertility. Man's essence deficiency causes impotence. It assists yang within yin, so it can treat impotence and notify kidney essence deficiency.

205. 雄 黄

雄黄 气味苦平寒,有毒。主治寒热鼠瘘,恶疮疽痔,死肌,杀精物恶鬼,邪气百虫毒,胜五兵,炼食之轻身,神仙。

《别录》云:雄黄出武都山谷,燉煌山之阳。武都氐羌也,是为仇池,后名阶州,地接西戎界。宕昌亦有而稍劣。燉煌在凉州西数千里。近来用石门谓之新坑,始兴石黄之好者耳。阶州又出一种水窟雄黄,生于山岩中有水流处,其色深红而微紫,体极轻虚,功用最胜。抱朴子云:雄黄当得武都山中出者纯而无杂,形块如丹砂,其赤如鸡冠,光明烨烨者,乃可用。有青黑色而坚者,名熏黄。有形色似真而气臭者,名臭黄,并不入服食,只可疗疮疥。金刚钻生于雄精之中,孕妇佩雄精,能转女成男。

雄黄色黄质坚,形如丹砂,光明烁烁,乃禀土金之气化,而散阴解毒之药也。水毒上行,则身寒热,而颈鼠瘘。雄黄禀土气而胜水毒,故能治之。肝血壅滞,则生恶疮而为疽痔,雄黄禀金气而平肝,故能治之。死肌乃肌肤不仁,精物恶鬼乃阴类之邪,雄黄禀火气而光明,故治死肌,杀精物恶鬼。邪气百虫之毒,逢土则解,雄黄色黄,故杀百虫毒。胜五兵者,一如硫黄能化金银铜铁锡也。五兵,五金也。胜五兵,火气盛也。炼而食之,则转刚为柔,金光内藏,故轻身神仙。

205. Xionghuang〔雄黄, realgar, Realgar〕

It is bitter in taste, mild, cold and toxic in property, and it is mainly used to treat cold and heat, scrofula, malign sores, carbuncle, hemorrhoids and necrotic muscles, expel severe pathogenic factors like ghosts, eliminate pathogenic qi, resolve various kinds of worm toxin and melt five kinds of important weapons. Taking the refined one will keep people healthy and as dexterous as immortals.

Ming Yi Bie Lu〔《名医别录》, *Miscellaneous Records of Famous Physicians*〕 says that Xionghuang (realgar) exists in the mountain valleys of Wudu (武都) and the sunny side of Dunhuang Mountain (敦煌山). Shiqiang (氐羌) in Wudu (武都), also called Qiuchi (仇池) and later renamed Jiezhou (阶州), borders Xirong (西戎). It also exists in Dangchang (宕昌) but it is a little inferior. Dunhuang (敦煌) is located thousands of Li west of Liangzhou (凉州). Xionghuang (realgar) produced in Shimen (石门) which is also called new cave, is of good quality, so it is often used in recent years. In Jiezhou (阶州), there is a kind of water cave Xionghuang (realgar). It grows in the mountain rocks where water flows by, deep red and slightly purple in color, extremely light in weight but the most powerful in function. *Bao Pu Zi*〔《抱朴子·仙药》, *Primitive and Natural Viewabout Magic Medicinals*〕 says that Xionghuang (realgar) produced from the mountains of Wudu (武都) is very pure, which is like Dansha〔丹砂, cinnabar, Cinnabaris〕in shape, its color as red as cockscomb and as bright as the sun. Only this kind of the herb can be used as medicinal. The one that is blue-black and hard is called Xunhuang (熏

黄）. The one that looks like the real in shape and color but is smelly is called Chouhuang（臭黄）which cannot be taken but only be used to treat sores and scabies. The diamond drill is made from Xiongjing［雄精, lucid realgar, Realgar Lucidum］, which can turn female fetus into male when worn by the pregnant woman.

Yellow in color, hard in texture, shaped like Dansha（cinnabar）and bright like the sun, Xionghuang（realgar）is a medicinal that receives the qi transformation of earth and metal and can dissipate yin and resolve toxin. The upward moving of the water toxin causes cold and heat in the body and the scrofula in the neck. It receives earth qi to predominate the water toxin, so it can treat these diseases. The stagnation of the liver blood causes malign sores which become carbuncle and hemorrhoids. It receives metal qi to pacify the liver, so it can treat these diseases. Necrotic muscles refer to the numbness of the skin, and the severe pathogenic factors like ghosts are the pathogens of yin. It receives fire qi to be bright, so it can treat necrotic muscles and expel the severe pathogenic factors like ghosts. Pathogenic qi and various kinds of worm toxin can be resolved when encountering earth. It is yellow in color, so it can resolve various kinds of worm toxin. Just like Shiliuhuang［石流黄, sulphur, Sulfur］, it can melt five kinds of important weapons, which refer to five metals, gold, silver, copper, iron and tin. It is exuberant in fire qi, so it can melt them. Taking refined Xionghuang（realgar）can convert hardness into softness and hide the metal light inside, so it can keep people healthy and as dexterous as immortals.

206. 雌 黄

雌黄 气味辛平,有毒。主治恶疮头秃,痂疥,杀毒虫虱,身痒邪气诸毒。炼之久服,轻身,增年不老。

> 雌黄与雄黄同产,雄黄生山之阳,雌黄生山之阴,一阴一阳,有似夫妇之道,故曰雌雄。

李时珍曰:雌黄、雄黄同产,但以山阴山阳受气不同分别,服食家重雄黄,取其得纯阳之精也。雌黄则兼有阴气,故不重。若治病,则二黄之功,亦相仿佛,大要皆取其温中搜肝,杀虫解毒,祛邪焉尔。

愚按：雄黄、雌黄气味宜同，今雄黄曰苦平，雌黄曰辛平，须知雄黄苦平而兼辛，雌黄辛平而兼苦，气味之同，难以悉举，故彼此稍异，以俟人之推测耳。

206. Cihuang [雌黄, orpiment ore, Orpimentum]

It is pungent in taste, mild and toxic in property, and it is mainly used to treat maglign sores and baldness, crust and scabies, kill toxic worms and louse, relieve itching, eliminate pathogenic qi and resolve various toxins. Taking the refined one for a long time will keep people healthy, prolong life and prevent aging.

Cihuang (orpiment ore) and Xionghuang [雄黄, realgar, Realgar] exist in the same places with the former on the shady side of the mountain and the latter on the sunny side. One is yin and the other is yang, just like the relationship between husband and wife, so they are called Cihuang (orpiment ore) and Xionghuang (realgar).

Li Shizhen (李时珍) said, "Xionghuang (realgar) and Cihuang (orpiment ore) exist in the same places, but they are differentiated by the sunny side or the shady side of the mountain where they receive different kinds of qi. Those who often take some supplements to regulate and nourish their bodies attach much importance to Xionghuang (realgar) for it obtains the essence of pure yang. Cihuang (orpiment ore,) also has yin qi, so it doesn't get this attention. However, in medicine, they almost have the same effects, which mainly include warming the middle, dispelling wind, killing worms, resolving toxin, and eliminating pathogen."

Note by Zhang Zhicong (张志聪): Xionghuang (realgar) and Cihuang (orpiment ore) most probably have the same taste and property. Nowadays it is said that the former is bitter and mild while the latter is pungent and mild. It should be known that being bitter and mild, Xionghuang (realgar) is also pungent in taste and that being pungent and mild, Cihuang (orpiment ore) is also bitter in taste. Their tastes are so close to each other that it is hard to differentiate them. Therefore, to say that they are slightly different from each other is just to encourage people to make further exploration and speculation.

207. 水 银

水银 气味辛寒,有毒。主治疥瘘痂疡白秃,杀皮肤中虱,堕胎,除热,伏金银铜锡毒,熔化还复为丹。久服神仙不死。

水银一名汞,一名灵液,又名姹女。古时出符陵平土,产于丹砂中,亦有别出沙地者。今秦州、商州、道州、邵武军、西羌、南海诸番、岭外州郡皆有。《陈霆墨谈》云:拂林国当日没之处,地有水银海,周遭四五十里,国人取之近海十里许,掘坑井数十,乃使健夫骏马皆贴金箔行,近海边日照金光晃耀,则水银滚沸,如潮而来,其势若粘裹,其人即回马疾驰,水银随赶。若行缓则人马具扑灭也,人马行速则水银势远力微,遇坑堑而溜积于中,然后取之。又,马齿苋干之十斤,可得水银八两,名曰草汞。

水银气味辛寒,禀金水之真精,为修炼之丹汞,烧硃则鲜红不渝,烧粉则莹白可爱,犹人身中焦之汁,化血则赤,化乳则白,此天地所生之精汁也。主治疥瘘痂疡白秃者,禀水精之气,能清热而养血也。杀皮肤中虱,堕胎者,禀金精之气,能肃杀而攻伐也,性寒故能除热,汞乃五金之精,故能杀金银铜锡毒。水银出于丹砂之中,而为阳中之阴。若熔化,则还复为丹,而为阴中之阳。一名灵液,又名姹女,乃天地所生之精汁,故久服神仙不死。

凡人误食水银则死。《本经》乃谓:久服神仙不死者,盖以古之神仙,取铅汞二物,用文武火候炼养久久,而成还丹,服之得以延年不老,指此言耳,非谓水银可以久服也。然其法久已失传,方士窃取其说以惑人,苟有服者,势在必死,载于典籍不一而足,不可以《本经》有是文而误试之。然谓《本经》六字竟是后之方士增加者,恐又不然也。

207. Shuiyin [水银, mercury, Hydrargyrum]

It is pungent in taste, cold and toxic in property, and it is mainly used to treat rash, fistula, crust, ulcer and white bald scalp, kill the lice in the skin, induce abortion, relieve fever, and remove the toxin in gold, silver, copper and tin. When melted, it will become Dansha [丹砂, cinnabar, Cinnabaris] again. Long-term taking of it will prolong life like immortals.

Shuiyin (mercury) is also called Gong [汞, mercury, Hydrargyrum],

Lingye [灵液, magic liquid] or Channü [姹女, beautiful lady]. In ancient times, it existed in the flat land of Fuling (符陵), originating from Dansha (cinnabar). It also existed in sandy land. Nowadays, it exists in Qinzhou (秦州), Shangzhou (商州), Daozhou (道州), Shaowujun (邵武军), Xiqiang (西羌), many foreign lands in the South China Sea and the areas in Lingnan (岭南). *Chen Ting Mo Tan* [《陈霆墨谈》, *Tittle-tattles by Chen Ting*] says that in the place where Fulin Country (拂林国) was submerged, there was Mercury Sea which was forty or fifty Li wide. To get the mercury, the locals dug dozens of wells about ten Li away from the sea and pasted gold foil on sturdy men and steeds. Sent to the seaside, they were shining with golden lights under the sun. The mercury sea was boiling and rolling towards them like the tide. At the moment when they were about to be stuck and wrapped by the mercury, the men ordered the steeds to gallop back, the mercury following behind. If the steeds ran too slowly, both the men and the steeds would be buried. If they ran fast enough, the mercury would become weaker and weaker as it ran farther and farther, finally falling into the wells. Then it could be fetched. Besides, ten Jin of Machixian [马齿苋, purslane, Portulacae Herba] can produce eight Liang of Shuiyin (mercury), thus called Caogong (草汞).

Pungent in taste and cold in property, Shuiyin (mercury) receives the true essence of metal and water. It is Danzhong (丹汞) which is used to be refined. It is bright red in color when it is burnt into Zhusha [朱砂, cinnabar, Cinnabaris], while it is white and lovely when it is transformed into Qingfen [轻粉, Calomel, Calomelas], just like the liquid in the middle energizer of the human body, which is red when it is transformed into the blood and white when it is transformed into human milk. Thus, it is the essence liquid created by the heaven and the earth. It can mainly treat rash, fistula, crust, ulcer and white bald scalp because it receives the qi of water essence to clear heat and nourish the blood. It can kill the lice in the skin and induce abortion because it receives the qi of metal essence to clear and downward, attack and quell. It is cold in property, so it can relieve fever. Gong [汞, mercury, Hydrargyrum] is the essence of five metals, so it can remove the toxin in gold, silver, copper and tin. Shuiyin (mercury) originating from Dansha (cinnabar) is yin within yang. If melted, it will become Dansha (cinnabar) again which is yang within yin. Shuiyin（mercury）, also called Lingye（灵液）or Chanü（姹女）, is the essence liquid created by the heaven and the earth, so long-term taking of it will prolong life like immortals.

The mortals will die if they eat mercury by mistake. *Shen Nong Ben Cao Jing*［《神农本草经》, *Shennong's Classic of Materia Medica*］says that long-term taking of it will prolong life like immortals. Probably it means that the ancient immortals refined Qian［铅, galenite, Galenitum］and Gong（mercury）for a long time by using both the mild fire and the strong fire to transform them back into Dansha（cinnabar）, which was taken to prolong life. Thus, it doesn't mean that it can be taken for a long time. However, this method has been lost for a long time, and the alchemists took advantage of the words in the book to confuse people. Those convinced to take it are bound to die. Many such examples are recorded in the classics, therefore we should not try it just because there are such statements in *Shen Nong Ben Cao Jing*［《神农本草经》, *Shennong's Classic of Materia Medica*］. There is the view that these six characters "久服神仙不死"（Long-term taking of it will prolong life like immortals）in *Shen Nong Ben Cao Jing*［《神农本草经》, *Shennong's Classic of Materia Medica*］ were added by later alchemists, which, I am afraid, is also not true.

208. 铁 落

铁落 气味辛平,无毒。主治风热恶疮,疡疽,疮痂,疥气在皮肤中。

铁落是锻铁匠砧上锤锻所落之铁屑。又,生铁打铸有花,如兰如蛾而落地者,俗谓之铁蛾,今烟火家用之。

铁名黑金,生于西北,五金中之属水者也。禀金气,故治风。禀水气,故治热。恶疮、疡疽疮,热也。痂疥气在皮肤中,风也。以火煅转乌之金,而清热毒之疮,故治恶疮、疡疽疮,以皮肤所落之金,而杀皮肤之虫,故治痂疥气在皮肤中。《素问·病能论》有生铁落饮,言其下气疾世。今人以铁锈磨涂疔肿,汤火伤,蜈蚣咬,喜儿疮,重舌脚肿,正治风热恶疮之义。

208. Tieluo［铁落, iron flakes, Ferrum Pulveratum］

It is pungent in taste, mild and non-toxic in property, and it is mainly used to treat wind-heat malign sores, ulcer and carbuncle, sore crust, and scabies the qi in the skin.

Tieluo (iron flakes) is the iron filings produced when ironsmith forges hammers on the anvil. In addition, in pig iron casting iron filings fall onto the ground like blue moths, popularly called Tiee (铁蛾). Nowadays, it is often used in cooking.

Tie [铁, iron ore, Ferri Mineral], named black metal, exists in the northwest of China. Among the five metals, it pertains to water. It receives metal qi to control wind and water qi to control heat. Malign sore, ulcer and carbuncle are all caused by heat, while crust and the scabies qi in the skin are caused by wind. It can treat malign sore, ulcer and carbuncle because it is forged by fire and can clear heat toxin. It can treat scabies qi in the skin because it falls from the surface of iron and can kill the worms in the skin. *Suwen: Bingnenglun* [《素问·病能论》, *Plain Questions: Discussion on the Manifestations of Diseases*] says that Shengtieluo Yin [生铁落饮, Iron Flakes Beverage] is effective in descending qi and treating diseases. Nowadays, iron rust is applied externally to treat furuncle and swelling, burns and scalds, the bite by centipede, child sore, double tongue and foot swelling. All these external applications are based on its effectiveness in treating wind-heat malign sores.

209. 猬 皮

猬皮 气味苦平,无毒。主治五痔,阴蚀,下血赤白五色,血汁不止,阴肿,痛引腰背。

猬处处山野中时有,俗名刺鼠。头嘴足爪俱似鼠,刺毛所豪猪,见人则卷缩,形如芡房及栗房,攒毛外刺,溺之即开。陶弘景曰:其脂烊铁中,入少水银则柔如铅锡。愚按:猬脂柔铁,即羚羊角碎金刚石之义。

猬形同鼠,毛刺若针,乃禀金水所生之兽,故能益肠解毒,清热平肝。主治五痔,益肠也。治阴蚀,解毒也。治下血赤白五色,血汁不止,清热也。治阴肿痛引腰背,平肝也。

209. Weipi〔猬皮，hedgehog hide，Corium Erinacei seu Hemiechini〕

It is bitter in taste，mild and non-toxic in property，and it is mainly used to treat five kinds of hemorrhoids，genital erosion，the vaginal bleeding with five colors and difficult to cease，genital swelling and the pain extending to the waist and the back.

The hedgehog often exists in mountains and wilds，popularly called the thorny rat. Its head，mouth，foot and paw are all like those of rat，its thorns and hairs like those of porcupine. When seeing people，it curls up like the shell of Qianshi〔芡实，Euryale，Euryale〕or Banli〔板栗，chestnut，Castaneae Semen〕. When it gathers its hairs together，its thorns will be exposed to the outside，but if put in the water，its hairs will stretch out again. Tao Hongjing （陶弘景）said，"Melt the fat of hedgehog in the iron and add a small amount of Shuiyin〔水银，mercury，Hydrargyrum〕，and the iron will become as soft as lead and tin." Note by Zhang Zhicong（张志聪）：The fat of hedgehog can soften the iron in much the same way that Lingyangjiao〔羚羊角，antelope horn，Cornu Saigae Tataricae〕can hit the diamond into pieces.

Physically similar to the rat with thorns like needles，the hedgehog is the kind of beast that receives metal water，so it can benefit the intestines，resolve toxin，clear heat and pacify the liver. It can mainly treat five kinds of hemorrhoids because it benefits the intestines，treat genital erosion because it resolves toxin，treat the vaginal bleeding with five colors and difficult to cease because it clears heat，and treat genital swelling and the pain extending to the waist and the back because it pacifies the liver.

210. 鳖 甲

鳖甲　气味咸平，无毒。主治心腹症瘕，坚积寒热，去痞疾，息肉，阴蚀，痔核，恶肉。

鳖，水中介虫也，江河池泽处处有之。水居陆生，穹脊连胁，与龟同类。夏日孚乳，其抱以影。《埤雅》云：卵生思抱，其状随日影而转，在水中上必有浮沫,名鳖津,人以此取之。《淮南子》曰:鳖无耳,以目听,名曰神守。陆佃云:鱼满三千六百,则蛟龙引之而飞,纳鳖守之则免,故一名神守。管子云:鳖畏蚊,生鳖遇蚊叮则死,老鳖得蚊煮而烂。熏蚊者,复用鳖甲,物性相报复,如是异哉。甲以九肋者为胜,入药以醋炙黄用。

鳖生池泽,随日影而转,在水中必有津沫上浮,盖禀少阴水气,而上通于君火之日。又,甲介属金,性主攻利,气味咸平,禀水气也。主治心腹症瘕,坚积寒热者,言心腹之内,血气不和,则为症为瘕,内坚积而身寒热。鳖禀少阴之气,上通君火之神,神气内藏,故治在内之症瘕坚积。又曰:去痞疾者,言症瘕坚积,身发寒热。若痞疾,则身无热寒,而鳖甲亦能去也。夫心腹痞积,病藏于内。若息肉,阴蚀,痔核,恶肉,则病见于外。鳖甲属金,金主攻利,故在外之恶肉阴痔,亦能去也。

210. Biejia [鳖甲, turtle carapace, Carapax Trionycis]

It is salty in taste, mild and non-toxic in property, and it is mainly used to treat the abdominal mass in the heart and abdomen, intractable accumulation and cold and heat, and eliminate stuffiness, polyp, genital erosion, hemorrhoid and necrotic muscles.

The turtle, a kind of animal with carapace in the water, exists in rivers, lakes and pools. Of the same species as tortoise, it is born on the land but lives in the water, its high arched spine connected with the ribs. In summer it spawns and its eggs are arranged according to the shadow of the sun. *Pi Ya* [《埤雅》, *A Supplement Book to Erya*] says that the turtle is oviparous and its eggs tend to stay together in a circle. Its shape rotates with the shadow of the sun. When it is in the water, there is floating foam on the surface, called the turtle fluid, which helps people to catch turtles. Huannanzi [《淮南子》, Huainanzi] says that the turtle has no ears and listens with eyes, also called the divine keeper. Lu Dianyun (陆佃云) said, "When the number of fish reaches three thousand and six hundred, the dragon will lead them to fly. However, if the turtle stays there, the fish will not fly way, thus called the divine keeper." Guan Zi (管子) said, "The turtle is afraid of mosquitoes. The newly-born ones could be bitten to death by mosquitoes while the old ones could become very soft when they are boiled together with them. Biejia (turtle carapace) is also used to drive mosquitoes away. Their properties restrain each other, which is very amazing. " The turtle with nine ribs is the best. It should be stir-fried yellow with vinegar for medical use.

The turtle exists in lakes and pools, whose eggs rotate with the shadow of the sun; when it is in the water, there is fluid foam on the surface; it receives the water qi from lesser yin and connects upwards with the sun of sovereign fire. In addition, the turtle carapace pertains to the metal which governs attacking and promoting. Salty in taste and mild in property, it receives water qi. It can mainly treat the abdominal mass in the heart and abdomen, intractable accumulation and cold and heat, because these diseases are caused by disharmony of the blood and qi in the heart and abdomen. The turtle receives the qi of water yin and connects upwards with the god of sovereign fire to store spirit qi internally. Thus, it can treat internal abdominal mass and intractable accumulation. Abdominal mass and intractable accumulation lead to cold and heat in the body while stuffiness doesn't. However, it can also eliminate stuffiness. Stuffiness in the heart and abdomen is a kind of disease hidden inside while polyp, genital erosion, hemorrhoid and necrotic muscles are the diseases that can be seen from outside. It pertains to metal which governs attacking and promoting, so it can treat these external diseases.

211. 蟹

蟹　气味咸寒,有小毒。主治胸中邪气热结痛,喎辟面肿,能败漆,烧之致鼠。

蟹,山东、淮阳、江浙、闽广近海诸处及水乡多有之。有螃蟹、郭索、横行、介士、无肠、公子诸名。雄者脐长,雌者脐圆,腹中之黄,应月盈亏,其性多躁,引声喷沫,至死乃已霜降前食物,故有毒,霜降后可食。

今人以蟹为肴馔,未尝以之治病,唯面有漆疮,多用蟹黄敷之。

211. Xie〔蟹, crab, Eriocheiris Caro et Viscera〕

It is salty in taste, cold and slightly toxic in property, and it is mainly used to treat the pathogenic qi in the chest, the pain caused by heat accumulation, the distorted mouth and the swollen face caused by lacquer. When broiled by fire, it can attract the mouse.

The crab exists in the offshore areas of Shandong (山东), Huaiyang (淮阳), Jiangzhe (江浙) and Minguang (闽广), and in rivers and lakes. It is also called Pangxie (螃蟹), Guosuo (郭索), Hengxing (横行), Jieshi (介士), Wuchang (无肠) and Gongzi (公子). The male has a long umbilicus while the female has a round one. The ovary and digestive glands of crab changes with the shape of the moon. It is easy to be agitated and often spits foam to avoid noises. Those that die before Frost's Descent are toxic. But it is edible after Frost's Descent.

Nowadays, Xie (crab) serves as a dish, and it is not used as medicinal. Only the ovary and digestive glands of crab is applied externally to treat the swollen face caused by lacquer.

212. 蟹 壳 附

蟹壳 附　烧存性,蜜调,涂冻疮及蜂虿伤,酒服治妇人儿枕痛,及血崩,腹痛,消积。《本草纲目》附。

今外科多用蟹壳,捣细筛末,为铁箍败毒散。大抵蟹壳为攻毒散风,消积行瘀之用。学者以意会之可也。

212. Xieqiao〔蟹壳, crabshell, Eriocheiris Crusta〕*supplement*

Broiled to preserve its property and mixed with honey, it is used to smear chilblain and bee sting, treat woman and child pillow pain when taken with liquor, metrorrhagia and abdominal pain, and disperse accumulation. Supplemented in *Ben Cao Gang Mu*〔《本草纲目》, *Compendium of Materia Medica*〕

Xieqiao (crabshell) is often used in surgery today. After it is pounded and sieved, it can be made into Tiegu Baidu San〔铁箍败毒散, Iron Hoop Toxin-Vanquishing Powder〕. It is mainly used to attack toxin, disperse wind, resolve accumulation and remove stasis. Scholars get to know about its effects in treating diseases based on their understanding of it.

213. 蚱蝉

蚱蝉 气味咸甘寒,无毒。主治小儿惊痫,夜啼,癫病寒热。

蝉者总名也,其类不一。二三月即先鸣,小而色黑者,名蜩母,今浙人谓之蛮虫。五月始鸣,大而色黑者,马蜩也。《毛诗》:五月鸣蜩。《月令》:仲夏之月,蝉始鸣即是。此种今浙人谓之老蝉,土音讹为老潜,又谓之蚕蝶。《本经》所谓蚱蝉者,正此蝉也。今时药中所用蝉蜕亦是此蝉之蜕。其头上有花冠者,曰冠蝉,又曰蜩螗。《毛诗》:如蜩如螗是也。小而色青绿者,曰茅蜩,又曰茅螽,今浙中谓之蜘蟟。秋月始鸣,小而色青紫者,曰蟪蛄。《庄子》:蟪蛄,不知春秋者是也。未立秋以前喑而不鸣,先谓之哑蝉,又曰喑蝉。入秋而鸣,时天候渐寒,故又谓之寒蝉,又曰寒蜩,又曰寒螀。《月令》:孟秋之月,寒蝉鸣,即是此种。其余颜色少异,音声略殊,尚有多名,形皆相似。方首广额,两翼六足,升高而鸣,鸣不以口而以胁,吸风饮露,溺而不粪,三十日而死,古时用蝉身,今时只用蝉蜕,不复用身。

蝉感秋气而生,应月周而去,禀金水之气化也。金能制风,水能清热,故主治小儿惊痫。昼鸣夜息,故止小儿夜啼。水火不交,则癫病寒热。蝉禀金水之精,能启下焦之水气,上合心包,故治癫病寒热。

蚱蝉生于夏月,寒蝉生于秋时,今概谓蝉感秋气而生,禀金水之气者,恐未是缪。仲醇曰:蚱蝉禀水土之精,风露之气化而成形。其鸣清响,能发音声。其体轻浮,能出疮疹。其味甘寒,能除风热。其性善蜕,能脱翳障,及女子生子不下。

213. Zhachan [蚱蝉, cicada, Cryptotympana atrata]

It is salty and sweet in taste, cold in property, and it is mainly used to treat infantile fright epilepsy, infantile night crying, depressive psychosis and cold and heat.

Chan [蝉, cicada, Cicadae] is the general name of the animal, which can be divided into different types. Those that begin to sing in the second and third lunar months, small in shape and black in color are called Zhumu (蜩母), nowadays also called Manchong (蛮虫) in Zhejiang (浙江). Those that begin to sing in the fifth lunar month, big in shape and black in color are called Matiao (马蜩). *Maoshi* [《毛诗》, *Mao Poems*] says that Tiao (蜩, cicada) begins to sing in the fifth lunar month. *Yueling* [《月令》, *The Phenology of the Lunar Month*] says that in midsummer, Chan (cicada) begins to sing. Nowadays, in Zhejiang (浙江) this type of Chan (cicada) is called Laochan (老蝉) which is incorrectly pronounced as Laoqian (老潜) by the local accent. It is also called Candie (蚕蝶). The so-called Zhachan (cicada) in *Sheng Nong Ben Cao Jing* [《神农本草经》, *Shennong's Classic of Materia Medica*] just refers to this type of Chan (cicada). It is Chantui [蝉蜕, cicada molting, Cicadae Periostracum] of this type that is used as medicinal nowadays. Those that have flower-like crowns on their heads are called Guanchan (冠蝉) or Tiaotang (蜩螗). *Maoshi* [《毛诗》, *Mao Poems*] says that it is like Tiao (蜩) or Tang (螗). Those that are small and green are called Maotiao (茅蜩) or Maoge (茅蠽), which are also called Zhiliao (蜘蟟) nowadays in Zhizhong (浙中). Those that begin to sing in autumn, small in shape and blue-purple in color are called Huigu (蟪蛄). *Zhuang Zi* [《庄子》, *Zhuangzi*] says that Huigu (蟪蛄) has no idea about the season. It keeps silent and does not sing before the beginning of autumn, and thus initially it is called Yachan (哑蝉) or Yinchan (喑蝉). It begins to sing when the autumn sets in. At this time, the weather is becoming colder and colder, and thus it is also called Hanchan (寒蝉), Hantiao (寒蜩) or Hanjiang (寒蠽). *Yueling* [《月令》, *The Phenology of the Lunar Month*] says that Hanchan (寒蝉) begins to sing in the first month of autumn, which just refers to this type of Chan (cicada). For the other types, their colors are almost the same, and their sounds are slightly different. Although traditionally named differently, they are similar in appearance. Chan (Cicada) has a square face, a broad forehead, two wings and six feet, flying to high places to sing and singing with hypochondrium instead of mouth. It breathes wind in and drinks dew. It only urinates but doesn't defecate and its life only lasts 30 days. Its body was used in ancient times while only Chantui (cicada molting) is used nowadays and its body is no longer used.

Born when sensing autumn qi and die after a cycle of a month, Chan (cicada) receives the qi transformation of metal and water. Metal can control wind and water can clear heat, so it can mainly treat infantile fright epilepsy. It sings in the daytime and rests at night, so it can stop infantile night crying. The non-interaction of water and fire causes depressive psychosis and cold and heat. Receiving the essence of metal and water, it can open the water qi of the lower energizer and combine it with pericardium, so it can treat depressive psychosis and chills and fever.

Zhachan（cicada）is born in summer while Hanchan（寒蝉）in autumn. Thus, it is said nowadays that Chan（cicada）is born after sensing autumn qi and receives the qi of metal and water, which, I'm afraid, probably is not false. Zhong Chun（仲醇）said, "Zhachan（cicada）receives the essence of water and earth and is shaped by the qi transformation of wind and dew." Its sound is clear and loud, so it can treat the loss of voice; its body is light, so it can erupt sores and rashes; its taste is sweet and its property is cold, so it can eliminate wind heat; it is good at molting, so it can remove nebula and treat woman retention of fetus.

214. 蝉 蜕 附

蝉蜕 附 气味咸甘寒,无毒。主治小儿惊痫,妇人生子不下。烧灰水服,治久痢。《别录》附。

李时珍曰:凡用蜕壳,沸汤洗去泥土、翅足,浆水洗过晒干用。

古人用身,后人用蜕。蜕者,褪脱之义。故眼膜翳障,痘瘄不起,皮肤隐疹,一切风热之证,取而用之。学者知蝉性之本原,则知蝉蜕之治疗矣。

214. Chantui [蝉蜕, cicada molting, Cicadae Periostracum] *supplement*

It is salty and sweet in taste, cold and non-toxic in property, and it is mainly used to treat child fright epilepsy and the woman retention of fetus. It is also used to treat chronic dysentery when burned into ashes and taken with water. Supplemented in *Ming Yi Bie Lu* [《名医别录》, *Miscellaneous Records of Famous Physicians*].

Li Shizhen（李时珍）said, "To use Chantui（cicada molting）as medicinal, first wash away dust, wings and feet in boiling water, then wash it in the sour millet water and finally dry it in the sun."

The ancients used the body of Chan （cicada） as medicinal while the later generations have used Chantui （cicada molting）. Molting means sloughing and casting off. Therefore， it can treat all the wind-heat syndromes， such as eye film nebula， failure in eruption of pox and rash， and skin urticaria. Scholars know the origin of the property of Chan （cicada），so they know what kind of diseases it can be used to treat.

215. 白僵蚕

白僵蚕　气味咸辛平，无毒。主治小儿惊痫夜啼，去三虫，灭黑䵟，令人面色好，男子阴痒病。

蚕处处可育，而江浙尤多，蚕病风死，其色不变，故名白僵，僵者死而不朽之谓。

《乘雅》云：今市肆多用中温死蚕，以石灰淹拌，令白服之，为害最深。若痘疹，必燥裂黑陷。若疮毒必黑烂内攻，不可不慎也。

僵蚕色白体坚，气味咸辛，禀金水之精也。东方肝木，其病发惊骇，金能平木，故主治小儿惊痫。金属乾而主天，天运环转，则昼开夜合，故止小儿夜啼。金主肃杀，故去三虫。水气上滋，则面色润泽，故主灭黑䵟而令人面色好。金能制风，咸能杀痒，故治男子阴痒之病。阴，前阴也。

蝉蜕、僵蚕，皆禀金水之精，故《本经》主治大体相同。但蝉饮而不食，溺而不粪。蚕食而不饮，粪而不溺，何以相同。《经》云：饮入于胃，上归于肺。谷入于胃，乃传之肺。是饮是食虽殊，皆由肺气之通调；则溺粪虽异，皆禀肺气以传化矣。又，凡色白而禀金气之品，皆不宜火炒。僵蚕具坚金之体，故能祛风攻毒。若以火炒，则金体消败，何能奏功。后人不体物理，不察物性，而妄加炮制者，不独一僵蚕已也。如桑皮炒黄，麻黄炒黑，杏仁、蒺藜皆用火炒。诸如此类，不能尽述，皆由不知药性之原，狃于习俗之所致耳。

215. Baijiangcan［白僵蚕，silkworm larva，Larva Bombycis］

It is salty and pungent in taste， mild and non-toxic in property， and it is mainly used to treat infantile fright epilepsy and night crying， eliminate three worms， reduce black moles， luster complexion and treat the genital itching in men.

Silkworm can be raised everywhere, but most of them are produced in Jiangzhe（江浙）. When they catch diseases and die quickly, their skin color does not change, thus called Baijiang［白僵, white corpse］which means dead but not rotten.

Ben Cao Cheng Ya［《本草乘雅》, *Explanation on Materia Medica from Four Aspects*］says that nowadays the silkworms which died of plague and was whitened by mixing with lime are often used in the market, which could lead to severe consequences. If it is used to treat pox and rash, they will become dry cracked and black, falling inward. If it is used to resolve sore toxin, the sore will become black and ulcerated, attacking inward. Therefore, people should be very cautious when using it.

White in color, salty and pungent in taste, and its body being hard, Baijiangcan（silkworm larva）receives the essence of metal and water. The diseases with the liver causes fright; metal can calm wood, so it can mainly treat infantile fright epilepsy. Metal pertains to Qian［乾, one of the Nine Palaces］and governs the heaven; the circular movement of the heaven leads to the changes of day and night, so it can stop infantile night crying. Metal is characterized by clearing and downward, so it can eliminate three worms. Water qi moves upward to moisten and luster complexion, so it can reduce black moles and luster complexion. Metal can control wind and saltiness can relieve itching, so it can treat the genital itching in men. Yin（阴）here refers to the external genitalia.

Both Chantu［蝉蜕, cicada molting, Cicadae Periostracum］and Baijiangcan（silkworm larva）receive the essence of metal and water, thus they can mainly treat almost the same diseases in *Shen Nong Ben Cao Jing*［《神农本草经》, *Shennong's Classic of Materia Medica*］. But Chan［蝉, cicada, Cicadae］drinks but it doesn't eat; it urinates but it doesn't defecate. Can［蚕, silkworm, Bombycis］eats but doesn't drink, defecates but doesn't urinate. How could they treat the same diseases? *Huang Di Nei Jing*［《黄帝内经》, *Huangdi's Internal Canon of Medicine*］says that when water is taken into the stomach, its essence qi is transported upwards into the lung; when food is taken into the stomach, its nutrient substance is transported into the lung. Therefore, eating and drinking, though different, are both regulated by lung qi; urination and defecation, though different, both receives lung qi for transportation and transformation. In addition, those white in color and receiving metal qi are not suitable to be stir-fried. Baijiangcan (silkworm larva) has the sturdy metallic body, so it can dispel wind and attack toxin. If stir-fried, it will lose the metallic body, how could it be effective in treating diseases? Baijiangcan (silkworm larva) is not the only one to be mistakenly processed by the later generations who don't explore the properties and qualities of these medicinals. For instance, Sangpi [桑皮, mulberry bark, Mori Cortex] is stir-fried to yellow, Mahuang [麻黄, ephedra, Ephedrae Herba] is stir-fried to black, and both Xingren [杏仁, apricot kernel, Armeniacae Semen] and Jili [蒺藜, tribulus, Tuibuli Fructus] are stir-fired. Those instances are too numerous to be dwelled on. The reason for these mistakes is that people don't know about the origin of medicinal property and are chained to customs.

216. 原蚕沙 附

原蚕沙 附　气味甘辛温,无毒。主治肠鸣,热中消渴,风痹,隐疹。《别录》附。

　　原蚕,晚蚕之母蚕也,故名原蚕,在头蚕之前先养数百,出蛾生子,俟头蚕茧后,然后育此子,为二蚕。是原蚕先得桑叶始发之纯精,故去风、清热、续绝之功最大,此沙极少。日华子释原蚕为晚蚕,此误释也。原蚕沙难得,今医俱用晚蚕沙。夫晚蚕即原蚕所育之二蚕也,与其用原蚕所育之二蚕,不若竟用头蚕之沙矣。品虽闲冷,不可不知。

　　按:《周礼》有禁原蚕之文。郑康成注云:原,再也,谓再养者为原蚕,自古已然。隐庵乃释为晚蚕之母蚕,正恐未的,古人于蚕蛾、蚕沙俱用。晚蚕者,盖取其得夏时火令深耳。

216. Yuancansha [原蚕沙, silkworm droppings, Bombycis Faeces] supplement

It is sweet and pungent in taste, warm and non-toxic in property, and it is mainly used to treat rumbling intestines, heat stroke, consumptive thirst, wind impediment, and urticaria. Supplemented in *Ming Yi Bie Lu* [《名医别录》, *Miscellaneous Records of Famous Physicians*].

The silkworm here refers to the mother of summer silkworms, thus called source silkworms. Before spring silkworms, hundreds of worms are raised and their moths give birth to them. After the spring worms cocoon, they give birth to source silkworms which actually are produced by the second hatch. It is the source silkworm that first obtains the pure essence of young mulberry leaves, so it is most effective in dispelling wind, clearing heat and prolonging menstruation. Yuancansha (silkworm droppings) are very rare. Ri Huazi (日华子) said that source silkworms were summer silkworms, which is wrong. Since it is hard to get it, nowadays Wancansha [晚蚕沙, silkworm droppings, Bombycis Faeces] is used in medicine. Summer silkworms are hatched by source silkworms. Therefore, it is better to use the droppings of spring silkworms rather than those hatched by source silkworms. Although it is seldom used, it should be known.

Note by Gao Shishi (高世栻): It is recorded in *Zhou Li* [《周礼》, *Rites of the Zhou*] that source silkworms are banned. Zheng Kangcheng (郑康成) made a commentary, "Yuan (原) means again, so source silkworms are the second hatched silkworms, which has been the case since ancient times." According to Yin Annai (隐庵乃), source silkworms are the mother of summer silkworms; as it was hard to get, both silkworm moth and Cansha [蚕沙, silkworm droppings, Bombycis Faeces] were used in ancient times. Summer silkworms get their name probably because they are hatched in later summer.

217. 樗 鸡

樗鸡 气味苦平,有小毒。主治心腹邪气,阴痿,益精强志,生子好色,补中轻身。

樗鸡出梁州、岐州、汴洛诸界尤多。生樗树上,形类蚕蛾而腹大,六足、重翼,外一重灰黄有斑点,内一重深红,五色相间。有一种头翅皆赤者,名红娘子。今樗鸡未之用也,而红娘子间有用者。

樗鸡生于木上,味苦色赤,禀木火之气化。主治心腹邪气者,禀火气以治心,禀木气以治腹也。治阴痿者,火气盛也。益精强志者,水火相济也。生子好色者,木生火也。补中轻身者,火生土也。

217. Chuji [樗鸡, red lady-bug, Huecchys Sanguinea]

It is bitter in taste, mild and slightly toxic in property, and it is mainly used to treat the pathogenic qi in the heart and abdomen and impotence, replenish essence, strengthen memory, enable women to conceive babies, increase sexuality, tonify the middle and keep people healthy.

Chuji (red lady-bug) mainly exists in Liangzhou (梁州), Qizhou (岐州) and Bianluo (汴洛). It is born on ailanthus, which is like the silk moth in shape and has a large belly, six feet and double wings. The outer wing is gray-yellow with spots, and the inner one is deep red with five-coloured stripes. There is a kind of animals which are like Chuji (red lady-bug) but with a red head and wings, so they are called Hongniangzi [红娘子, red cicada, Huechys]. Nowadays, Chuji (red lady-bug) is seldom used while Hongniangzi (red cicada) is used occasionally.

Born on the wood, bitter in taste and red in color, Chuji (red lady-bug) receives the qi transformation of wood and fire. It can mainly treat the pathogenic qi in the heart and abdomen because it receives fire qi to treat the diseases in the heart, and receives wood qi to treat the diseases in the abdomen. It can treat impotence because it is exuberant in fire qi. It can replenish essence and strengthen memory because fire and water coordinate with each other. It enables women to conceive babies and increase sexuality because wood generates fire, and it can tonify the middle and keep people healthy because fire generates earth.

218. 䗪虫

䗪虫 气味咸寒,有毒。主治心腹寒热洗洗,血积症瘕,破坚,下血闭,生子大良。䗪音蔗。

䗪虫《本经》名地鳖。《别录》名土鳖,以其形扁如鳖也。又名簸箕虫,亦以其形相似也。陆农师云:䗪逢申日则过街,故又名过街。生人家屋下土中湿处及鼠壤中,略似鼠妇而圆,大寸余,无甲有鳞。李时珍云:处处有之,与灯蛾相牝牡。

《金匮》方中治久病结积,有大黄䗪虫丸。又治疟痞,有鳖甲煎丸。及妇人下瘀血汤方并用之。今外科、接骨科亦用之。乃攻坚破积,行血散疟之剂。学者以意会之可也。

218. Zhechong〔䗪虫, ground beetle, Corydiidae〕

It is salty in taste, cold and toxic in property, and it is mainly used to treat the cold and heat in the heart and abdomen with chilliness and shivering and the abdominal mass due to blood accumulation, break hard mass and precipitate blood block. It is very effective in promoting the conception of babies. "䗪" is pronounced as zhe（蔗）.

Zhechong（ground beetle）is called Dibie（地鳖）in *Shen Nong Ben Cao Jing*〔《神农本草经》, *Shennong's Classic of Materia Medica*〕and Tubie（土鳖）in *Ming Yi Bie Lu*〔《名医别录》, *Miscellaneous Records of Famous Physicians*〕, for it is as flat as Bie（鳖）. It is also called "dustpan bug" due to their similarity in shape. Lu Nongshi（陆农师）said, "Zhechong（ground beetle）crosses the street on Shenri（申日）, thus also called Guojie〔过街, crossing the street〕." It is born in the wet soil below houses and the soil of the rat's hole. It looks somewhat like a Shufu〔鼠妇, wood louse, Armadilidium〕, round, about one Cun in length, having no shell but scaly." Li Shizhen（李时珍）said, "It exists everywhere. Together with the tiger moth, they are females and males."

In *Jin Gui Yao Lue*〔《金匮要略》, *Synopsis of Golden Chamber*〕, Dahuang Zhechong Wan〔大黄䗪虫丸, Rhubarb and Ground Beetle Pill〕is used to treat the binding and accumulation due to chronic diseases; Biejiajian Wan〔鳖甲煎丸, Turtle Shell Decocted Pill〕is used to treat malaria and stuffiness. Zhechong（ground beetle）is used together with Xiayuxue Tang〔下瘀血汤, Stasis-Precipitating decoctions〕for women. Nowadays, it is also used in surgery and orthopedics. It is a formula that can attack hard mass and break accumulation, move the blood and dissipate chronic malaria. Scholars get to know about its effects in treating diseases based on their understanding of it.

219. 虻 虫

虻虫 气味苦,微寒,有毒。主逐瘀血,破血积坚痞,症瘕寒热,通利血脉,及九窍。

虻虫一名蜚虻,大如蜜蜂,腹凹褊,微黄绿色,牲啖牛马血。

虻乃吮血之虫,性又飞动,故主逐瘀血积血,通利血脉、九窍。《伤寒论》:太阳病,表不解,随经瘀热在里,抵当汤主之。内用虻虫、水蛭、大黄、桃仁。近时儿医治痘不起发,每加牛虻,此外未之用也。

219. Mangchong〔虻虫, tabanus, Tabanus〕

It is bitter in taste, slightly cold and toxic in property, and it is mainly used to expel static blood, break blood accumulation, hard mass and stuffiness, treat abdominal mass and cold and heat, promote the blood vessels and relieve the nine orifices.

Mangchong (tabanus), also known as Feimang (蜚虻), is as big as a bee, with a concave and flat abdomen, a little yellow-green in color. It feeds on the cattle and horse blood.

Mangchong (tabanus) is a kind of blood-sucking insect which is able to fly, so it can mainly expel static blood, break blood accumulation and promote the blood vessels and the nine orifices. *Shang Han Lun*〔《伤寒论》, *Treatise on Exogenous Febrile Diseases*〕says that as for greater yang syndrome, the exterior is not resolved and the stagnated heat stays in the interior with the channel; it should be treated with the decoction made up of Mangchong (tabanus), Shuizhi〔水蛭, leech, Hirudo〕, Dahuang〔大黄, rhubarb, Rhei Radix et Rhizoma〕and Taoren〔桃仁, peach kernel, Persicae Semen〕. In recent times, pediatricians always use Mangchong (tabanus) to treat pox when it fails to rise and erupt. Except that, it is seldom used.

220. 蛞 蝓

蛞蝓 气味咸寒,无毒。主治贼风喎僻,跌筋,及脱肛,惊痫,挛缩。蛞蝓音阔俞。

蛞蝓即蜒蚰也,大者如人手指,肥泽有涎,头有二角,行则角出,惊之则缩,以其身涎涂蜗蚣、蝎虿毒,疼痛即止。

蜒蚰感雨湿之气而生,故气味咸寒。主定惊清热,解毒输筋。寇宗奭曰:蛞蝓能解蜈蚣毒。近时治咽喉肿痛,风热喉痹,用簪脚捵之,内入喉中,令吞下,即愈。

220. Kuoyu〔蛞蝓,slug,Limax〕

It is salty in taste, cold and non-toxic in property, and it is mainly used to treat the distorted mouth due to abnormal weather, sinew injury from falls, prolapse of rectum, fright epilepsy and contracture. "蛞蝓" is pronounced as kuoyu(阔俞).

Kuoyu (slug) is popularly known as Yanyou (蜒蚰). The big one is like a human finger, fat, moist and having saliva. It has two tentacles on its head, emerging when it moves and contracting when it is scared. Its saliva can relive pain when applied to the toxins of centipede and scorpion.

Kuoyu (slug) is born after sensing the qi of rain and dampness, so it is bitter in taste and cold in property. It can mainly stabilize fright, clear heat, resolve toxin, and relax sinews. Kou Zongshi (寇宗奭) said that Kuoyu (slug) could resolve centipede toxin. In recent times, it is used to treat sore swollen throat and wind-heat pharyngitis. Pick it up with the end of hairpin, put it into the throat, swallow it, and the diseases can be cured very soon.

221. 蜗 牛

蜗牛 附气味咸寒,有小毒。主治贼风喎辟,跌跌,大肠脱肛,筋急,及惊痫。《别录》附。

蛞蝓,蜗牛一种二类,背负壳者,名蜗牛,无壳者,名蛞蝓,主治功用相同。

蜗牛一名蜗蠃,感雨湿化生而成介虫之类,气味咸寒,能清热解毒。甲虫属金,能去风定惊。大肠属阳明,寒则收缩,热则纵驰,故主治如此。

221. Woniu〔蜗牛, snail, Eulota〕

It is salty in taste, cold and slightly toxic in property, and it is mainly used to treat the distorted mouth due to the abnormal weather, bent hands and feet causing falls, large intestinal prolapse of rectum, the tension of the sinews, and fright epilepsy. Supplemented in *Ming Yi Bie Lu*〔《名医别录》, *Miscellaneous Records of Famous Physicians*〕.

Kuoyu〔蛞蝓, slug, Limax〕and Woniu (snail) are two types of the same species. Those who bear shells are named Woniu (snail), those without shells Kuoyu (slug). They have the same effects in treating diseases.

Woniu (snail), also called Woying (蜗蠃), is born after sensing rain and dampness and grows into a kind of beetle. It is salty in taste and cold in property, so it can clear heat and resolve toxin. The beetle pertains to metal, so it can expel wind and stabilize fright. The large intestine which pertains to yang brightness contracts when it feels cold and expands when it feels hot, so it is mainly used to treat the large intestinal prolapse of rectum.

222. 露蜂房

露蜂房 气味甘平,有毒。主治惊痫瘛疭,寒热邪气,癫疾,鬼精蛊毒,肠痔。火熬之良。

蜂房是胡蜂所结之窠,悬于树上,得风露者,故名露蜂房,乃水土所结成。大者如瓮,小者如桶,十一二月采之。

蜂房水土结成,又得雾露清凉之气,故主祛风解毒,镇惊清热。仲祖鳖甲煎丸用之,近医用之治齿痛,褪管,攻毒,解毒,清热祛风。学者以意会之可也。

222. Lufengfang〔露蜂房, honeycomb of paper wasps, Nidus Polistis Mandarini〕

It is sweet in taste, mild and non-toxic in property, and it is mainly used to treat fright epilepsy, convulsion, the chills and fever due to pathogenic qi, epilepsy, the diseases caused by the strange pathogenic factors like ghosts, relieve parasitic toxin, and treat intestinal hemorrhoids. It is more effective when boiled by fire.

Fengfang [蜂房, hornet's nest, Vespae Nidus] is the nest built by wasps, which is hung on the tree and exposed to wind and dew, thus called Lufengfang (honeycomb of paper wasps). It is made of water and soil, bigger ones like urns and small ones like barrels. It can be collected in the eleventh and twelfth lunar months.

Fengfang (hornet's nest) is made of water and soil and receives the cool qi of fog and dew, so it can mainly expel wind, resolve toxin, stabilize fright, and clear heat. It is used in Biejiajian Wan [鳖甲煎丸, Turtle Shell Decocted Pill] by Zhang Zhongjing (张仲景). Nowadays, doctors use it to treat toothache, remove fistula, attack toxin, resolve toxin, clear heat, and expel wind. Scholars get to know about its effects in treating diseases based on their understanding of it.

223. 乌贼鱼骨

乌贼鱼骨 气味咸,微温,无毒。主治女子赤白漏下经汁,血闭,阴蚀肿痛,寒热症瘕,无子。

乌贼鱼生海中,形若革囊,口在腹下,八足聚生于口旁,无鳞有须,皮黑肉白。其背上只生一骨,厚三四分,两头小,中央阔,色洁白,质轻脆,如通草,重重有纹,以指甲可刮为末。腹中血及胆正黑如墨汁,可以书字,但逾年则迹灭,唯存空纸尔。其骨《素问》名乌鲗骨,今名海螵蛸。

乌贼骨禀金水之精,金能平木,故治血闭肿痛,寒热症瘕。水能益髓,故治赤白漏下,女子无子。《素问》:治年少时,有所大脱血,或醉入房,中气竭肝伤,故月事衰少不来,病名血枯,治以四乌鲗骨,一茹蘆为末,丸以雀卵,大如小豆,每服五丸,饮以鲍鱼汁。

223. Wuzei Yugu [乌贼鱼骨, cuttlefish bone, Sepiae Endoconcha]

It is salty in taste, slightly warm and non-toxic in property, and it is mainly used to treat red and white metrostaxis, amenorrhea, genital erosion, swelling and pain, cold and heat, abdominal mass and infertility.

The cuttlefish exists in the sea and is like a leather bag in shape. Its mouth is under the belly with its eight feet around the mouth. It has whiskers but no scales; its skin is black and its meat white. There is only one bone on its back, three to four Fen in thickness, small at both ends but wide in the middle, which is white, light and crisp, just like Tongcao〔通草, rice-paper plant pith, Tetrapanacis Medulla〕. The bone has layers of stripes and can be scraped into powder by nails. The blood in the abdomen and the bile are as black as ink, which can be used to write. However, after a year, the writing will disappear, only blank paper left. The bone is named Xiezeigu（写鲗骨）in *Huang Di Nei Jing: Su Wen*〔《黄帝内经·素问》, *Huangdi's Internal Classic: Plain Questions*〕, and today it is called Haipiaoshao〔海螵蛸, cuttlefish bone, Sepiae Endoconcha〕.

Wuzei Yugu（cuttlefish bone）receives the essence of metal and water. Metal can restrain wood, so it can treat amenorrhea, swelling and pain, cold and heat and abdominal mass. Water can replenish marrow, so it can treat red and white metrostaxis, and infertility. *Huang Di Nei Jing: Su Wen*〔《黄帝内经·素问》, *Huangdi's Internal Classic: Plain Questions*〕says that the excessive loss of blood when the patient was young or sexual intercourse after drinking of wine which exhausts center qi and impairs the liver, consequently lead to scanty menstruation or amenorrhea, which is called Xueku〔血枯, amenorrhea〕; to treat it, Wuzei Yugu（cuttlefish bone）and Rulü〔茹蘆, Indian madder, Herba Rubiae〕, with the ratio of 4∶1, are mixed up with bird eggs and made into pills as large as a red bean. The patient can take five pills each time and then drink some abalone soup.

224. 文　蛤

文蛤　气味咸平，无毒。主治恶疮蚀，五痔。

文蛤生东海中，背上有斑文，大者圆三寸，小者圆五六分。沈存中《笔谈》云：文蛤即今吴人所食花蛤也，其形一头小，一头大，壳有花斑者是。《开宝》《药性》有五倍子，亦名文蛤，乃是蜀中盐肤子树上之虫窠也，以象形而称之，与水中所产文蛤不同。

蛤乃水中介虫，禀寒水之精，故主治恶疮蚀。感燥金之气，主资阳明大肠，故治五痔。五痔解，见黄芪条下。

《伤寒太阳篇》曰：病在阳,应以汗解之,反以冷水噀之,若灌之,其热被却不得去,弥更益烦,肉上粟起,意欲饮水,反不渴者,服文蛤散。文蛤五两为末,每服方寸匕,沸汤下,甚效。文蛤外刚内柔,象合离明,能燥水湿,而散热邪也。

224. Wenge [文蛤, meretrix clam shell, Concha Meretricis]

It is salty in taste, mild and non-toxic in property, and it is mainly used to treat malign sore erosion and five kinds of hemorrhoids.

Wenge (meretrix clam shell) exists in East China Sea, with spots on its back. The bigger ones are three Cun round and the small ones five or six Fen round. In *Meng Xi Bi Tan* [《梦溪笔谈》, *Dream Pool Essay*], Shen Cunzhong (沈存中) said, "Wenge (meretrix clam shell) is just clam eaten by people in Wu (吴) nowadays; it is big at one end and small at the other, with colored spots on its shell. In *Kai Bao Ben Cao* [《开宝本草》, *Materia Medica of the Kaibao Era*] and *Yao Xing Fu* [《药性赋》, *Properties of the Medicines*], Wubeizi [五倍子, sumac gallnut, Galla Chinensis Galla] is also called Wenge (meretrix clam shell)). However, it is actually worm's nest on the Chinese sumac fruit tree in Shuzhong (蜀中). Due to their similar physical appearance, it is also called Wenge (文蛤), which is actually quite different from Wenge (meretrix clam shell) produced in the sea.

As a kind of beetle existing in the sea, Wenge (meretrix clam shell) receives the essence of cold water, so it can mainly treat malign sore erosion. It senses qi of dry metal and mainly supports the large intestine of yang brightness, so it can treat five kinds of hemorrhoids. As for the method to treat five kinds of hemorrhoids, please refer to the entry of Huangqi [黄芪, astragalus, Astragali Radix].

Shang Han Lun: Tai Yang Pian [《伤寒太阳篇》, *Treatise on Exogenous Febrile Diseases: Great Yang*] says that when the disease is at the initial yang channel, diaphoresis should be adopted as the correct therapy. But the patient was showered with cold water. Consequently, the pathogenic heat cannot come out from the sweat glands as the cold water hampers the activity. Besides, the patient would become more vexed and has millet papules on the skin. He would like to have a drink of water, but he doesn't feel thirsty. In this case, he should take

Wenge San［文蛤散, Meretrix Clam Shell Powder］which includes five Liang of Wenge（meretrix clam shell）powder. The patient can take one Fangcunbi of powder each time with boiled water. It is very effective. Wenge（meretrix clam shell）, which is rigid externally and soft internally, just like Liming［离明, fire light］, can dry water dampness and dissipate heat pathogen.

225. 发 髲

发髲 气味苦温,无毒。主治五癃,关格不通,利小便水道,疗小儿惊,大人痉,仍自还神化。髲音备。

发髲,近于头皮之发也。剪下者为整发,梳栉而下者为乱发。发髲以皂荚水洗净,入瓶内固济,煅存性用,谓之血余。《别录》复有乱发,大义与发髲相同,不必别出。

古之发髲,取男子年近二十岁以上,无疾患,颜貌红白者,从顶心剪切,煅研入丸药膏中用。今时以剃下短发入用,似于髲字之义更合。

发者,血之余。血者,水之类。水精奉心,则化血也。又,《经》云:肾之合骨也,其荣发也。是发乃少阴心肾之所主,故气味苦温,苦者火之味,温者火之气也,水火相济,则阴阳和合,故主治五癃,及关格不通。又曰:利小便水道者,言禀肾气而益膀胱,则利小便。禀心气而益三焦,则利水道也。心虚则惊,肾虚则痉。发乃少阴心肾之所主,故疗小儿惊,大人痉。小儿天癸未至,故病惊。大人天癸已至,故病痉也。发髲炼服,能益水精而资血液,故曰:仍自还神化。谓仍能助水精而上奉心藏之神,以化其血也。凡吐血、衄血之证,皆宜用血余也。

225. Fabei［发髲, human hair, Capillus］

It is bitter in taste, warm and non-toxic in property, and it is mainly used to treat five kinds of ischuria, anuria and vomiting, disinhibit urination and dredge water passage, treat the infantile fright and tetany in adults, and enable people to have magic transformation. "髲" is pronounced as Bei（备）.

Fabei（human hair）refers to the hair root near the scalp. The hair that has been cut off is called "neat hair", and the one that has been combed off is called "messy hair". The one that is washed with Zaojia［皂荚, gleditsia,

Gleditsiae Fructus] water, bonded in the bottle and calcined without destroying the nature is called Xueyu [血余, hair, Crinis]. Besides Fabei (human hair), Luanfa [乱发, hair, Crinis] is also recorded in *Ming Yi Bie Lu* [《名医别录》, *Miscellaneous Records of Famous Physicians*]. However, their properties and usages are almost the same, so there is no need to record them separately.

In ancient times, Fabei (human hair) was taken from a man over 20 years old, having no disease and with a fair and rosy complexion. It was cut off from the top center of the head, calcined and ground into pills and medicinal pastes for medical use. Nowadays, short hair is used, which seems to be more appropriate to the meaning of "髪" (Bei).

The hair is the surplus of the blood, which belongs to the category of water. Water essense is supplied to the heart and transformed into the blood. Besides, *Huang Di Nei Jing* [《黄帝内经》, *Huangdi's Internal Classic*] says that the kidney coordinates with bones and its splendor is reflected on the hair. The hair is governed by the heart and kidney of lesser yin, so it is bitter in taste and warm in property. Bitterness is the taste of fire and warmness is the qi of fire. The coordination between fire and water leads to the combination and harmonization of yin and yang, so Fabei (human hair) can mainly treat five kinds of ischuria, anuria and vomiting. It receives kidney qi and replenishes the bladder, so it can disinhibit urination. It receives heart qi and replenishes the triple energizer, so it can dredge water passage. The heart deficiency causes fright, and the kidney deficiency causes tetany. The hair is governed by the heart and kidney of lesser yin, so it can treat the infantile fright and tetany in adults. For children, as Tiangui (reproduction-stimulating essence) hasn't appeared, they are infected with fright while for adults, as it has appeared, they are infected with tetany. Fabei (human hair), calcined and taken, can replenish water essence and nourish the blood. Therefore, it can enable people to have the magic transformation. As Fabei (human hair) can assist water essence and supply the spirit stored in the heart to be transformed into blood, it is suitable to be used to treat such diseases as hematemesis and epistaxis.

卷下 本经下品

Volumn 3　Low-Grade Medicinals

226. 附 子

附子 气味辛温,有大毒。主治风寒咳逆邪气,寒湿踒躄拘挛,膝痛不能行走,破症坚积聚,血瘕金疮。

附子以蜀地绵州出者为良,他处虽有,为薄不堪用也。绵州邻县八,唯彰明出附子,彰明领乡二十,唯赤水、廉水、昌明、会昌四乡出附子,而又推赤水一乡出者为最佳。其初种而成者,为乌头,形如乌鸟之头也。其附母根而生,虽相须实不相连者,为附子,如子附母也。旁生支出而小者,名侧子。种而独生无所附,长三四寸者,名天雄。附子之形以蹲坐正节,而侧子少者为上,有节多乳者次之。形不正而伤缺风皱者为下。其色以花白者为上,黑色者次之,青色者为下,俗呼黑附子,正以其色黑,兼以别于白附之子名耳。

附子禀雄壮之质,具温热之性,故有大毒。《本经》下品之药,大毒、有毒者居多,《素问》所谓毒药攻邪也。夫攻其邪而正气复,是攻之即所以补之。附子味辛性温,生于彰明赤水,是禀大热之气,而益太阳之标阳,助少阳之火热者也。太阳阳热之气,不循行于通体之皮毛,则有风寒咳逆之邪气。附子益太阳之标阳,故能治也。少阳火热之气,不游行于肌关之骨节,则有寒湿踒躄拘挛,膝痛不能行走之证。附子助少阳之火热,故能治也。症坚积聚,阳气虚而寒气内凝也。血瘕,乃阴血聚而为瘕。金疮,乃刀斧伤而溃烂。附子具温热之气,以散阴寒,禀阳火之气,以长肌肉,故皆治之。

《经》云:草生五色,五色之变,不可胜视。草生五味,五味之美,不可胜极。天食人以五气,地食人以五味。故在天时,宜司岁备物;在地利,在五方五土之宜。附子以产彰明、赤水者为胜,盖得地土之专精。夫太阳之阳,天一之水也,生于膀胱水府,而彰明于上。少阳之阳,地二之火也,生于下焦之火,而赤日行天。据所出之地,曰彰明、曰赤水者,盖亦有巧符者矣。学者欲知物性之精微,而五方生产之宜,与先圣命名之意,亦当体认毋忽。今陕西亦莳植附子,谓之西附,性辛温,而力稍薄,不如生于川中者,土厚而力雄也。又,今药肆中零卖制熟附子,皆西附之类。盖川附价高,市利者皆整卖,不切片卖,用者须知之。

凡人火气内衰,阳气外驰,急用炮熟附子助火之原,使神机上行而不下殒,环行而不外脱,治之于微,奏功颇易。奈世医不明医理,不识病机,必至脉脱厥冷,神去魄存,方谓宜用附子。夫附子治病者也,何能治命? 甚至终身行医,而终身视附子为蛇蝎。每告人曰:附子不可服,服之必发狂,而九窍流血;服之必发火,而痈毒顿生;服之必内烂五脏,今年服之,明年毒发。嗟嗟! 以若医而遇附子之证,何以治之。肯后利轻名而自谢不及乎? 肯自居庸浅而荐贤以补救乎? 必至今日药之,明日药之,神气已变,然后覆之,斯时虽有仙丹,莫之能救。贤者于此,或具热衷,不忍立而视其死,问投附子以救之,投之而效,功也。投之不效,亦非后人之过。前医唯恐后医奏功,衹幸其死,死后推过,谓其死,由饮附子而死。噫,若医而有良心者乎,医不通经旨,牛马而襟裾,医云乎哉。

如用附子,本身有一两余者,方为有力。侧子分两须除去之,土人欲增分两,用木杯将侧子敲平于上,故连侧子重一两五六钱者,方好。土人又恐南方得种,生时以戎盐淹之,然后入杯敲平。是附子本无咸味,而以盐淹之,故咸也。制附子之法,以刀削去皮脐,剖作四块,切片,用滚水连泡二次,去盐味、毒味,晒半燥,于铜器内炒熟用之。盖上古司岁备物,火气司岁,则备温热之药。《经》曰:司岁备物,专精者也。非司岁备物,气散者也。后世不能如上古之预备,故有附子火炮之说。近世皆以童便煮之,乃因讹传讹,习焉不知其非耳。

226. Fuzi〔附子, aconite, Radix Aconiti Praeparata〕

It is pungent in taste, warm and severely toxic in property, and it is mainly used to relieve wind-cold and the cough with dyspnea caused by pathogenic qi, treat limp and the spasm of legs due to cold-dampness and inability to walk due to the pain of the knees, break the abdominal mass, accumulation and the blood conglomeration, and heal the incised wounds.

Those growing in Mianzhou（绵州）of Shu（蜀）area are of good quality, while those growing in some other places are too inferior in quality to use. There are eight counties neighboring Mianzhou（绵州）, among which only Zhangming（彰明）produces it. Zhangming（彰明）includes twenty townships, among which only Chishui（赤水）, Lianshui（廉水）, Changming

（昌明）and Huichang（会昌）produce it, and Chishui（赤水）is the place to produce the best quality of it. The one planted originally is called Wutou［乌头, root of Szechwan aconita, Radix Aconiti］which looks like the head of a blackbird. The one growing up on the parent root, despite mutual reinforcement but disconnection, is called Fuzi（aconite）, the same as a child attached to his mother. The one growing sideways and smaller is called Cezi（侧子）. The one growing lonely without attaching to anything, three or four Cun in lengths is called Tianxiong［天雄, tianxiong conite, Aconiti Radix Lateralis Tianxiong］. Fuzi（aconite）with the shape of squat-like sitting steadily, fewer knots and less Cezi（侧子）is regarded as the best quality; the one with many knots and much sap as inferior quality; the one which is deformed and has missing parts or wrinkled skins is of the lowest quality. The one with white color is of top quality, and the black is next to it, and the green is of the lowest quality, which is popularly called Heifuzi［黑附子, black sliced aconite, Aconiti Radix Lateralis Denigrata］, distinguishing itself from Baifuzi［白附子, typhonium, Typhonii Rhizoma］in name.

Fuzi（aconite）, strong and violent in nature and warm in property, is severely toxic. The low-grade medicinals recorded in *Shen Nong Ben Cao Jing*［《神农本草经》, *Shennong's Classic of Materia Medica*］are mostly toxic or severely toxic, as *Su Wen*［《素问》, *Plain Questions*］says that the toxic medicinals attack pathogens. So it attacks pathogens and restores healthy qi because attacking is tonifying. Fuzi（aconite）, pungent in taste and warm in property, growing in Chishui（赤水）of Zhangming（彰明）, receives great heat qi, replenishes branch yang from greater yang and assists the fire-heat of lesser yang. The yang heat qi of greater yang may cause the pathogenic qi of wind-cold and the cough with dyspnea if it cannot circulate through the skin and the hair of the whole body. Fuzi（aconite）is effective for the syndromes because it replenishes the branch yang from greater yang. The fire-heat qi of lesser yang may cause the syndromes of limp and the spasm of legs due to cold-dampness and inability to walk due to the pain of knees if it cannot run through the muscles and the joints of the whole body. Fuzi（aconite）is effective for the syndromes because it assists the fire-heat of lesser yang. The obstinate conglomeration and accumulation are caused by the internal congealing cold due to yang qi deficiency; the blood conglomeration is the movable abdominal mass formed by the yin-blood gathering; the incised wounds are ulceration caused by the knife or ax wound. Fuzi (aconite) is effective for all syndromes above because it has warm-heat qi to dissipate the yin cold and receives yang-fire qi to engender muscles.

Huang Di Nei Jing [《黄帝内经》, *Huangdi's Internal Classic*] says, "The grasses have five kinds of colors and the change of these five colors cannot be fully observed. The grasses have five kinds of flavors and the deliciousness of these flavors cannot be completely tasted. The heaven feeds the human with five qi, and the earth feeds the human with five flavors." So it should get herbs and food abided by the yin-yang transformation at the right time and it makes use of the advantages of the five directions and five color soils at the right place. Fuzi (aconite), growing in the areas of Zhangming (彰明) and Chishui (赤水), has better quality because it receives the exclusive essence of their directions and soils. The yang of greater yang is the water of Heaven One (天一), comes from the water home of bladder and is manifested in the upper. The yang of lesser yang is the fire of Earth Two (地二), comes from the fire of the lower energizer and runs in the sky like the sun. Zhangming (彰明) and Chishui (赤水) are the places where it comes out, the names of them happen to be in accordance with the properties of it. If scholars try to know the nature of it comprehensively and profoundly, they should understand precisely the advantages of the five geographical directions and the significance of the name given by the sage. Fuzi (aconite), nowadays planted in Shaanxi, is called Xifu (西附) which is pungent in taste and warm in property, slightly inferior in effect to that growing in Sichuan which is more effective due to the fertility of the soil. The cooked Fuzi (aconite) sold at retail in the drug stores is all Xifu (西附) and the like. Chuanfu (川附) is usually sold as a whole by the merchants, without slicing because of the high price. Users should know this.

People whose fire qi declines internally and yang qi runs externally should be treated immediately with the blast-fried Fuzi (aconite) to assist the origin of fire and make spirit mechanism go upward instead of causing detriment to the lower body and circulate instead of deserting outward. The treatment of mild cases with it can achieve the desirable effect easily. Unfortunately, understanding neither the principles of medicine nor the pathogenesis, physicians don't think it should be used until the appearance of the syndromes such as the missing pulse, the reversal cold and the corporeal soul without spirit. So it can treat diseases only, how can it save life? Some physicians consider it as viper even if they carry on lifelong medical practice. Every time they told people: Do not take it, or he would go crazy with nine orifices bleeding, get inflamed with welling-abscess, erupt poison the following year with the putrefied five zang-organs. When encountering the syndrome which should be treated with Fuzi (aconite), what should physicians do? Are they willing to admit their inability to use the medicinal without caring about fame and fortune? Or will they confess their incompetence and recommend other able physicians to redeem the case? They will definitely treat the patient today and again tomorrow until his spirit qi has changed. Then they will repeat the same practice. At that time, even the elixir can not save life. If the sage with devotion encounters this situation, he will never let him die and try Fuzi (aconite) to save the life; if it works, it will be his contribution, otherwise it's not his fault. The former physicians may be afraid of the latter's success, and then he would rather wish the patient to die and shift responsibility onto the use of Fuzi (aconite). If the physician of this kind has the conscience, he should feel ashamed that he doesn't command the medical knowledge. How can a beast in human attire be a physician and save people?

When used, the one of more than one Liang in weight is effective. The weight of Cezi (侧子) should be removed. If trying to increase its weight, the local people usually use the wood cup to beat Cezi (侧子) flat on it. So the one together with Cezi (侧子) of one Liang and five or six Qian in weight is just good. The local people are afraid of the southerners planting it, they macerate it with Rongyan [戎盐, halite, Halitum] when it is raw and then beat it flat in the cup. So Fuzi (aconite) actually has no salty taste. It is salty because it is macerated in Rongyan (halite). The method of making it is to cut off the navel with a knife, cut it into four pieces, slice them, soak them in the boiling water twice to remove the taste of salt and poison, make them semi-dry in the sun and fry them in a copper vessel. Therefore, the preparation of herbs and food is abided by the yin-yang transformation of the year in ancient times, when fire qi dominates in the year, the drugs in warm property should be prepared. *Huang Di Nei Jing* [《黄帝内经》, *Huangdi's Internal Classic*] says, "To prepare drugs according to the qi that dominates in the year, the drugs have absorbed the essence from the heaven and the earth." Those that do not abide by the yin-yang transformation of the year are not pure. The later generations can not prepare herbs and food as well as ancient people, so there is a method of storing it by blast-frying. In recent times, the false message that it is boiled with a child's urine has been spread, and people have just got used to it without knowing it is wrong.

227. 天　雄

天雄　气味辛温,有大毒。主治大风,寒湿痹,历节痛,拘挛缓急,破积聚邪气,金疮,强筋骨,轻身健行。

附子种在土中,不生侧子,经年独长大者,故曰雄也。土人种附子,地出天雄,便为不利,如养蚕而成白僵也。时俗咸谓一两外者为天雄,不知天雄长三四寸许,旁不生子,形状各异。

天雄、附子,《本经》主治稍异,而旨则同,故不加释。

李士材曰:天雄之用,与附子相仿,但功力略逊耳。李时珍曰:乌头、附子、天雄皆是补下焦命门阳虚之药,补下所以益上也。若是上焦阳虚,即属心脾之分,当用参芪,不当用天雄也。乌附天雄之尖皆是向下,其气下行,其脐乃向上,生苗之处。寇宗奭言其不肯就下,张元素言其补上焦阳虚,皆是误认尖为上耳。唯朱震亨以为下部之佐者得之,而未发出此义。卢子由曰:天以体言,雄以用言,不杂于阴柔,不惑于邪乱。若夫风寒湿痹证,及积聚邪气、金疮,嫌于无阳者,乃得行险而不失其正。

227. Tianxiong [天雄, Tianxiong Conite, Aconiti Radix Lateralis Tianxiong]

It is pungent in taste, warm and severe toxic in property, and it is mainly used to treat great wind, the impediment due to cold and dampness, multiple arthralgia, the mild and emergent spasm of the limbs, break abdominal mass and pathogenic qi, heal incised wounds, strengthen the sinews and the bones, keep healthy and make people walk sturdily.

Fuzi [附子, aconite, Radix Aconiti Praeparata] growing ripe in soil without Cezi (侧子) is called Tianxiong (Tianxiong Conite). The local people see it as bad luck that it turns out to be Tianxiong (Tianxiong Conite) when planting Fuzi (aconite), just like turning out to be the stiff silkworms in raising silkworms. It is commonly known that the one weighing more than one Liang is Tianxiong (Tianxiong Conite), but fail to know that it is three or four Cun long with no lateral structure attached and has a variety of shapes.

Tianxiong (Tianxiong Conite) and Fuzi (aconite) mentioned in *Shen Nong Ben Cao Jing* [《神农本草经》, *Shennong's Classic of Materia Medica*] is slightly different in effects and actions, but the same purposes, so no notes added.

Li Shicai (李士材) said, "Compared with Fuzi (aconite), it has similar functions but it is less effective." Li Shizhen (李时珍) said, " Wutou [乌头, root of Szechwan aconita, Radix Aconiti], Fuzi (aconite) and Tianxiong (Tianxiong Conite) are all the drugs tonifying yang-deficiency of the lower energizer life gate, so tonifying the lower to boost the upper." It is Ginseng and Astragalus not Tianxiong (Tianxiong Conite) that should be used when tonifying the yang-deficiency of the upper energizer which mainly refers to the heart and the spleen. The tips of these three plants face downward, which makes qi go down, while the hilum of them faces upward, where the young plants grow. Kou Zongshi (寇宗奭) said that it does not benefit the lower; Zhang Yuansu (张元素) said that it tonifies the yang-deficiency of the upper energizer, both of them mistakenly believe that the tip part is better. Only Zhu Zhenheng (朱震亨) held a different opinion that the tip assists the bottom, but the opinion wasn't claimed. Lu Ziyou (卢子由) said, "Tian refers to the body, Xiong refers to the use, it does not mix with the soft yin and involves in evil and chaos." It is a risky but correct choice to use Tianxiong (Tianxiong Conite) to treat the impediment due to wind, cold and dampness, break the abdominal mass and pathogenic qi, heal incised wounds and tonify yang-deficiency.

228. 乌 头 附

乌头 附　气味辛温,有毒。主治诸风,风痹,血痹,半身不遂,除寒冷,温养脏腑,去心下坚痞,感寒酸痛。《洁古珍珠襄》附。

乌头乃初种而未旁生附子者。乌头如芋头,附子如芋子,本一物也,其形如乌之头,因以为名。各处皆有,以川中出者入药,故医家谓之川乌。

李士材曰:大抵寒证用附子,风证用乌头。

228. Wutou［乌头, root of Szechwan aconita, Radix Aconiti］*supplement*

It is pungent in taste, warm and toxic in property, and it is mainly used to treat various wind syndromes, wind impediment, blood impediment and hemiplegia, expell cold, warm and nourish the zang-fu organs and eliminate hardness and the abdominal mass below the heart and the aching pain caused by catching cold. Supplemented in *Jie Gu Zhen Zhu Xiang*［《洁古珍珠襄》, *Pouch of Pearls*］.

Wutou（root of Szechwan aconita）is the first-planted taproot without the lateral roots of Fuzi［附子, aconite, Radix Aconiti Praeparata］. The relationship between the former and the latter is just like that between taro and young taro, therefore they are actually the same. Wutou（root of Szechwan aconita）looks like the head of crow, thus getting its name. It grows everywhere; however, those growing in Sichuang（四川）can be used as medicinal, so it is also called Chuangwu（川乌）by doctors.

Li Shicai（李士材）said, "Generally speaking, Fuzi（aconite）can mainly treat the cold syndromes while Wutou（root of Szechwan aconita）can mainly treat the wind syndromes."

229. 乌 喙 附

乌喙 附　气味辛温,有大毒。主治中风,恶风洗洗出汗,除寒湿痹,咳逆上气,破积聚寒热。其汁煎之,名射罔,杀禽兽。《别录》附。

《本经》名乌头,《别录》名乌喙,今时名草乌,乃乌头之野生者,处处有之。其根外黑内白,皱而枯燥。其性大毒,较之川乌更烈,与前条洁古所言者,不可一例用也。

草乌头今杭人多植于庭院,九月开花淡紫娇艳,与菊同时,谓之鹦鸪菊,又谓之双鸾菊,鸳鸯菊,僧鞋菊,皆以花之形状名之。根有大毒,与川中所出之乌头大别。古时或名乌头,或名乌喙,随时所称,未有分别。后人以形正者,有似乌乌之头;其两岐相合而生者,有似乌乌之喙,以此别之。然形状虽殊,主治则一,亦可不必分别。隐庵以乌头判属川乌,以乌喙判属草乌,盖恐后人以混称误用,或致伤人故耳。虽属强分,其用心大有益于天下后世。

乌喙虽亦名乌头,实乃土附子也。性劣有毒,但能搜风胜湿,开顽痰,破坚积,治顽疮,以毒攻毒,不能如附子益太阳之标阳,助少阳之火热,而使神机之环转,用者辨之。

草乌之毒甚于川乌,盖川乌由人力种莳,当时则采。草乌乃野生地上,多历岁月,故其气力尤为勇悍。犹之芋子,人植者无毒可啖,野生者有毒不可啖,其理一也。又,川乌先经盐淹杀其烈性,寄至远方,为日稍久,故其毒少减。草乌未经淹制,或兼现取宜,其毒之较甚也。卢不远曰:人病有四痹风痿厥。草乌力唯宣痹风。阳行有四,曰升降出入。草乌力唯从升出,但阳喜独行而专操杀业。如刚愎人所当避忌。采乌头捣汁煎之,名曰射罔。猎人以付箭镞射鸟兽,中者立死,中人亦立死。《日华本草》云:人中射罔毒,以甘草、蓝汁、小豆叶、浮萍、冷水、荠苨皆可解,用一味御之。

229. Wuhui［乌喙, root of Szechwan aconita, Radix Aconiti］ *supplement*

It is pungent in taste, warm and severely toxic in property, and it is mainly used to treat wind stroke, the shivering and sweating caused by aversion to wind, the cough with dyspnea, descend adverse-rising qi, eliminate the impediment due to cold and dampness and break accumulation-gathering, cold and heat. The decoction of its sap is called Shewang（射罔）, killing birds and beasts. Supplemented in *Ming Yi Bie Lu*［《名医别录》, *Miscellaneous Records of Famous Physicians*］.

It is called Wutou（乌头）in *Shen Nong Ben Cao Jing*［《神农本草经》,

Shennong's Classic of Materia Medica], Wuhui (乌喙) in *Ming Yi Bie Lu* [《名医别录》, *Miscellaneous Records of Famous Physicians*] and Caowu (草乌) nowadays, which is the wild Wutou (乌头) and grows everywhere. Its root is black outside and white inside, wrinkled and dry. It is severely toxic in property, even more toxic than Chuanwu (川乌) and different in use from the one listed by *Jie Gu Zhen Zhu Xiang* [《洁古珍珠囊》, *Pouch of Pearls*] in the previous item.

Nowadays, it is usually planted in the gardens of Hangzhou (杭州). It blossoms with pale purple flowers which are delicate and charming in the ninth lunar month, the same time as chrysanthemum (菊). It is called Yinggeju (鹦鸽菊), Shuangluanju (双鸾菊), Yuanyangju (鸳鸯菊), and Sengxieju (僧鞋菊), all based on the flower forms. Its root is severely toxic, quite different from Wutou [乌头, root of Szechwan aconita, Radix Aconiti] growing in Chuanzhong (川中). In ancient times, it was called Wutou (乌头) or Wuhui (乌喙) in different periods without distinction. People later on distinguished the two in the way that the one with perfect form similar to the head of blackbird is called Wutou (乌头); the one with two tips growing connected just like the mouth of blackbird is called Wuhui (乌喙). Though different in forms, these two have the same function in treatment, thus there is no need to distinguish them. Yin An (隐庵) used different forms to judge which one is Chuanwu (川乌) and which one is Caowu (草乌) because he was afraid that the people later on might mistake them by names and use them improperly to hurt people. Though his distinction is a little irrational, his intention greatly benefits the later world.

Though Wuhui (root of Szechwan aconite) is also called Wutou (乌头), it is Tufuzi (土附子) in fact. Though its property is inferior and toxic, it can track wind, predominate dampness, resolve stubborn phlegm, break hardness and accumulation, treat stubborn sores and attack toxin with toxin. However, unlike Fuzi (aconite), it cannot replenish the branch yang from greater yang or assist the fire-heat of lesser yang to make vital activity move around. So people should distinguish it when it is used.

It is more toxic than Chuanwu (川乌) because the latter one is planted by people and collected at the proper time while the former one grows wildly on the ground for a long time, so its qi and strength are very strong and fierce. Just like Yuzi〔芋子, dasheen seed, Semen Colocasiae Esculentae〕, the one planted by people without toxicity can be eaten; the one growing wildly with toxicity cannot be eaten. This is the first reason. Second, Chuanwu（川乌）is usually soaked in salt to curb its strength and then delivered to the distant places. As time goes by, its toxicity becomes weaker. On the contrary, Caowu（草乌）is collected on the spot without salt-soaking, so its toxicity is stronger. Lu Buyuan（卢不远）said, "There are four kinds of diseases for humans: impediment, wind, flaccidity and syncope. Caowu（草乌）is devoted to diffusing impediment and expelling wind. There are four moving patterns of yang: ascending, descending, exiting and entering. Caowu（草乌）has the function of ascending and exiting. But yang qi is very strong and prefers to move straight in one pattern, just like the killers being good at killing. So the one who has tough and brave temper should avoid taking Caowu（草乌）." The decoction of the sap of Wutou（root of Szechwan aconita）is called Shewang（射罔）. Hunters apply it to the metal arrowhead to shoot birds and beasts. The one being shot will die on the spot. When shooting people, the one shot will die on the spot too. *Ri Hua Ben Cao*〔《日华本草》, *Rihuazi's Materia Medica*〕says that Gancao〔甘草, licorice, Glycyrrhizae Radix〕, sap of Daqingye〔大青叶, isatis leaf, Isatidis Folium〕, Xiaodouye〔小豆叶, mung bean leaf, Phaseoli Radiati Semen Folium〕, Fuping〔浮萍, duckweed, Spirodelae Herba〕, cold water and Jini〔荠苨, apricot-leaved adenophora, Adenophorae Trachelioidis Radix〕can remove the toxin of Shewang（射罔）in the human body. One of these medicinals can inhibit the toxin of Caowu（草乌）in formula.

230. 大 黄

大黄 气味苦寒,无毒。主下瘀血,血闭寒热,破症瘕积聚,留饮宿食,荡涤肠胃,推陈致新,通利水谷,调中化食,安和五脏。

大黄《本经》谓之黄良,后人谓之将军,以其有伐邪去乱之功力也。古时以出河西、陇西者为胜,今蜀川河东,山陕州郡皆有,而以川中锦纹者为佳。八月采根,根有黄汁,其性滋润,掘得者,竿于树枝上,经久始干。

大黄味苦气寒,色黄臭香,乃肃清中土之剂也。其性走而不守,主下瘀血血闭。气血不和,则为寒为热,瘀血行而寒热亦除矣。不但下瘀血血闭,且破症瘕积聚,留饮宿食。夫留饮宿食,在于肠胃,症瘕积聚,陈垢不清,故又曰:荡涤肠胃,推陈致新。夫肠胃和,则水谷通利,陈垢去,则化食调中,故又曰:通利水谷,调中化食也。《玉机真藏论》云:五脏者,皆禀气于胃。胃者,五脏之本也。胃气安则五脏亦安,故又曰:安和五脏。

愚按:大黄抑阳养阴,有安和五脏之功,故无毒,而《本经》名曰黄良。但行泄大迅,下瘀破积,故别名将军,而列于下品。

西北之人,土气敦厚,阳气伏藏,重用大黄,能养阴而不破泄。东南之人,土气虚浮,阳气外泄,稍用大黄,即伤脾胃,此五方五土之有不同也。又,总察四方之人,凡禀气厚实,积热留中,大黄能养阴,而推陈致新,用之可也。若素禀虚寒,虽据证,当用大黄,亦宜量其人而酌减,此因禀质之有不同也。至伤寒阳明篇中,三承气汤,皆用大黄。大承气、调胃承气与芒消同用,所以承在上之火热而调其肠胃,使之下泄也。小承气但用大黄,不用芒消,所以行肠胃之燥结也。燥结行而阴阳上下内外皆和。今人不知伤寒精义,初起但发散而消食,次则平胃而挨磨,终则用大黄以攻下,不察肌表经脉之浅深,不明升降出入之妙义。胸隔不舒,便谓有食,按之稍痛,更云有食。外热不除,必绝其谷,肠虚不便,必下其粪,处方用药,必至大黄而后已。夫禀质敦厚,或感冒不深,虽遭毒害,不即殒躯,当一二日而愈者,必至旬日,当旬日而愈者,必至月余。身愈之后,医得居功。若正气稍虚,或病邪猖獗,亦以此医治之,此医但知此法,鲜不至死。噫,医所以寄死生,可以盲瞽不明者,而察秋毫之末乎?不思结纲,但知羡鱼,耻也。旁门管窥,居之不疑,耻更甚焉。

230. Dahuang〔大黄, rhubarb, Radix et Rhizoma Rhei〕

It is bitter in taste, cold and non-toxic in property, and it is mainly used to treat blood-stasis, blood block, cold and heat, break abdominal mass and accumulation-gathering, eliminate retention of fluid and indigestion, activate the stomach and intestines, bring forth the new by reducing the old, dredge and promote water and food, regulate the middle and digest food, and harmonize the five zang-organs.

It is called Huangliang（黄良）in *Shen Nong Ben Cao Jing*［《神农本草经》, *Shennong's Classic of Materia Medica*］. People later on called it Jiangjun（将军）for it has the function of quelling evil and eliminating disorder. In ancient times, the one growing in Hexi（河西）and Longxi（陇西）is of better quality. Now it exists in the counties of Shuchuan（蜀川）, Hedong（河东）and Shanshan（山陕）, among which the one with brocade pattern in Chuangzhong（川中）is good. Collected in the eighth lunar month, its root has yellow sap and moistening nature. Those who dig it out dry it by hanging it on the tree branches, which will last for a long time.

Bitter in taste, cold in property, yellow in color and fragrant in smell, it is the medicinal of purifying the center earth. It can mainly treat blood stasis and blood block because its nature is moving and not defending. The disharmony of qi and blood causes cold and heat. Once the blood stasis is moved, cold and heat will be eliminated. It can also break abdominal mass and accumulation-gathering and eliminate the retention of fluid and indigestion. The retention of fluid and indigestion stay in the stomach and intestines, and abdominal mass and accumulation-gathering are caused by too much stale grime. Therefore, it can also activate the stomach and intestines and bring forth the new by reducing the old. The harmony of the stomach and intestines brings the dredging and promotion of water and food; the elimination of stale grime promotes the regulation of the middle and food digestion. Therefore, it can also dredge and promote water and food, regulate the middle and digest food. *Yu Ji Zhen Cang Lun*［《玉机真藏论》, *Discussion on Genuine-Zang Pulses*］says that the five zang-organs all receives the qi from the stomach, thus the stomach is the root of the five zang-organs. The harmony of stomach qi ensures the harmony of the five zang-organs. Therefore, it can also harmonize the five zang-organs.

Note by Zhang Zhicong（张志聪）: Inhibiting yang and nourishing yin, it has the function of harmonizing the five zang-organs. So it is non-toxic and called Huangliang（黄良）in *Shen Nong Ben Cao Jing*［《神农本草经》, *Shennong's Classic of Materia Medica*］. However, it is much more effective in discharging immediately, precipitating stasis and breaking accumulation, so it is also called Jiangjun（将军）

and listed in the third grade.

The people living in the northwest are rich in earth qi and have hidden yang qi. For them, taking a lot of Dahuang (rhubarb) can nourish yin and avoid discharging. The people living in the southeast are deficient and floating in earth qi and have out-discharging yang qi. For them taking a little of Dahuang (rhubarb) may damage the spleen and the stomach. This is due to the differences among the five directions and five color soils. Observing people from four directions, those who are rich in qi and have accumulated heat in the middle can take Dahuang (rhubarb) because it can nourish yin and bring forth the new by reducing the old; those who are endowed with deficiency and cold, though there is evidence that they can take Dahuang (rhubarb), should take it in the reduced amount according to their specific situation because different people have different endowments. In *Shang Han Yang Ming Pian* [《伤寒阳明篇》, *Yangming Pian of Decoction Treatise on Cold Damage*], there are three kinds of Purgative Decoction which all use Dahuang (rhubarb). Major Purgative Decoction and Stomach-Regulating Purgative Decoction are used with Mangxiao [芒消, mirabilite, Natrii Sulfas] together. So this combination can bear the fire heat of the upper body, regulate the stomach and intestines and discharge the fire heat downward. Minor Purgative Decoction contains Dahuang (rhubarb) instead of Mangxiao (mirabilite), so it can relieve the dryness accumulation in the stomach and intestines. The relief of dryness accumulation contributes to the harmony of yin and yang in the upper and the lower and in the internal and the external. Nowadays, people don't understand the essence of treating the cold damage. When it first occurs, physicians may use the method of dissipating and promoting digestion. Then, they may harmonize the stomach and activate the function of the stomach. Finally they may use Dahuang (rhubarb) to attack to discharge it without observation of the situation of fleshy exterior and meridians and understanding of the ingenious meaning of ascending, descending, exiting and entering. If a person feels uneasy about the chest and diaphragm, they will diagnose that he has food accumulation. If the person reacts with pressed pain, they will be even more certain about their diagnosis. To relieve the external heat, they definitely stop the food intake. To treat the constipation due to the intestine deficiency, they definitely discharge stool. To comply to the formula, they definitely use Dahuang (rhubarb). The one taking Dahuang (rhubarb) who has rich endowment or gets mild cold, though poisoned but not killed, will recover ten days later. As a fact, if he doesn't take Dahuang (rhubarb), he may recover one or two days later. The one who should recover ten days later may postpone to one month if taking Dahuang (rhubarb). The physician will take the credit for his recovery. If the one deficient in qi and attacked by the strong disease pathogen is treated by the same physician using the same method, he is sure to die. If the physicians know the proper use of this medicinal, then how many people's lives can be saved? Since physicians are the people who can master others' lives, how can the blind and the deaf perceive these subtle changes? It's shameful that they just desire the credit without effective practice and it's even more shameful that they only have narrow and one-sided views about the medicinal and adhere stubbornly to them.

231. 半 夏

半夏 气味辛平,有毒。主治伤寒寒热,心下坚,胸胀咳逆,头眩,咽喉肿痛,肠鸣,下气,止汗。

半夏青齐江浙在处有之。二月生苗,一茎高八九寸,茎端三叶,三三相偶,略似竹叶,其根圆白,五月八月采根晒干,不厌陈久。

《月令》:五月半夏生,盖当夏之半也。《脉解篇》云:阳明者,午也。五月盛阳之阴也。半夏生当夏半,白色味辛,禀阳明燥金之气化。主治伤寒寒热者,辛以散之也。阳明胃络上通于心,胃络不通于心,则心下坚。胸者,肺之部,阳明金气上合于肺。金气不和于肺,则胸胀咳逆。半夏色白属金,主宣达阳明之气,故皆治之。金能制风,故治头眩,以及咽喉肿痛。燥能胜湿,故治肠鸣之下气而止汗也。

231. Banxia〔半夏, pinellia, Rhizoma Pinelliae〕

It is pungent in taste, mild and toxic in property, and it is mainly used to treat the cold damage manifested by cold and heat, the lumps below the heart, chest distension, the cough with dyspnea, vertigo, swelling and the sore throat and borborygmus. It can promote qi to flow downwards and stop sweating.

Banxia (pinellia), growing commonly in Shandong, Jiangsu and Zhejiang, sprouts in February. Its stem is high in eight or nine Cun with three leaves on the top, which is symmetrical in three and the shape is a little like that of bamboo leaves. Its root, round and white, collected in the fifth and eighth lunar month and dried in the sun is suitable to be stored for a long time.

Yue Ling [《月令》, *Monthly Order*]: Banxia (pinellia) grows in May, as it has passed the mid-summer. *Mai Jie Pian* [《脉解篇》, *Explanations of Channels*] said, "The yang brightness is in predominance in Wu." Yang has reached its peak in the fifth lunar month and Yin begins to emerge. Banxia (pinellia), growing at mid-summer, white in color and pungent in taste, receives the qi transformation of yang brightness and dryness metal. It can mainly treat the cold damage manifested by cold and heat because its pungent taste can dissipate it. The stomach meridian of yang brightness connects the heart; otherwise, the lumps below the heart will appear. The chest is the place where the lung resides. The yang brightness metal qi turns upwards and joins with the lung; otherwise, the chest distension and the cough with dyspnea will appear. Banxia (pinellia), white in color and pertaining to metal, mainly promotes the qi of yang brightness, so it can treat the two diseases above. It can treat vertigo and swelling and sore throat because metal dominates over wind. And it can treat borborygmus, promote qi to flow downwards and stop sweating too, because dryness predominates over dampness.

232. 连 翘

连翘　气味苦平,无毒。主治寒热鼠瘘瘰疬,痈肿恶疮,瘿瘤结热,蛊毒。

　　连翘出汴京及河中、江宁、润淄、泽兖、鼎岳、南康诸州皆有之,而以蜀中者为胜。有大翘、小翘二种。大翘生下湿地,叶如榆叶,独茎赤色,稍间开花黄色可爱,秋结实,形如莲,内作房瓣,气甚芳馥,根黄如蒿根。小翘生岗原之上,叶茎花实皆似大翘,但细小耳。实房黄黑,内含黑子,根名连轺,须知大翘用实不用根,小翘用根不用实。

连翘味苦性寒,形象心肾,禀少阴之气化。主治寒热鼠瘘瘰疬者,治鼠瘘瘰疬之寒热也。夫瘘有内外二因,内因曰鼠瘘,外因曰瘰疬,其本在脏,其末在脉。

此内因而为水毒之瘰，故曰鼠瘰也。陷脉为瘰，留连肉腠，此外因而寒邪薄于肉腠之瘰，故曰瘰疬也。是鼠瘰起于肾脏之毒，留于心主之血脉。瘰疬因天气之寒，伤人身之经脉。连翘形象心肾，故治鼠瘰瘰疬也。痈肿恶疮，肌肉不和。瘿瘤结热，经脉不和。连翘味苦，其气芳香，能通经脉而利肌肉，故治痈肿恶疮，瘿瘤结热也。受蛊毒者在腹，造毒者在心。苦寒泄心，治造毒之原。芳香醒脾，治受毒之腹，故又治蛊毒。

《灵枢·寒热论》岐伯曰：鼠瘰寒热之毒气也，留于脉而不去者也。其本在于水脏，故曰鼠。上通于心主之脉，颈腋溃烂，故曰瘰。鼠瘰寒热之毒气者，言鼠瘰水毒而为寒，上合心包而为热也。主治寒热鼠瘰者，治鼠瘰之寒热也。今人不解《本经》，祇事剿袭，以寒热二字句逗，谓连翘主治寒热，出于神农之言。凡伤寒中风之寒热，一概用之，岂知风寒之寒热起于皮肤，鼠瘰之寒热起于血脉，风马牛不相及也。嗟嗟，为医者可不知《内经》乎。《灵枢》论营卫血气之生始，出入脏腑经脉之交合贯通，乃医家根本之学，浅人视为针经而忽之，良可惜也。

李时珍曰：连翘状似人心，两片合成，其中有仁甚香，乃少阴心经，厥阴包络气分主药。诸痛痒疮疡皆属心火，故为十二经疮家圣药，而兼注手足少阳、手阳明之经气分之热也。

232. Lianqiao [连翘, fruit of weeping forsythia, Fructus Forsythiae]

It is bitter in taste, mild and non-toxic in property, and it is mainly used to treat cold and heat, mouse fistula, scrofula, abscess, severe sore, goiter, tumor, heat stagnation and parasitic toxin.

It grows in Bianjing (汴京) and the areas of Hezhong (河中), Jiangning (江宁), Runzi (润淄), Zeyan (泽兖), Dingyue (鼎岳) and Nankang (南康). The one growing in Shuzhong (蜀中) is of better quality. There are two kinds of it, the big one and the small one. The big one grows in marsh land. Its leaves are like dwarf elm leaves, and it has only one stem in red color. It blossoms with yellow and lovely flowers next to each other and bears fruits in autumn in the shape of lotus, forming ovary inside, with fragrant smell. Its root is yellow in color just like the sweet wormwood root. The small one grows upon the mountains and plains. Its leaf, stem, flower and fruit are all similar to those of the big one but smaller in size. Its ovary is yellow-black with black seeds inside. Its root is called Lianyao (连轺). It should be known that the fruit of the big one is used as medicinal rather than the root while the root of the small one is used rather than the fruit.

Bitter in taste and cold in property, it is in the form of heart and kidney and receives the qi transformation of lesser yin. It can mainly treat cold and heat, mouse fistula and scrofula, which means it can treat the cold and heat caused by mouse fistula and scrofula. There are two reasons causing fistula. The one caused by the internal reason is mouse fistula; the one caused by the external reason is scrofula. Its root lies in the zang-organ and its end lies in vessel. The fistula caused by the internal reason of the water toxin is called mouse fistula. Some fistula sinks in the vessel and connects the interstices of the flesh. The fistula caused by the external reason of cold evil staying in the interstices of the flesh is called scrofula. The mouse fistula stems from the toxin of the kidney but stays in the blood and vessel governed by heart. Scrofula, due to the cold weather, can damage the meridian. Lianqiao (fruit of weeping forsythia) can treat mouse fistula and scrofula because it is in the form of the heart and the kidney. The swollen abscess and the severe sore manifest the disharmony of muscles and flesh; goiter, tumor and heat stagnation manifest the disharmony of the meridian. It can treat swollen abscess, severe sore, goiter, tumor and heat stagnation because its bitter taste and fragrant smell can dredge meridian and benefit the flesh and muscles. The parasitic toxin damages the abdomen but it is produced by the heart. It can treat parasitic toxin because bitterness and coldness can discharge heart, the origin of toxin, and fragrance can enliven the spleen treating the poisoned abdomen.

In *Ling Shu: Han Re Lun* [《灵枢·寒热论》, *Miraculous Pivot*, *Cold and Heat Diseases*], Qi Bo said, "This is the disease of scrofula with fistula caused by the toxin of cold and heat that accumulates in the vessels and is difficult to be removed. The one with its root cause lying in the water zang-organ is called mouse. The one connecting upward with vessels governed by the heart and causing the ulceration of the neck and armpit is called fistula. The scrofula with fistula caused by the toxin of cold and heat means that the one caused by the water toxin belongs to cold and the one connecting upward with the heart belongs to heat."

That it can mainly treat cold and heat and mouse fistula means it can treat the cold and heat of mouse fistula. Modern people don't understand the meaning of *Shen Nong Ben Cao Jing* [《神农本草经》, *Shennong's Classic of Materia Medica*], just garble the words, put cold and heat as an independent meaning group and allege that Agricultural God said that Lianqiao (连翘) could mainly treat the cold and heat. So it is used to treat the cold and heat of cold damage and stroke. However, it is unknown that the cold and heat of wind-cold starts from the skin while the cold and heat of mouse fistula starts from the blood and vessels. These two syndromes are totally different from each other. How can the doctors not know *Huang Di Nei Jing* [《黄帝内经》, *Huangdi's Internal Classic*]? *Ling Shu* [《灵枢》, *Miraculous Pivot*] talks about the engendering and beginning of nutrient-defense, blood and qi and connection and unobstruction of the zang-fu organs and meridian, which is the fundamental study for the people who practise. Those with short vision consider it as the principle for acupuncture thus ignoring it. What a pity!

Li Shizhen (李时珍) said, "Composed of two pieces, Lianqiao (fruit of weeping forsythia) is in the form of heart with fragrant kernels inside. So it is the main qi aspect medicinal of heart meridian of lesser yin and the pericardium meridian of reverting yin. All painful and itching sores pertain to heart fire. So it is the efficacious medicine to treat the sores of the twelve meridians and also treat the heat of qi aspect of meridian of the hand and foot lesser yang and the hand yang brightness meridian."

233. 翘 根

翘根　气味甘寒平,有小毒。主治下热气,益阴精,令人面悦好,明目。久服轻身耐老。

《本经》翘根生嵩高平泽,二月八月采,陶隐居曰:方药不用,人无识者。王好古曰:此即连翘根也。张仲景治伤寒瘀热在里,身色发黄,用麻黄连轺赤小豆汤。注云:连轺即连翘根。今从之。

233. Qiaogen〔翘根，root of weeping forsythia，Radix Forsythiae〕

It is sweet in taste，cold，mild and slightly toxic in property，and it is mainly used to relieve heat qi，replenish yin and essence，luster the face and improve vision. Long-term taking of it can keep healthy and prevent aging.

Shen Nong Ben Cao Jing〔《神农本草经》，*Shennong's Classic of Materia Medica*〕says，"It grows in mountains，lakes and swamps and can be collected in the second lunar month and the eighth lunar month." Tao Yinju（陶隐居）said，"It is no longer used in formula，and nobody can recognize it." Wang Haogu（王好古）said，"It is the root of Lianqiao（fruit of weeping forsythia）." Zhang Zhongjing（张仲景）used Ephedra，Forsythia and Rice Bean Decoction to treat cold damage and the stagnated heat in the interior and yellow body. Note：Lianyao in this formula is just the root of Lianqiao（fruit of weeping forsythia），and this formula is used since then.

234. 桔　梗

桔梗　气味辛，微温，有小毒。主治胸胁痛如刀刺，腹满，肠鸣幽幽，惊恐悸气。

　　桔梗近道处处有之，二三月生苗，叶如杏叶而有毛，茎如笔管，紫赤色，高尺余，夏开小花紫碧色，秋后结实。其根外白中黄有心，味辛而苦；若无心味甜者，荠苨也。

　　桔梗根色黄白，叶毛，味辛，禀太阴金土之气化。味苦性温，花茎紫赤，又禀少阴火热之气化。主治胸胁痛如刀刺者，桔梗辛散温行，能治上焦之胸痛，而旁行于胁，复能治少阳之胁痛而上达于胸也。腹满，肠鸣幽幽者，腹中寒则满，肠中寒则鸣。腹者土也，肠者金也。桔梗禀火土金相生之气化，能以火而温腹满之土寒，更能以火而温肠鸣之金寒也。惊恐悸气，少阴病也。心虚则惊，肾虚则恐，心肾皆虚则悸。桔梗得少阴之火化，故治惊恐悸气。

　　愚按：桔梗治少阳之胁痛，上焦之胸痹，中焦之肠鸣，下焦之腹满。又，惊则气上，恐则气下，悸则动中，是桔梗为气分之药，上中下皆可治也。张元素不参经义，谓桔梗乃舟楫之药，载诸药而不沉。今人熟念在口，终身不忘。夫以元素杜撰之言为是,则《本经》几可废矣。医门豪杰之士,阐明神农之《本经》,轩岐之《灵》《素》,仲祖之《论》《略》,则千百方书,皆为糟粕。设未能也,必为方书所囿,而蒙蔽一生矣,可畏哉。

234. Jiegeng〔桔梗, platycodon grandiflorum, Radix Platycodi〕

It is pungent in taste, slightly warm and slightly toxic in property, and it is mainly used to treat the pain of the chest and rib-side like being stabbed by a knife, abdominal fullness, rumbling intestines like deer crying, fright, fear and palpitation.

It grows everywhere nearby and sprouts in the second lunar month or the third lunar month. Its leaf is like the apricot leaf with hair on it. Its stem is like the barrel of a pen in the color of purple and in the height of more than one Chi. It blossoms with small flowers, purple and green, in summer and bears fruits in late autumn. Its root is white inside, yellow outside and hard in the center and has the pungent and bitter taste. The sweet one without hardness in the center is Jini〔荠苨, apricot-leaved adenophora, Adenophorae Trachelioidis Radix〕.

It has a yellow-white root, hairy leaves and pungent taste, and receives the qi transformation of metal and earth from greater yin. It has bitter taste, warm property and purple-red flowers and stems, and receives the qi transformation of fire-heat from lesser yin. It can mainly treat the pain of the chest and rib-side like being stabbed by a knife because its pungent taste disperses and its warm property moves, which can treat the chest pain of the upper energizer. Since it can move to the rib-side, it can also treat the pain of rib-side of lesser yang reaching upward to the chest. The cold in the abdomen causes fullness, and the cold in the intestines causes rumbling. The abdomen pertains to earth and the intestines to metal. It can treat abdominal fullness and rumbling intestines like deer crying because it receives the qi transformation of mutual generation among fire, earth and metal, using fire to warm the earth-cold of abdominal fullness let alone the metal-cold of rumbling intestines. Fright, fear and palpitation are the syndromes of lesser yin disease. The heart deficiency causes fright; the kidney deficiency causes fear; the deficiency in the heart and the kidney causes palpitation. It can treat fright, fear and palpitation because it receives fire transformation of lesser yin.

Note by Zhang Zhicong（张志聪）：It can treat the pain of rib-side of lesser yang, the chest impediment of the upper energizer, the rumbling intestines of the middle energizer and the abdominal fullness of the lower energizer. Besides, fright makes qi move upward; fear makes qi move downward; palpitation stirs the middle. As a medicinal of qi aspect, it can treat the syndromes of the upper, middle and lower parts of the body because it is the medicinal of qi aspect. Zhang Yuansu（张元素）didn't get the original meaning of *Shen Nong Ben Cao Jing* [《神农本草经》, *Shennong's Classic of Materia Medica*] and spoke of it as boat medicinal which can hold the other medicinals without sinking them. Nowadays, people are so familiar with his statements that they will never forget it, which is talked about too much by people and remembered forever. If his fabricated statements were regarded as true, then *Shen Nong Ben Cao Jing* [《神农本草经》, *Shennong's Classic of Materia Medica*] would be almost useless. All great figures in the traditional Chinese medicine wrote a lot of books trying to explain *Shen Nong Ben Cao Jing* [《神农本草经》, *Shennong's Classic of Materia Medica*] by Agriculture God, *Ling Shu* [《灵枢》, *Miraculous Pivot*] by Yellow Emperor, *Su Wen* [《素问》, *Plain Questions*] by Qi Bo, *Shang Han Lun* [《伤寒论》, *Treatise on Cold Damage Diseases*] and *Jin Gui Yao Lue* [《金匮要略》, *Synopsis of the Golden Chamber*] by Zhang Zhongjin. If his fabricated statements were regarded as true, all these books would be dross. For the incompetent and inexperienced doctors, they are bound to be restricted and cheated by these low-quality formula books all their life. How terrible it is!

235. 白头翁根

白头翁根　气味苦温，无毒，主治温疟，狂狷寒热，症瘕积聚，瘿气，逐血，止腹痛，疗金疮。

白头翁高山田野处处有之，正月生苗，叶如杏叶，上有细白毛，茎头着花紫色，如木槿花，近根有白茸，根紫色深，如蔓菁，其苗有风则静，无风而摇，与赤箭、独活同也。陶隐居曰：近根处有白茸，状如白头老翁，故以为名。寇宗奭曰：白头翁生河南洛阳界，于新安山野中，屡尝见之。山中人卖白头翁丸，言服之寿考。不失古人命名之义。

白头翁，无风而摇者，禀东方甲乙之气，风动之象也。有风则静者，得西方庚辛之气，金能制风也。主治温疟者，温疟之邪，藏于肾脏，禀木气则能透发母邪也。狂猲寒热，温疟病也。治症瘕积聚，瘿气，逐血者，禀金气则能破积聚而行瘀也。止腹痛，乃腹中之痛，有由于积滞者，积滞去，故痛止也。疗金疮，是和血行瘀之效。

235. Baitouweng Gen [白头翁根, pulsatilla, Radix Pulsatillae]

It is bitter in taste, warm and non-toxic in property, and it is mainly used to treat warm malaria, mania, chills and fever, abdominal mass, accumulation-gathering and goiter, expel blood stasis, relieve abdominal pain and cure the incised wounds.

It grows everywhere in high mountains and fields and sprouts in the first lunar month. Its leaves are like apricot leaves and have thin and white hair. There is purple flower on the top of its stem which is like Mujinhua [木槿花, rose-of-Sharon, Hibisci Syriaci Flos] and there is white fuzz near the root. Its root is dark purple in color, similar to that of Manjing [蔓菁, turnip, Brassicae Rapae Tuber et Folium]. Its seedlings are motionless when there is wind but waving when there is no wind, which is similar to Chijian [赤箭, gastrodia, Gastrodiae Rhizoma] and Duhuo [独活, pubescent angelica, Angelicae Pubescentis Radix]. Tao Hongjin (陶弘景) said, "There is white fuzz near the root and it looks like an old man with white hair, so it got this name." Kou Zongshi (寇宗奭) said, "It grows in Luoyang (洛阳) of Henan (河南) and is often in the mountains and fields of Xin'an (新安). People in the mountain sell its pellet and say taking it can prolong life, which is in accordance with the ancients' intention of naming it."

It, waving without wind, receives the qi of Jiayi of the east, which indicates the image of the wind movement. It, motionless in the wind, receives the qi of Gengxin of the west and metal can control wind. It can mainly treat warm malaria because the pathogen of warm malaria hides in the kidney and Baitouweng [白头

翁, pulsatilla, Radix Pulsatillae] receives wood qi to expel the root of the pathogen. Mania and chills and fever both belong to warm malaria. It can treat abdominal mass, accumulation-gathering and goiter, and expel blood stasis because it receives metal qi to break accumulation-gathering and move stasis. It can relieve abdominal pain because it can eliminate accumulation and stagnation which cause abdominal pain. It can cure the incised wounds because it can harmonize blood and move stasis.

236. 甘 遂

甘遂 气味苦寒,有毒。主治大腹,疝瘕,腹满,面目浮肿,留饮宿食,破症坚积聚,利水谷道。

　　甘遂始出太山及代郡,今陕西、江东、京口皆有。苗似泽漆,茎短小而叶有汁,根皮色赤,肉色白,作连珠状,大如指头,实重者良。

　　土味曰甘,径直曰遂。甘遂味苦,以其泄土气而行隧道,故名甘遂。土气不和,则大腹。隧道不利,则疝瘕。大腹则腹满,由于土不胜水,外则面目浮肿,内则留饮宿食。甘遂治之,泄土气也。为疝为瘕则症坚积聚。甘遂破之,行隧道也。水道利则水气散,谷道利则宿积除,甘遂行水气而通宿积,故利水谷道。

　　《乘雅》论:甘遂其为方也,为大,为急。其于剂也,为通,为泄。但气味苦寒,偏于热,为因寒则非所宜矣。

236. Gansui [甘遂, kansui, Radix Kansui]

It is bitter in taste, cold and toxic in property, and it is mainly used to treat greater abdomen, hernia, movable abdominal mass, abdominal fullness, the dropsy of the face and eyes, the retention of fluid and the undigested food, break fixed abdominal mass, hardness and accumulation, and promote water passage and digestion.

　　Firstly recorded to be growing in Taishan Mountain (太山) and Daijun (代郡), now it grows in Shaanxi (陕西), Jiangdong (江东) and Jingkou (京口). Its seedling is like Zeqi [泽漆, sun spurge, Herba Euphorbiae Helioscopiae]. Its stem is short and small, its leaves are juicy, the skin of its root is red and its flesh is white. It is in the form of the string of beads and as big as fingers. Those with heavy fruits are good.

The taste of earth is considered to be sweet and the straightness is called Sui （遂）. Its bitter taste discharges earth qi and disinhibits urination and defecation, so it is called Gansui (kansui). The disharmony of earth qi leads to greater abdomen. Dysfunction of the stomach and intestines leads to hernia and movable abdominal mass. The greater abdomen causes abdominal fullness. As earth fails to restrict water, people will have the dropsy of the face and eyes externally and the retention of fluid and the undigested food internally. It can treat these symptoms because it can discharge earth qi. Hernia and movable abdominal mass causes fixed abdominal mass, hardness and accumulation. It can break them and disinhibit urination and defecation. With the water passage promoted, water qi will be dispelled while with digestion promoted, the retention of fluid and the undigested food will be eliminated. It can promote the function of the stomach and intestines because it can move water qi and dredge the retention of fluid and the undigested food.

In *Cheng Ya* [《乘雅》, *Explanation on Materia Medica from Four Aspects*], it argues that when used in a prescription, it can treat the severe and acute diseases. When used in a formula, it can be used to dredge and discharge. However, as its taste is bitter and its property is cold, it is suitable for the febrile diseases and shouldn't be used to treat the diseases caused by coldness.

237. 天南星

天南星 气味苦温,有大毒。主治心痛寒热,结气积聚,伏梁,伤筋痿拘缓,利水道。

《本经》之虎掌,今人谓之天南星,处处平泽有之。四月生苗,状如荷梗,高一二尺,一茎直上,茎端有叶如爪,岐分四步,岁久则叶不生,而中抽一茎,作穗直上如鼠尾,穗下舒一叶如匙,斑烂似素锦,一片裹茎作房。穗上布蕊满之,花青褐色,子如御粟子,生白熟则微红,久又变为蓝色。其根形圆,色白,大如半夏二三倍。曰虎掌者,因叶形似之;曰天南星者,以根形圆白,如天上南方之大星,取以为名也。

天南星色白根圆,得阳明金土之气化,味苦性温,又得阳明燥烈之气化,故有大毒。主治心痛寒热结气者,若先入心而清热,温能散寒而治痛结也。积聚、伏梁者,言不但治痛结无形之气,且治有形之积聚、伏梁。所以然者,禀金气而能攻坚破积也。伤筋痿拘缓者,言筋受伤而痿拘能缓也。大小筋受伤而驰长为痿,犹放纵而委弃也。大筋受伤而软短为拘,犹缩急而拘挛也。阳明主润宗筋,束骨而利机关,故伤筋痿拘能缓。缓,舒缓也。利水道者,金能生水,温能下行也。

气味苦温,有大毒。主治心痛寒热,结气积聚,伏梁,伤筋痿拘缓,利水道。

237. Tiannanxing〔天南星, root or herb of brooklet anemone, Radix seu Herba Anemones Rivularis〕

It is bitter in taste, warm and severely toxic in property, and it is mainly used to treat heartache, cold and heat, qi stagnation, accumulation-gathering, visceral lump, the damage of sinews and flaccidity and spasms, and promote the water passage.

Originally called Huzhang（虎掌）in *Shen Nong Ben Cao Jing*〔《神农本草经》, *Shennong's Classic of Materia Medica*〕, now it is called Tiannanxing (root or herb of brooklet anemone). It grows in lakes and swamps. It bears seedlings in the fourth lunar month in the shape of lotus stalk and in the height of one or two Chi. It has one stem growing straight upward, on the top of which there are leaves in the form of paws. The leaves have four parts and will not grow for a long time. From the bottom of the stem, a new stem will grow, bearing the ears upward in the appearance of mouse tail. Beneath the ears, there is one leaf in the form of spoon with white silk-like spots, wrapping the stem to form the ovary. Its ear is fully covered by pistil and its flower is green and brown. Its seed is like the seed of Yusu（御粟）, white when it is raw and slightly red when it is ripe and blue when it grows for a long time. Its root is round and white, two or three times the size of Banxia〔半夏, pinellia, Rhizoma Pinelliae〕. It is called Huzhang（虎掌）because its leaves are like tiger paws. It is called Tiannanxing (root or herb of brooklet anemone) because its root is round and white just like a big star in the south.

White with the round root, it receives the qi transformation of metal and earth from yang brightness; bitter in taste, warm in property, it receives the qi transformation of dryness from yang brightness; so it is severely toxic. It can mainly treat heartache, cold and heat, and qi stagnation because bitterness enters the heart to eliminate heat and warmth can dissipate cold to treat pain and stagnation. It can treat not only the pain and stagnation caused by invisible qi but also the visible accumulation-gathering and visceral lump. It has this effect because it receives metal qi to eliminate hardness and accumulation. It can treat the damage of sinews, flaccidity and spasm. The damaged, long and hard little sinew which functions slackly without restriction is considered as the syndrome of flaccidity; the damaged, short and soft big sinew which functions stiffly with compression is considered as the syndrome of spasm. It can treat the damage of sinews, flaccidity and spasm because yang brightness dominates to nourish sinews and bundles bone to benefit joints. To treat means to relieve. It can promote the water passage because metal can generate water and warmth can lower water.

238. 大　戟

大戟　气味苦寒,有小毒。主治蛊毒,十二水,腹满急痛,积聚,中风皮肤疼痛,吐逆。

大戟始出常山,今近道皆有之,多生平泽,春生红芽,渐长丛高,茎直中空,叶长狭如柳,折之有白汁,三四月开黄紫花,根皮有紫色,有黄白色,浸于水中,水色青绿。杭州紫大戟为上,江南土大戟次之,北方绵大戟根皮柔韧于如绵而色白,甚峻利能伤人。

大戟生于西北,茎有白汁,味苦气寒,皮浸水中,其色青绿,乃禀金水木相生之气化。水能生木,则木气运行,故主治蛊毒。治蛊毒者,土得木而达也。金能生水,则水气运行,故主治十二水。十二经脉环绕一身,十二水者,一身水气不行而肿也。腹满急痛,积聚,言蛊毒之病,则腹满急痛,内有积聚,大戟能治之。中风皮肤疼痛,言十二水之病,则身中于风而皮肤疼痛,大戟亦能治之。吐逆者,腹满急痛,积聚,则土气不和。中风皮肤疼痛,则肌表不通,皆致吐逆,而大戟皆能治之也。

238. Daji〔大戟, root of Peking euphorbia, Radix Euphorbiae Pekinensis〕

It is bitter in taste, cold and slightly toxic in property, and it is mainly used to treat the parasitic toxin, the twelve waters, abdominal fullness and the sharp pain, accumulation-gathering, stroke, the skin pain and vomiting.

Firstly recorded to be growing in Changshan（常山）, now it grows in the place nearby and mostly in the plain wetland. It bears red sprouts in spring and grows taller in bundles. Its stem is straight and empty inside. Its leaves are long and thin just like willow leaves and when snapped, white sap flows out. It blossoms yellow-purple flowers. The skin of its root is purple or yellow-white in color, which, once immersed in the water, will turn water into blue-green. The purple one growing in Hanzhou（杭州）is of the best quality; followed by the earth one growing in Jiangnan（江南）in quality; the one growing in the north, white in color and with soft and tough root skin which is like silk, is sharp enough to hurt people.

It grows in the northwest with white sap in the stem, bitter in taste and cold in property. Its skin can make the water become blue-green when immersed in it. All of these is because it receives the qi transformation of mutual generation among metal, water and wood. It can mainly treat the parasitic toxin because water generates wood to promote wood qi to move and earth will be free under the assistance of wood. It can mainly treat the twelve waters because metal generates water to promote water qi to move. The twelve meridians run through the whole body. The twelve waters is the syndrome that the water qi in the twelve meridians is blocked and causes the swelling of the whole body. It can treat abdominal fullness, the sharp pain and accumulation-gathering because these syndromes are caused by the worm toxin. It can treat stroke and the skin pain because these syndromes are caused by the twelve waters. It can treat vomiting because this syndrome is caused by the disharmony of the earth qi due to abdominal fullness, the sharp pain and accumulation-gathering and the block of fleshy exterior due to stroke and the skin pain.

239. 泽 漆

泽漆　气味苦,微寒,无毒。主治皮肤热,大腹水气,四肢面目浮肿,丈夫阴气不足。

泽漆《本经》名漆茎,李时珍云:《别录》、陶氏皆言泽漆是大戟苗。日华子又言是大戟花,其苗可食。然大戟苗泄人,不可为菜。今考《土宿本草》及《宝藏论》诸书并云:泽漆是猫儿眼睛草,一名绿叶绿花草,一名五凤草。江湖原泽平陆多有之,春生苗,一科分枝成丛,柔茎如马齿苋,绿叶如苜蓿叶,叶圆而黄绿,颇似猫睛,故名猫儿眼。茎头凡五叶中分,中抽小茎五枝,每枝开细花,青绿色,复有小叶承之,齐整如一,故又名五凤草,绿叶绿花草。茎有白汁黏人,其根白色,有硬骨,以此为大戟苗者,误也。据此则泽漆是猫儿眼睛草,非大戟苗也。今方家用治水盅、脚气有效,尤与《神农》本文相合,自汉人集《别录》,误以名大戟苗,故诸家袭之尔。

愚按:泽漆与大戟同类,而各种用者,须知之。

李时珍曰:泽漆利水功类大戟,人又见其茎有白汁,遂误以为大戟,大戟根苗皆有毒泄人,而泽漆根硬,不可用苗,亦无毒,可作菜食,而利丈夫阴气,甚不相侔也。

泽漆五枝五叶,白汁白根,禀金土之精,故能制化其水,盖金生水而土制水也。气味苦寒,故主治皮肤热,土能制水,故治大腹水气,四肢面目浮肿,金能生水,故治丈夫阴气不足。《金匮》有泽漆汤,治咳逆上气,咳而脉浮者,厚朴麻黄汤主之,咳而脉沉者,泽漆汤主之。

239. Zeqi［泽漆, sun spurge, Herba Euphorbiae Helioscopiae］

It is bitter in taste, slightly cold and non-toxic in property, and it is mainly used to treat the heat in the skin, the retention of fluid in the abdomen, the dropsy of the face, limbs and eyes, and impotence.

It is called Qijin（漆茎）in *Shen Nong Ben Cao Jing*［《神农本草经》, *Shennong's Classic of Materia Medica*］. Li Shizhen（李时珍）said, "It is said to be the seedling of Daji［大戟, root of Peking euphorbia, Radix Euphorbiae Pekinensis］in *Ming Yi Bie Lu*［《名医别录》, *Miscellaneous Records of Famous*

Physicians] and by Tao Shi（陶氏）."Ri Huazi（日华子）also said that it was the flower of Daji（root of Peking euphorbia）, and its seedling can be eaten. However, the seedling of Daji（root of Peking euphorbia）causes diarrhea, so it cannot be served as dish. Nowadays referring to several books such as *Tu Xiu Ben Cao*［《土宿本草》, *Tu Xiu Materia Medica*］and *Bao Zang Lun*［《宝藏论》, *Treasure Theory*］, it is said that Zeqi（泽漆）is Mao'er Yanjingcao［猫儿眼睛草, Nepalese polygonum, Polygoni Nepalensis Herba］, also called Lüye Lühuacao（绿叶绿花草）or Wufengcao（五凤草）. It grows in waters or on the flat land and bears seedlings in spring which bears several branches in cluster. Its soft stem is like Machixian［马齿苋, purslane, Portulacae Herba］. Its green leaves are like the leaves of Muxu［苜蓿, alfalfa, Medicaginis Herba］, round in shape and yellow-green in color, much like cats' eyes. So it is called Mao'eryan［猫儿眼, Nepalese polygonum］. The top of the stem bears five little stems from the middle of five leaves respectively. Each of these little stems bears thin and blue-green flowers with little leaves supporting them and each flower looks like the same. So it is also called Wufengcao（五凤草）and Lüye Lühuacao（绿叶绿花草）. Its stem has the white and sticky sap and its root is white in color and hard in texture. Owing to this, it is often mistaken as the seedling of Daji（root of Peking euphorbia）. Therefore, it is Mao'er Yanjingcao（Nepalese polygonum）rather than the seedling of Daji（root of Peking euphorbia）. Now it is used to treat water tympanites and the weak foot effectively which is in accordance with the description in *Shen Nong Ben Cao Jing*［《神农本草经》, *Shennong's Classic of Materia Medica*］. Since it is called the seedling of Daji（root of Peking euphorbia）in *Ming Yi Bie Lu*［《名医别录》, *Miscellaneous Records of Famous Physicians*］compiled in Han Dynasty collected by Han people, a lot of medical experts just mistakenly follow suit.

Note by Zhang Zhicong（张志聪）：Zeqi（sun spurge）and Daji（root of Peking euphorbia）belong to the same genus. However, people should know every respective use of them.

Li Shizhen（李时珍）said, "Just like Daji（root of Peking euphorbia）, Zeqi（sun spurge）also has the function of draining water, and people mistake it as Daji（root of Peking euphorbia）when seeing the white sap in its stem.

However, both the root and the seedlings of Daji（root of Peking euphorbia）are toxic and cause diarrhea while the root of Zeqi（sun spurge）is hard and nontoxic, and its seedlings cannot be used as medicinal but can be served as dish. It can treat impotence. So these two are different from each other in use."

With five stems, five leaves, a white sap and a white root, it receives the essence of metal and earth. Therefore, it can control and generate water, because metal generates water and earth controls water. It can treat the heat in the skin because of its bitter taste and cold property. It can treat the retention of fluid in the abdomen and the dropsy of the face, limbs and eyes because earth controls water. It can treat impotence because metal generates water. There is Sun Spurge Decoction in *Jin Gui*［《金匮》, *Synopsis of the Golden Chamber*］. When treating the cough with dyspnea and descending adverse-rising qi, Officinal Magnolia and Ephedra Decoction is mainly used to treat the cough with the floating pulse and Sun Spurge Decoction is mainly used to treat the cough with the deep pulse.

240. 常　山

常山　气味苦寒,有毒。主治伤寒寒热,热发温疟,鬼毒,胸中痰结,吐逆。

常山又名恒山,出益州及汉中,今汴西、淮浙、湖南州郡皆有。生山谷间,茎高三四尺,圆而有节,其叶似茗,两两相对,二月作白花,青萼,五月结实青圆。常山者,根之名也。状似荆根,细实而黄者,谓之鸡骨常山,用之最胜,其苗别名蜀漆。古时根苗皆入药用,今时但用常山,不用蜀漆,犹之赤箭、天麻,但用天麻,无有用赤箭者,盖以其苗不复远市耳。

恒山,北岳也。后以汉文帝讳恒,遂改名常山。此草名常山,亦名恒山。李时珍疑其始出于常山,故得此名,余以此思常山之草,盖禀西北金水之化而气出于东南。主治伤寒之寒热者,从西北之阴而外出于阳也。热发温疟者,乃先发热之温疟。温疟病藏于肾,常山从西北而出于东南,则温疟可治也。神气乃浮,则鬼毒自散。阳气外行,则胸中痰结自消,痰结消而吐逆亦平矣。

愚按:伤寒寒热,言伤寒之病,先寒后热也。热发温疟,言温疟之病,先热发而后寒也。言不尽意,以意会之。

《阴阳离合论》云:圣人南面而立,前曰广明,后曰太冲,太冲之地,名曰少阴,少阴之上,名曰太阳,是太阳之气根于少阴,主于肤表。常山从少阴而达太阳之气以外出,所谓因于寒,欲如运枢,起居如惊,神气乃浮者,是也。

240. Changshan〔常山, root of antifebrile dichroa, Radix Dichroae〕

It is bitter in taste, cold and toxic in property, and it is mainly used to treat the cold and heat due to the cold damage, the fever caused by warm malaria, the severe toxin like a ghost, the retention of phlegm in the chest and vomiting.

Also called Hengshan（恒山）and originally growing in Yizhou（益州）and Hanzhong（汉中）, now it grows in the counties of Bianxi（汴西）, Huaizhe（淮浙）and Hunan（湖南）. It grows in mountain valleys with stems in the height of three or four Chi, it is round and has joints. Its leaves are similar to tea, forming opposing pairs. It blossoms with white flowers and green calyxes in the second lunar month and bears green and round fruits in the fifth lunar month. Changshan（root of antifebrile dichroa）is the name of the root which is similar to Jinggen〔荆根, vitex root, Viticis Negundinis Radix〕in shape. The one that is thin, full and yellow is called Jigu Changshan〔鸡骨常山, alstonia, Alstoniae Ramulus et Folium〕which is of the best quality and its seedling is also called as Shuqi〔蜀漆, dichroa, Ramulus et Folium Dichroae〕. In ancient times, both roots and seedlings were used as medicinals. Nowadays, only Changshan（root of antifebrile dichroa）is used, just like Chijian（赤箭）and Tianma〔天麻, gastrodia, Gastrodiae Rhizoma〕of which only Tianma（gastrodia）is used. So its seedlings fade away from the market.

The name of Hengshan Mountain（恒山）, Northern Sacred Mountain, was changed into Changshan Mountain（常山）because Emperor Wen of the Han Dynasty took the character of "恒"（Heng）as a taboo. This grass is called Changshan（root of antifebrile dichro）and also called Hengshang（恒山）. Li Shizhen（李时珍）suspected that it firstly grew in Changshan（常山）, so it got its name. Accordingly, I thought this grass from Changshan（常山）receives the transformation of metal and water in the northwest and makes qi present in the southeast. It can mainly treat the cold and heat due to the cold damage because it comes from yin in the northwest and comes out of yang. The fever caused by warm malaria refers to the warm malaria with fever as the start of the syndrome. It can treat warm malaria because warm malaria hides in the kidney and it comes from the northwest and goes out from the southeast. Spirit qi disperses and the severe toxin like a ghost is removed. Yang qi runs outside and retention of phlegm in the chest is dispersed naturally and thus vomiting is treated.

Note by Zhang Zhicong（张志聪）: The cold and heat due to the cold damage refers to the syndrome of cold damage with chills occurring prior to fever. The fever caused by warm malaria refers to the syndrome of malaria with fever occurring prior to chills. As the words do not fully explain the meaning, we should depend on our senses to understand it.

Yin Yang Li He Lun [《阴阳离合论》, *Separation and Combination of Yin and Yang*] says, "When sages stand facing the south, the front is called Guangming, and the back is called Taichong. The place where Taichong starts is called Shaoyin and the place above Shaoyin is called Taiyang. The qi of Taiyang starts from Shaoyin and prodominates the skin." Changshan（常山）makes the qi of greater yang from Shaoyin manifest on the skin. It is so called that in cold weather, Yang qi flows in the body just like a door-hinge rotating in the door-mortar. Any rash action in daily life will disperse spirit qi.

241. 蜀 漆

蜀漆 气味辛平,有毒。主治疟及咳逆寒热,腹中坚症痞结,积聚邪气,蛊毒鬼疰。

常山之茎,名蜀漆,其功用亦与常山相等。

蜀漆能通金水之气,以救火逆,又能启太阳之阳,以接助其亡阳,亦从阴出阳之药也。故《伤寒·太阳篇》云:伤寒脉浮,医以火迫劫之,亡阳必惊狂,起卧不安者,桂枝去芍药加蜀漆牡蛎龙骨救逆汤主之。又,《金匮论》云:疟多寒者,名曰牝疟。蜀漆散主之。李时珍曰:常山、蜀漆有劫痰截疟之功,须在发散表邪,及提出阳分之后,用之得宜,神效立见。用失其法,真气必伤。

愚谓:疟乃伏邪,有留于脏腑募原之间,而为三阴疟者;有藏于肾脏,而为先热后寒之温疟者;有气藏于心,而为但热不寒之瘅疟者。常山主通少阴太阳之气,从阴出阳,自内而外,则邪随气出,所谓有故无殒。若邪已提出阳分。而反用攻利之剂,岂不妄伤正气乎。李蕲阳数十年苦心始成《纲目》,而其间发明议论,有与经旨不合者,长于纂集,而少于参究故也。

241. Shuqi〔蜀漆, dichroa, Ramulus et Folium Dichroae〕

It is pungent in taste, mild and toxic in property, and it is mainly used to treat malaria, the cough with dyspnea, chills and fever, abdominal hard mass and fullness, the accumulation, pathogenic qi, parasitic toxin and Guizhu〔鬼疰, multiple infixation abscess〕.

The stem of Changshan〔常山, root of antifebrile dichroa, Radix Dichroae〕 is called Shuqi(dichroa) which has the same effects as Changshan(root of antifebrile dichroa) does.

It can free the qi of metal and water to redeem the malpractice of heat therapy and initiate the yang of greater yang to prolong and aid the yang exhaustions, so it is the medicinal bringing out yang from yin. Therefore, *Shang Han: Tai Yang Pian*〔《伤寒·太阳篇》, *Greater Yang of Treatise on Cold Pathogenic Diseases*〕 says, "Doctors use fire to distress and deteriorate cold damage and floating pulse, thus frightening yang exhaustion and causing restless life and sleep. Cinnamon Twig Minus Peony Plus Dichroa Leaf, Dragon Bone, Oyster Shell Counterflow Decoction can be used to treat the syndrome above." Also, *Jin Kui Lun*〔《金匮论》, *On the Golden Chamber*〕 says, "Malaria with more cold is called female malaria which can be treated by Shuqi(dichroa) powder." Li Shizhen(李时珍) said, "Changshan(root of antifebrile dichroa) and Shuqi(dichroa) have the effect of deteriorating the phlegm and preventing attack of malaria. They can be used properly and effectively only after the exterior pathogen is dissipated and yang is brought out. Once they are used improperly, genuine qi will be damaged."

In my humble opinion, malaria is the latent pathogen. The one staying in the zang-fu organs and membrane source is triple-yin malaria. The one hiding in the kidney with fever occurring prior to chills is warm malaria. The one with qi hiding in the heart is heat malaria which has fever but no chills. Changshan(root of antifebrile) mainly frees the qi of greater yang and lesser yin, and brings out yang from yin. From the internal to the external, the pathogen comes out with qi; owing to this, no harm is caused. If yang is already drawn out of pathogen and the purgative formula is used, healthy qi surely will be damaged. Li Qiyang（李蕲阳）devoted several decades to the completion of *Ben Cao Gang Mu*［《本草纲目》, *Compendium of Materia Medica*］. During this period, some comments uttered by him were different from the description in *Huang Di Nei Jing*［《黄帝内经》, *Huangdi's Internal Classic*］because he was better at compiling books than making research.

242. 葶苈子

葶苈子　气味辛寒,无毒。主治症瘕积聚,结气,饮食寒热,破坚逐邪,通利水道。

葶苈子始出藁城平泽田野间,汴东、陕西、河北州郡亦有之,近以彭城、曹州者为胜。春初生苗,叶高六七寸,似荠,故《别录》名狗荠。根白色,枝茎俱青,三月开花微黄,结角子扁小,如黍粒微长,黄色,《月令》:孟夏之月靡草死。许慎、郑元注皆云:靡草、狗荠、葶苈之属是也。

葶苈花实黄色,根白味辛,盖禀土金之气化。禀金气,故主治症瘕积聚之结气。禀土气,故主治饮食不调之寒热。破坚逐邪,金气盛也。通利水道,土气盛也。

李杲曰:《本草十剂》云:泄可去闭,葶苈、大黄之属二味,皆大苦寒,一泄血闭,一泄气闭,盖葶苈之苦寒,气味俱厚,不减大黄,又性过于诸药,以泄阳分肺中之闭,亦能泄大便,为体轻象阳故也。《别录》云:久服令人虚。朱丹溪谓:葶苈属火性急,善遂水,病人稍涉,虚者宜远之,且杀人,甚健何必久服而后虚也。

李时珍曰:葶苈子有甜苦二种,正如牵牛黑白二色,急缓不同。又如葫芦甘苦二味,良毒亦异,大抵甜者下泄之性缓,虽泄肺而不伤胃,苦者下泄之性急,既泄肺而兼伤胃,故古方多以大枣辅之。若肺中水气膹满急者,非此不能除,但水去则止,不可过剂,既不久服,何至杀人。淮南子云:大戟去水,葶苈愈胀,用之不节,反及成病,亦在用之有节与不耳。

242. Tinglizi［葶苈子, lepidium/descurainiae, Lepidii/Descurainiae Semen］

It is pungent in taste, cold and non-toxic in property, and it is mainly used to treat abdominal mass, accumulation-gathering, qi stagnation, diet and cold and heat, break hardness, expel the pathogenic factors and dredge and promote the water passage in the body.

Firstly recorded to be growing in the lakes, swamps, and fields of Gaocheng（藁城）and in the counties of Biandong（汴东）, Shaanxi（陕西）and Hebei（河北）, nowadays the one growing in Pengcheng（彭城）and Caozhou（曹州）is of better quality. It bears seedlings in early spring and its leaves are in the height of six or seven Cun, similar to Ji［荠, shepherd's purse, Capsellae Bursa-Pastoris Herba］, so it is called Gouji（狗荠）in *Ming Yi Bie Lu* ［《名医别录》, *Miscellaneous Records of Famous Physicians*］. Its root is white and its twig and stem are green. It blossoms with light yellow flowers in the third lunar month and bears flat, small and yellow pods which are just like the grains of Shu（黍）, but a little longer. *Yue Ling*［《月令》, Monthly Order］ said, "Micao（靡草）dies in the fourth lunar month in summer." Both Xu Shen（许慎）and Zheng Yuanzhu（郑元注）said, "Both Micao（靡草）and Gouji（狗荠）belong to the genus of Tingli（lepidium/descurainiae）."

It has yellow flowers and fruits, white root and pungent taste because it receives the qi transformation of earth and metal. It can mainly treat the qi stagnation caused by abdominal mass and accumulation-gathering because it receives metal qi. It can mainly treat the cold and heat due to improper diet because it receives earth qi. It can break hardness and expel the pathogenic factors because of the exuberance of metal qi. It can dredge and promote the water passage in the body because of the exuberance of earth qi.

Li Gao（李杲）said, " *Ben Cao Shi Ji*［《本草十剂》, *Ten Formulas of Materia Medica*］ says that discharging can remove block. Both Tingli（lepidium/descurainiae）and Dahuang［大黄, rhubarb, Rhei Radix et Rhizoma］, two kinds of medicinals, have severely bitter taste and cold property, the former discharging the blood block and the latter the qi block. For Tingli（lepidium/descurainiae）, it is rich in bitter taste and cold property which are no less than those of Dahuang（大黄）and it is better than many other meidicinals in nature. It can discharge the block of the lung qi in the upper body and relieve constipation because it is light in weight just like yang."*Ming Yi Bie Lu*〔《名医别录》, *Miscellaneous Records of Famous Physicians*〕says, "Long-term taking of it causes deficiency." Zhu Danxi（朱丹溪）said, "It pertains to fire with immediate effect, good at expelling the water pathogen. So patients should just take a bit of it. The one with deficiency should avoid taking it. It can kill people, so the one with good health should not take it for a long time or it may cause deficiency."

Li Shizhen（李时珍）said, "There are two kinds of Tinglizi（lepidium/descurainiae）with different properties, one sweet and the other bitter, just like the situation that there are two kinds of Qianniu〔牵牛, morning glory, Pharbitidis Semen Album〕, one white with immediate effect and the other black with mild effect, also like Hulu〔葫芦, bottle gourd, Lagenariae Depressae Fructus〕, one sweet and non-toxic and the other bitter and toxic. Generally speaking, the sweet one has the mild effect of discharging downward, so it discharges the lung but doesn't hurt the stomach; the bitter one has the immediate effect of discharging, so it not only discharges the lung but also hurts the stomach. Accordingly Dazao〔大枣, jujube, Jujubae Fructus〕is often used as adjuvant in ancient formula. Only Tinglizi（lepidium/descurainia）can treat rushing, fullness and the tension of the water qi in the lung. Once the water is removed, this formula shouldn't be used. It cannot be overtaken or taken for a long time. Thus it will not kill people." Huai Nanzi（淮南子）said, "Daji（root of Peking euphorbia）discharges water and Tingli（lepidium/descurainia）removes swelling. Once they are used improperly, they may cause diseases. Thus, the key point here is whether they can be used properly or not."

243. 莞 花

莞花 气味苦寒,有毒。主治伤寒温疟,下十二水,破积聚,大坚症瘕,荡涤胸中留澼饮食,寒热邪气,利水道。荛音饶。

　　荛花始出咸阳、河南、中牟,今所在有之,以雍州者为胜,苗似胡荽,茎无刺,花细黄色,六月采花阴干。

《诊要经终论》云:五月六月,天气高,地气盛,人气在头。荛花气味苦寒,花开炎夏,禀太阳本寒之气,而合太阳之标阳,故苦寒有毒。伤寒者,寒伤太阳。荛花气合标阳,故治伤寒。温疟者,病藏于肾,荛花气禀寒水,故治温疟。膀胱水气藉太阳阳热而运行于周身,则外濡皮毛,内通经脉。水气不行,则为十二经脉之水。荛花合太阳之阳,故下十二水,且破阴凝之积聚,及大坚之症瘕。太阳之气,从胸膈以出入,故荡涤胸中之留澼痰饮类也。不但荡涤胸中留澼,且除饮食内停之寒热邪气。水气得阳热以运行,故利水道。

　　按:《伤寒论》云:伤寒表不解,心下有水气,干呕,发热而咳。若微利者,小青龙汤加荛花,如鸡子大,熬令赤色。大如鸡子,形圆象心也。熬令赤色,取意象火也。是荛花气味虽属苦寒,而有太阳之标阳,恐后世不能司岁备物,故加炮制如是尔。

243. Raohua［荛花, canescent, Flos Wikstroemia Canescens］

It is bitter in taste, cold and toxic in property, and it is mainly used to treat cold damage, warm malaria, and the twelve waters, break accumulation-gathering, hard mass and abdominal mass, resolve the retention of the undigested food, cold and heat and pathogenic qi, and promote the water passage. Rao（荛）is pronounced as Rao（饶）.

　　Firstly recorded to be growing in Xianyang（咸阳）, Henan（河南）and Zhongmu（中牟）, now it grows everywhere and those in Yongzhou（雍州）are of better quality. Its seedling is similar to Husui［胡荽, coriander, Coriandri Herba cum Radice］, its stalk has no thorns, its flower is thin and yellow in color which is collected in the sixth lunar month and dried in shade. *Zhen Yao Jing Zhong Lu*［《诊要经终论》, *Discussion on the Essentials of Diagnosis and Exhaustion of the Twelve Channels*］says, "In the fifth lunar month and the sixth lunar month, heaven qi rises, earth qi is exuberant and human qi is in the head." Bitter in taste, cold in property and blossoming in hot summer, it receives the cold qi of greater yang when it follows the root and combines with the branch yang from greater yang, so it is bitter, cold and toxic. As for cold damage, cold does harm to greater yang. Raohua (canescent) can treat cold damage because its qi harmonizes with the branch yang. The warm malaria hides the pathogenesis in the kidney. It can treat warm malaria because its qi receives the cold water. The water qi of the bladder moves around the whole body with the assistance of the yang heat of greater yang, so it nourishes the skin and hair externally and dredges the channels internally. The failure of water qi to move causes the twelve waters. It can eliminate the twelve waters and break accumulation-gathering, hard mass and abdominal mass because it harmonizes with the yang of greater yang. The qi of greater yang comes in and out of the chest and diaphragm, so it can remove the retention of the undigested food and phlegm-rheum in the chest. Besides, it also can eliminate cold and heat and the pathogenic qi caused by the retention of the undigested food. It can promote the water passage because water qi can move with the help of the yang heat.

Note by Gao Shishi (高世栻): *Shang Han Lun* [《伤寒论》, *Treatise on Cold Pathogenic Diseases*] says, "If cold damage cannot be released exteriorly, there will be water qi below the heart and patients will retch and cough due to fever. Boil the mixture of Minor Green-Blue Dragon Decoction and Raohua (canescent) in the size of an egg to red. People who have the mild diarrhea can take the decoction. Its egg-big size represents the form of heart. The boiled red color signifies the meaning of fire. Though it is bitter in taste and cold in property, it pertains to the branch yang from greater yang. For fear that people later on can not prepare it according to the qi that dominates in the year, so it is processed in this way."

244. 芫 花

芫花 气味辛温,有小毒。主治咳逆上气,喉鸣喘,咽肿,短气,蛊毒鬼疟,疝瘕痈肿,杀虫鱼。

芫花《本经》名去水,言其功也。《别录》名毒鱼,言其性也。根名黄大戟,言其似也。俗人因其气恶,又名头痛花。近道处处有之。春生苗,茎紫色,长一二尺,叶色青,厚则黑。二月开花,有紫、赤、黄、碧、白数种,根色黄白如桑根，小人争斗者，取其叶挪擦皮肤，辄作赤肿，如被伤以诬人。和盐擦卵，能染其壳，若赭色。

草木根荄之在下者，性欲上行，花实之在上者，性复下降，此物理之自然也。芫花气味辛温，花开赤白，禀金火之气化，主行心肺之气下降，故治咳逆上气，喉鸣而喘，以及咽肿而短气。禀火气，故治虫毒鬼疟。禀金气，故治疝瘕痈肿。辛温有毒，故杀虫鱼。

244. Yuanhua〔芫花，immature flower of lilac daphne，Flos Genkwa〕

It is pungent in taste, warm and slightly toxic in property, and it is mainly used to treat the cough with dyspnea, descend adverse-rising qi, treat laryngeal stridor and dyspnea, the swelling of the throat, shortness of breath, parasitic toxin, severe malaria, hernia, movable abdominal mass, abscess and swelling, and kill worms and fish.

It is called Qushui（去水）in *Shen Nong Ben Cao Jing*〔《神农本草经》, *Shennong's Classic of Materia Medica*〕based on its function and called Duyu（毒鱼）in *Ming Yi Bie Lu*〔《名医别录》, *Miscellaneous Records of Famous Physicians*〕based on its property. Its root is called Huangdaji（黄大戟）based on its form. It is also popularly called Toutonghua（头痛花）because it stinks. It grows everywhere nearby. It bears seedlings in spring, and its stem is purple in color and in the length of one or two Chi. Its leaves are green and the thick ones are black. It blossoms in the color of purple, red, yellow, bluish green and white in the second lunar month. Its root is yellow-white similar to the root of Sanggen〔桑根, mulberry, Mori Radix〕. When fighting with others, the treacherous people may rub its leaves on their skin which soon becomes red and swelling. In this case, they can accuse their opponents of hurting them. Rubbing it with salt on the egg can dye its shell into the color of dark red.

For plants, if their roots are at the bottom, they have the nature of going upward; if their flowers and fruits are on the top, they have the nature of going downward, which is the natural rule. Pungent in taste, warm in property and with red and white flowers, it receives the qi transformation of metal and fire. It can treat the cough with dyspnea, laryngeal stridor and dyspnea, the swelling of the throat and shortness of breath and descend adverse-rising qi because it promotes the qi of the heart and the lung to go downward. It can treat the parasitic toxin and severe malaria because it receives fire qi. It can treat hernia, movable abdominal mass and abscess and swelling because it receives metal qi. It can kill worms and fish because of its pungent taste and warm and toxic property.

245. 萹 蓄

萹蓄 气味苦平,无毒。主治浸淫疥瘙疽痔,杀三虫。

萹蓄一名扁竹,处处有之,多生道旁,春时蔓延布地,苗似瞿麦,叶细绿如竹弱,茎促节,节紫赤似钗股。三月开细红花,如蓼蓝花状,结细子,炉火家烧灰炼霜用。

《金匮要略》曰:浸淫疮从口流向四肢者,可治。从四肢流来入口者,不可治。盖口乃脾窍,脾属四肢,萹蓄禀火气而温土,故主治脾湿之浸淫。充肤热肉之血,不淡渗于皮毛,则为疥瘙。萹蓄禀东方之木气,故主治疥瘙,浸淫可治,则疽痔亦可治矣。疥瘙可治,则三虫亦可治矣。缘其禀木火之气,通利三焦,从经脉而达于肌腠皮肤,故主治如此。

245. Bianxu [萹蓄, common knotgrass herb, Herba Polygoni Avicularis]

It is bitter in taste, mild and non-toxic in property, and it is mainly used to treat immersion, scabies, itch, abscess and hemorrhoids and kill three worms.

It is also called Bianzhu (扁竹), growing everywhere and mainly beside the road. It sprawls along the ground in spring. Its seedling looks like Qumai [瞿麦, dianthus, Dianthi Herba], and its leaves are thin and as green as Zhuruo (竹弱). Its stem has joints which are purple-red similar to Hairpin shares. It blossoms with thin and red flowers in the third lunar month which are like those of Liaolan (蓼蓝). It bears thin seeds which are used to burn and refine cream by the alchemist.

Jin Gui Yao Lue [《金匮要略》, *Synopsis of Golden Chamber*] says, "The immersion sore which spreads from the mouth to the limbs can be treated. The one that spreads from the limbs to the mouth can not be treated. The mouth is the spleen orifice and the spleen pertains to the limbs. Since Bianxu（common knotgrass herb）receives fire qi to warm earth, it can mainly treat immersion caused by spleen dampness. If the blood which circulates within the skin and warms the flesh cannot nourish the skin and hair, it will cause scabies and itch. Since Bianxu（common knotgrass herb）receives the wood qi of the east, it can treat scabies and itch. If immersion can be treated, accordingly, abscess and hemorrhoids can be treated too. If scabies and itch can be treated, accordingly, three worms can be killed too. That is because Bianxu（common knotgrass herb）receives the qi of wood and fire, frees the triple energizer and moves from the meridians to the interstices of the flesh and skin."

246. 商陆根

商陆根 气味辛平,有毒。主治水肿,疝瘕,痹熨,除痈肿,杀鬼精物。

　　商陆所在有之,春生苗,高二三尺,茎青赤,极柔脆,叶如牛舌而长,夏秋开花作朵,根如萝卜似人形者有神。有赤白二种,白根者,花白。赤根者,花赤。白者入药,赤者甚有毒,不可服,服之见鬼神。俗名章柳,相传刻其根为人能通鬼神也。

商陆禀金土之气化,故气味辛平,以根花白者为良。主治水肿者,辛走气,土胜水,气化则水行,水散则肿消也。治疝瘕者,疝瘕乃厥阴肝木之病,而金能平之也。痹熨,犹言熨痹,肌腠闭痹。商陆熨而治之,火温土也。除痈肿者,金主攻利也。杀鬼精物者,金主肃杀也。

246. Shanglugen［商陆根, phytolacca, Radix Phytolaccae］

It is pungent in taste, mild and toxic in property, and it is mainly used to treat edema, hernia and movable abdominal mass, compress impediment, eliminate abscess, swelling and the strange pathogenic factors like ghosts.

　　It grows in a lot of places and sprouts in spring which is two or three Chi high. Its stem is green-red, soft and crisp. Its leaves are as long as the cow's tongue. It blossoms in summer and autumn. Its root looks like a carrot and the one similar to a person is good. There are two types, one with the white root and white flowers and the other with the red root and red flowers. The white one can be used as medicinal while the red one is severely toxic and should not be taken. Once taken, people may see ghosts and gods. It is popularly called Zhangliu (章柳) and the legend has it that carved into human shape, it can connect the ghosts and gods.

Receiving the qi transformation of metal and earth, it has pungent taste and mild property and the one with the white root and flowers is of good quality. It can mainly treat edema because the pungent taste can dispel qi and earth restricts water. The qi transformation promotes the water movement which can alleviate swelling. It can treat hernia and movable abdominal mass because these two are the diseases of Jueyin liver-wood and metal can pacify it. Impediment, also called the compressing impediment, here refers to the impediment of muscle and striae. It compresses to treat it because fire warms earth. It can eliminate abscess and swelling because metal governs attacking and tonifying. It can eliminate the strange pathogenic factors like ghosts because metal governs clearing and downward.

247. 藜 芦

藜芦　气味辛寒,有毒。主治蛊毒,咳逆,泄痢,肠澼,头疡,疥瘙,恶疮,杀诸虫毒,去死肌。

藜芦一名山葱,所在山谷有之。茎下多毛,三月生苗,高五六寸,茎似葱,根色青紫,外有黑皮裹茎,宛似棕榈,根长四五寸许,黄白色。

藜芦气味辛寒,其根黄白,外皮黑色,禀土金水相生之气化。土气运行,则能治蛊毒。金气流通,则能治咳逆。水气四布,则能治泄痢肠澼也。治头疡疥瘙,金制其风也。治恶疮,水济其火也。杀诸虫毒,土胜湿而解毒也。土主肌肉,故又去死肌。

247. Lilu〔藜芦, root and rhizome of black falsehellebore, Radix et Rhizoma Veratri〕

It is pungent in taste, cold and toxic in property, and it is mainly used to treat parasitic toxin, the cough with dyspnea, diarrhea, dysentery, head ulcer, scabies, pruritus and malign sore, remove various worm toxins, and eliminate the numbness of muscles.

It is also called Shancong（山葱）, growing in the mountain valleys. There is a lot of hair at the bottom of its stem. It sprouts in the third lunar month which is five or six Cun tall. Its stem is similar to Cong（葱）with the blue-purple root and wrapped by the black skin which is like Zonglü［棕榈, trachycarpus, Trachycarpi］. Its root is four or five Cun long with the color of yellow-white.

Pungent in taste, cold in property, its root being yellow-white and its external skin being black, it receives the qi transformation of mutual generation among earth, metal and water. It can treat parasitic toxin because earth qi moves. It can treat the cough with dyspnea because metal qi flows. It can treat dysentery and diarrhea because water qi spreads. It can treat head ulcer, scabies and pruritus because metal controls wind. It can treat malign sore because water coordinates with fire. It can remove various worm toxins because earth restricts dampness to remove toxin. It can eliminate the numbness of muscles because earth governs muscles.

248. 旋覆花

旋覆花 气味咸温,有小毒。主治结气,胁下满,惊悸,除水,去五脏间寒热,补中,下气。

旋覆花《本经》名金沸草,《尔雅》名盗庚,近道皆有,多生水边及下湿地。二月以后生苗,长一二尺,茎柔细,叶似柳,六月至七八月开花,状如金钱菊,浅黄色,中心细白茸作丛,花圆而覆下,故名旋覆。相传叶上露水滴地即生,故繁茂。

花名旋覆者,花圆而覆下也。草名金沸者,得水露之精,清肺金之热沸也。又名盗庚者,开黄花白茸,于长夏金伏之时,盗窃庚金之气也。气味咸温,有小毒。盖禀太阳之气化,夫太阳之气,从胸胁以出入,故主治胸中结气,胁下胀满,太阳不能合心主之神气以外出,则惊。寒水之气动于中,则悸。旋覆花能旋转于外而覆冒于下,故治惊悸。太阳为诸阳主气,气化则水行,故除水。五脏如五运之在地,天气旋覆于地中,则五脏之寒热自去矣。去五脏间寒热,故能补中。治结气、胁满、惊悸、除水,故能下气也。

248. Xuanfuhua〔旋覆花，Inula flower，Flos Inula Japonica〕

It is salty in taste, warm and slightly toxic in property, and it is mainly used to treat qi stagnation, the fullness below hypochondrium, the palpitation due to fright, eliminate water-rheum and the cold and heat in the five zang-organs, tonify the middle and descend qi.

It is called Jinfeicao〔金沸草，Inula Herb，Herba Inulae〕in *Shen Nong Ben Cao Jing*〔《神农本草经》，*Shennong's Classic of Materia Medica*〕and Daogeng（盗庚）in *Er Ya*〔《尔雅》，*On Elegance*〕，growing in the places nearby, usually by the water and in the wetland. It sprouts after the second lunar month which is one or two Chi long. Its stem is soft and thin, and its leaves are similar to those of the willow. It blossoms from the six lunar month to the seventh or eighth lunar month. Its flower is light yellow in the form of chrysanthemums. The thin and white fuzz in the center is in clusters, and the petals are round and covering the underneath, so it is called Xuanfu（Inula flower）. The legend has it that even the dew on leaves which falls down to the ground can make it grow, so it thrives easily.

The flower is called Xuanfu（Inula flower）, for it is round and covering the underneath. The grass is called Jinfei（Inula Herb）, for it receives the essence of dew to clear the severe heat of lung-metal. It is also called Daogeng（盗庚）, for it produces yellow flowers and white fuzz in the sixth lunar month of metal latence and steals the qi of Geng-metal. Salty in taste and warm and slightly toxic in property, it receives the qi transformation of greater yang. The qi of greater yang moves through the chest and hypochondrium, so it can mainly treat the stagnation of qi in the chest and the fullness below hypochondrium. That greater yang cannot harmonize with the spirit qi which is governed by the heart and moves out will cause fright. That qi of cold water moves in the middle of the body will cause palpitation. It can treat the palpitation due to fright because it rotates outward and covers the underneath. It can eliminate water-rheum because greater yang is the governing qi among these yangs and qi transformation makes water move. The five zang-organs is just like the five-motions on earth. The heaven qi rotates in the earth, so the cold and heat in the five zang-organs disappears naturally. Since it can eliminate the cold and heat in the five zang-organs, it can tonify the middle. Since it can treat qi stagnation, the fullness below hypochondrium and the palpitation due to fright, and eliminate water-rheum, it can descend qi.

249. 青 葙

青葙 气味苦微寒,无毒。主治邪气,皮肤中热,风瘙身痒,杀三虫。子,气味同,主治唇口青。

　　青葙处处有之,乃野鸡冠也。子名草决明,花叶与鸡冠无二,但鸡冠花穗或团或大而扁,此则稍间出穗状如兔尾,水红色,亦有黄白色者,穗中细子黑而光亮,亦与鸡冠子及苋子无异。

　　青葙开花结实于三秋,得秋金清肃之气,故主清邪热,去风瘙,杀三虫。《辨脉篇》曰:唇口反青,四肢漐习者,此为肝绝也。青葙花开黄白,结黑子于深秋,得金水相生之化,以养肝木,故子治唇口青。肝气得其生化,故今时又用以明目。

249. Qingxiang [青葙, celosia, Celosiae Caulis, Folium et Radix]

It is bitter in taste, slightly cold and non-toxic in property, and it is mainly used to treat pathogenic qi, the heat in the skin, the pruritus due to wind and kill three worms. Its seed, with the same taste, is mainly used to treat the bluishness of the lips and mouth.

　　It grows everywhere, and it is actually the wild type of Jiguan [鸡冠, cockscomb, Celosiae Cristatae Flos]. Its seed is called Caojueming [草决明, cassis seed, Semen Cassiae], and its flowers and leaves are the same as those of Jiguan (cockscomb). However, the latter one's flower spikes are clustering or big and flat while the former one's are occasionally in the shape of a rabbit's tail, cerise, sometimes yellow-white in color. The thin seeds in the flower spikes are black and shining, the same as those of Jiguan (cockscomb) and Xianzi (苋子).

It blossoms and bears fruits in the ninth lunar month and receives the qi of the autumn-metal purification, so it can mainly clear the pathogenic heat, eliminate the pruritus due to wind and kill three worms. *Bian Mai Pian* [《辨脉篇》, *Differentiation of Pulse*] says, "The syndrome that the lip and the mouth are blue and the limbs are wet indicates the exhaustion of liver qi. Blossoming in yellow and white and bearing black seeds in late autumn, it receives the transformation of mutual generation between metal and water to nourish liver-wood so its seed can treat the bluishness of lips and mouth. The liver qi obtains its generation and transformation, so it is also used to improve vision nowadays."

250. 贯众根

贯众根 气味苦,微寒,有毒。主治腹中邪热气,诸毒,杀三虫。

贯众所在山谷有之,多生山阴近水处,数根丛生,交相贯穿,故《本经》名贯节,又名百头。形如大瓜,直而多枝,皮黑肉赤,黑须丛簇。春生赤苗,圆叶锐茎,黑毛布地,冬夏不死,四月花白,七月实黑。

贯众气味苦寒,色多赤黑,盖禀少阴水火之气。主治腹中邪热气,诸毒,禀水气也。杀三虫,禀火气也。

250. Guanzhonggen [贯众根, roots of rhizome of male fern, Rhizoma Dryopteris Crassirhizomae]

It is bitter in taste, slightly cold and toxic in property, and it is mainly used to treat the pathogenic heat qi in the abdomen, remove various toxins and kill three worms.

Guanzhong [贯众, rhizome of male fern, Rhizoma Dryopteris Crassirhizomae] grows in mountains and valleys mostly near the hill shadows and water. Its roots grow in dense tufts and intersect with another, so it is also called Guanjie (贯节) and Baitou (百头) in *Shen Nong Ben Cao Jing* [《神农本草经》, *Shennong's Classic of Materia Medica*]. It looks like a big melon with straight stalk and many branches, and it has black skin, red flesh and black hair in tufts. It grows red seedlings in spring, its leaves round, its stalk straight, and its black hair spreading around the ground. It doesn't die in summer and winter, blossoms white in the fourth lunar month, and bears black fruits in the seventh lunar month.

Bitter in taste, cold in property and mostly red-black in color, it receives the qi of water and fire from lesser yin. It mainly treats the pathogenic heat qi in the abdomen and various toxins because it receives water qi; it kills three worms because it receives fire qi.

251. 蛇含草

蛇含草　气味苦,微寒,无毒。主治惊痫寒热,邪气除热,金疮疽痔,鼠瘘恶疮,头疡。

　　蛇含草始出益州山谷,今处处有之,生土石上或下湿地,蜀中人家亦种之辟蛇。一茎五叶或七叶。有两种,细叶者,名蛇含,一名紫背龙牙。大叶者,名龙含。含,一作衔。含、衔二字义同通用。陶隐君曰:当用细叶、有黄花者。李时珍曰:龙含亦入疮膏用。抱朴子曰:蛇含膏连已断之指。

蛇含草始出西川,气味苦寒,花开黄色。西川,金也。苦寒,水也。黄色,土也。禀土金水之气化,金能制风,则惊痫之寒热可治也。寒能清热,则邪气之热气可除也。土能生肌,则金疮可治也。禀土金水之气,而和在下之经脉,则治疽痔。禀土金水之气,而和在上之经脉,则治鼠,恶疮,头疡。

251. Shehancao [蛇含草, klein cinquefoil herb with root, Herba Potentillae Kleinianae cum Radice]

It is bitter in taste, slightly cold and non-toxic in property, and it is mainly used to treat fright epilepsy, cold and heat and pathogenic qi, clear heat, and treat the incised wounds, carbuncle, hemorrhoids, scrofula, malign sore and head ulcer.

Firstly recorded to be growing in the mountain valleys of Yizhou (益州), now it grows everywhere, on the ground and stones or marsh land. People in Shuzhong (蜀中) plant it to drive snakes away. One stalk has five or seven leaves. There are two types. The one with thin leaves is called Shehan (蛇含)

and also called Zibei Longya（紫背龙牙）. The other one with big leaves is called Longhan（龙含）. Han（含）can be used as Xian（衔）and these two characters have the same meaning, so they are interchangeable in use. Tao Hongjing（陶弘景）said, "Those with thin leaves and yellow flowers should be used." Li Shizhen（李时珍）said, "Longhan（龙含）can be used as paste dealing with sores." Bao Puzi（抱朴子）said, "The paste made of Shehancao（klein cinquefoil herb with root）can reconnect the broken fingers."

Firstly it was recorded to be growing in the west of Sichuang, bitter in taste, cold in property and with yellow flowers. The west of Sichuang pertains to metal. Bitterness and cold pertain to water. The yellow color pertains to earth. It can treat the cold and heat caused by fright epilepsy, because it receives the qi transformation of earth, metal and water and metal can control wind. It can clear the heat caused by pathogenic qi because cold can clear heat. It can treat the incised wounds because earth can promote granulation. It can treat carbuncle and hemorrhoids because it receives the qi of earth, metal and water and harmonizes with the meridians of the lower body. It can treat scrofula, malign sore and head ulcer, because it receives the qi of earth, metal and water and harmonizes with the meridians of the upper body.

252. 狼毒根

狼毒根　气味辛平,有大毒。主治咳逆上气,破积聚,饮食寒热,水气,恶疮,鼠瘘疽蚀,鬼精蛊毒,杀飞鸟走兽。

狼毒始出陇西秦亭山谷及奉高、太山诸处,今陕西州郡及辽石州亦有之。叶似商陆,茎叶上有毛,其根皮色黄,肉色白,以实重者为良,轻浮者为劣。陶隐居曰:宕昌亦出之,乃言只有数亩地生,蝮蛇食其根,故为难得,今用出汉中及建平云。

狼毒草有大毒,禀火气也。气味辛平,茎叶有毛,入水则沉,禀金气也。禀金气,故主治肺病之咳逆上气。金能攻利,故破积聚。破积聚,则饮食壅滞而为寒为热之病,亦可治矣。水气,水寒之气也。水气而濡,则有恶疮、鼠瘘、疽蚀,并鬼精蛊毒之病。狼毒禀火气而温脏寒,故皆治之。又言其毒能杀飞鸟走兽,草以狼名,殆以此故。李时珍曰:观其名,则知其毒矣。

252. Langdugen〔狼毒根, Chinese stellera root, fischer euphorbia root, Radix Stellerae Chamaejasmis seu Euphorbiae Fischerianae〕

It is pungent in taste, mild and severely toxic in property, and it is mainly used to treat the cough with dyspnea, descend adverse-rising qi, break accumulation-gathering, treat the cold and heat due to the improper diet, edema, malign sore, scrofula, and abscess erosion, remove ghost and the parasitic toxins and kill birds and animals.

Firstly recorded to be growing in the mountain valleys of Qingting (秦亭) in Longxi (陇西) and in Fenggao (奉高) and Taishan Mountain (太山), now it also grows in the areas of Shaanxi (陕西) and Liaoshi (辽石). Its leaves are similar to those of Shanglu〔商陆, phytolacca, Radix Phytollaccae〕and there is hair on its stems and leaves. Its root-skin is yellow, and its flesh is white. Those with heavy fruits are good, while those with light fruits are worse. Tao Hongjing (陶弘景) said, " It also grows in Dangchang (宕昌). It is said that it only grows on several Mu of land there and its roots are usually eaten by snakes, so it is hard to get. Now those growing in Hanzhong (汉中) and Jianping (建平) are used. "

Severely toxic, it receives fire qi. Pungent in taste and mild in property, with leaves and stems having hair, it sinks in water and receives metal qi. It can mainly treat the cough with dyspnea and descend adverse-rising qi, because it receives metal qi. Metal can purge diarrhea, so it can break accumulation-gathering. Accordingly it can treat the cold and heat due to the food stagnation. Edema refers to water-cold qi. The moistening of edema causes malign sore, scrofula, abscess erosion and ghost and the parasitic toxins. It can treat all of them because it receives fire qi and warms the cold of zang. It is named after the wolf, so it is also said that it can kill birds and animals. Li Shizhen (李时珍) said, " Its toxic property can be deduced based on its name. "

253. 狼牙根

狼牙根 气味苦寒,有毒。主治邪气热气,疥瘙恶疡,疮痔,去白虫。

狼牙《本经》名牙子,《别录》名狼齿,《吴普本草》名犬牙,又名抱牙。始出淮南川谷及冤句,今江东州郡所在有之,其根黑色,若兽之齿牙,故有诸名。

狼性灵知,此草根如兽之齿牙,而专以野狼名者,疑取其上下灵通之义,寒水之气上行,则能散在表之邪气热气,以及皮肤之疥瘙恶疡。苦寒之气下泄,则能除在下之疮痔,以及在内之白虫。《金匮要略》曰:少阴脉滑而数者,阴中即生疮,阴中蚀疮烂者,狼牙汤洗之。此草气味苦寒,禀性纯阴,故能治少阳之火热疮烂也。

253. Langyagen〔狼牙根，rose root，Radix Indigofera pseudotinctoria〕

It is bitter in taste, cold and toxic in property, and it is mainly used to treat pathogenic qi and heat qi, scabies, pruritus, severe sore and hemorrhoids and kill tapeworms.

It is called Yazi（牙子）in *Shen Nong Ben Cao Jing*〔《神农本草经》, *Shennong's Classic of Materia Medica*〕, Langchi（狼齿）in *Ming Yi Bie Lu*〔《名医别录》, *Miscellaneous Records of Famous Physicians*〕, Quanya（犬牙）or Baoya（抱牙）in *Wu Pu Ben Cao*〔《吴普本草》, *Wu Pu's Studies of Materia Medica*〕. Firstly recorded to be growing in the mountain valleys of Huainan（淮南）and Yuanju（冤句）, now it grows in the areas of Jiangdong（江东）. Its root is black and similar to the animal's tooth, thus getting its name.

The wolf is intelligent in nature. Its root looks like the animal's tooth, named in particular after the wolf probably to denote the meaning of being connected spiritually both up and down. The upward movement of the qi of the cold water can dispel external pathogenic qi and heat qi and treat scabies, pruritus, the severe sore of the skin. The downward discharging of the qi of the bitter cold can eliminate the hemorrhoids of the lower body and kill the tapeworms in the body. *Jin Gui Yao Lue*〔《金匮要略》, *Synopsis of Golden Chamber*〕says, "Those who have the slippery and rapid pulse of lesser yin often get the sores in the vulva. Langyagen（rose root）can be used to wash the ulcerated eroding sores in the vulva. It is bitter in taste, cold in property and pure yin in nature, so it can treat the fire-heat sore ulceration of lesser yang."

254. 羊蹄根

羊蹄根 气味苦寒,无毒。主治头秃疥瘙,除热,女子阴蚀。

羊蹄一名牛舌草,一名秃菜。羊蹄以根名,牛舌以叶名,秃菜以治秃疮名也。所在有之,近水及下湿地极多,秋深则生,凌冬不死,春发苗,高三四尺,叶大者长尺余,如牛舌之形,入夏起台,开青白花,花叶一色,成穗结子,夏至即枯,根长近尺,赤黄色如大黄胡萝卜之形,故一名羊蹄大黄,俗人谓之土大黄。子名金荞麦。烧炼家用以制铅汞。

羊蹄,水草也,生于川川泽及近水湿地。感秋气而生,经冬不凋,至夏而死,盖禀金水之精气所生。金能制风,故治头秃疥瘙。水能清热,故除热。苦能生肌,故治阴蚀。

254. Yangtigen〔羊蹄根,root of Japanese dock,Radix Rumicis〕

It is bitter in taste, cold and non-toxic in property, and it is mainly used to treat the bald scalp sore, scabies and pruritus, clear heat and treat the vulva ulcer.

The Japanese dock is also called Niushecao (牛舌草) and Tucai (秃菜). It is named Yangti (羊蹄) for its root, Niushe (牛舌) for its leaf and Tucai (秃菜) for its effect in treating the bald scalp sore. It grows in lots of places mostly by the water and in marsh land. It begins to grow in late autumn, survives winter and sprouts in spring. It is three or four Chi high, and the bigger leaves are more than one Chi in size just like the shape of beef tongue. It begins to blossom blue-white flower in summer with the same color as its leaves. It has ears, bears seeds and withers as soon as the Summer Solstice day comes. Its root is one Chi high in red-yellow color which looks like the big yellow carrot. So it is also called Yangti Dahuang (羊蹄大黄), also popularly known as Tudahuang (土大黄). Its seed is called Jinqiaomai (金荞麦). Alchemists use it to make lead and mercury.

The Japanese dock is a kind of water weed, growing in the mountain, swamp and marsh land near the water. It grows sensing autumn qi, survives winter without withering and doesn't die until the Summer Solstice Day. It is generated by the essence qi of metal and water. It can treat the bald scalp sore, scabies and pruritus, because metal can control wind. It can clear heat because water can clear heat. It can treat the vulva ulcer because bitterness can promote granulation.

255. 羊踯躅花

羊踯躅花　气味辛温,有大毒。主治贼风在皮肤中淫淫痛,温疟,恶毒,诸痹。

羊踯躅近道诸山皆有之,茎高三四尺,叶似桃叶,夏开花五出,蕊瓣皆黄色,羊食其花叶,即踯躅而死,故又名闹羊花。

羊踯躅花色黄,气味辛温,禀火土金相生之化。羊乃火畜而兼土金,南方赤色,其畜羊,火也。在辰为未,土也。在卦为兑,金也。此花大毒,亦禀火土金之化,羊食之,则同气相感而受其毒,是以踯躅而死。金主皮毛,土主肤肉,火主血脉,主治贼风在皮肤中淫淫痛,治金主之皮毛,土主之肤肉,乃以毒而攻毒也。疟邪随经内薄,治温疟恶毒,治火主之经脉也。诸痹乃皮脉肉之痹,而踯躅亦治之也。

按:闹羊花羊食之则死,缘此花有毒故也,谓同气相感而受毒,此说似属蛇足,不必参究至此。李时珍曰:此物有大毒,曾有人以其根入酒饮,遂至于毙。《和剂局方》治中风瘫痪,伏虎丹中亦用之,不多服耳。

255. Yangzhizhu Hua［羊踯躅花, flower of yellow azalea, Rhododendri Mollis Flos］

It is pungent in taste, warm and severely toxic in property, and it is mainly used to treat the wandering pain caused by the invasion of abnormal weather into the skin, warm malaria, severe toxin and various impediments.

It grows in the mountains nearby with the stems in the height of three or four Chi and leaves similar to the peach leaves. It blossoms in five petals, and its petal and pistil are both yellow. Once the goat takes its flowers and leaves, it will walk to and fro and die. So it is also called Naoyanghua (闹羊花).

Yellow in color, pungent in taste and warm in property, it receives the transformation of mutual generation among fire, earth and metal. The goat is the animal correspondent to fire and pertains to earth and metal. Those growing in the south of redness represent fire. In terms of the time, it refers to the period of the day from 1 pm to 3 pm which pertains to earth. In terms of the divinatory symbols, it refers to Dui (兑) which pertains to metal. Its flower has severe toxin and also receives the transformation of fire, earth and metal. So when the goat takes it, it will walk to and fro and die because the goat will be harmed by the similarity with it. Metal governs the skin and hair, earth governs the skin and flesh, fire governs the blood and meridian. It can mainly treat the wandering pain caused by the invasion of abnormal weather into the skin, because it can treat the skin and hair governed by metal and the skin and flesh governed by earth through the method of attacking toxin with toxin. The malarial pathogen becomes weaker in meridian. It can treat warm malaria and severe toxin because it can treat the meridian governed by fire. Various impediments refer to the impediments of the skin, meridian and flesh, which can also be treated by it.

Note by Gao Shishi (高世栻): The reason why the goat will die after eating it is that its flowers have toxin. The statement that the goat is harmed by the interaction with it because they have the same qi is just like adding something superfluous and useless, so there is no need to think about it deeply. Li Shizhen (李时珍) said, "It is severely toxic. Once a person takes the mixture of its root and liquor, he will die. It is used to treat stroke and paralysis in *He Ji Ju Fang* [《和剂局方》, *Formulary of the Bureau of Pharmacy*] and also used in Fuhudan (伏虎丹). However, it should not be taken too much."

256. 瓜 蒂

瓜蒂 气味苦寒,有毒,主治大水,身面四肢浮肿,下水,杀蛊毒,咳逆上气,及食诸果,病在胸腹中,皆吐下之。

蒂今作蒂,反蒂一名苦丁香,乃甜瓜蒂也。《别录》云:瓜蒂生蒿高平泽,七月七日采,阴干。今则甜瓜一种,北土中州处处皆莳植矣。三月下种,延蔓而生叶,大数寸,五六月开黄花,六七月瓜熟,其类最繁,有圆有长,有尖有扁,大或径尺,小或一捻,或有棱,或无棱,或色或青、或绿、或黄斑、或糁斑、或白路、或黄路,其瓤或白或红,其子或黄或赤,或白或黑。《王祯农书》云:瓜品甚多,不可枚举,以状得名者,有龙肝、虎掌、兔头、狸首、羊髓、蜜筒之称。以色得名者,有乌瓜、白团、黄觚、白觚、小青、大斑之别。然其味不出乎香甜而已,雷敩曰:凡使勿用白瓜蒂,要取青绿色,瓜气足时,其蒂自然落在蔓上者,采得系屋东有风处吹干用。

今浙中之香瓜即甜瓜也。诸瓜之中唯此瓜最甜,故名甜瓜。亦唯此瓜有香,故谓之香瓜,余瓜不尔也。今人治黄疸初起,取其蒂烧灰存性,用少许吸鼻中,流出黄水而愈,极验。

甜瓜生于嵩高平泽,味甘,臭香,色黄。盖禀天地中央之正气,其瓜极甜,其蒂极苦,合火土相生之气化,故主治大水,及身面四肢浮肿。所以然者,禀火土之气,达于四旁,而能制化其水湿,故又曰:下水。土气运行,故杀蛊毒。苦主下泄,故治咳逆上气。苦能上涌,又主下泄,故食诸果病在胸腹中者,皆可吐下之也。

愚按:苦为阴,甘为阳,此系蔓草,性唯上延,以极苦之蒂,生极甜之瓜,直从下而上,从阴而阳,故《伤寒》《金匮》方作为吐剂。

256. Guadi [瓜蒂, fruit pedicel of muskmelon, Pedicellus Melo Fructus]

It is bitter in taste, cold and toxic in property, and it is mainly used to treat the dropsy of the body, face and four limbs caused by severe edema, promote urination, kill the parasitic toxin and treat the cough with dyspnea, descend adverse-rising qi and treat the disease in the chest and abdomen caused by eating various fruits and help vomit and defecate them.

The Chinese character "蔕" (Di) nowadays is replaced by "蒂" (Di). Guadi (fruit pedicel of muskmelon) is also called Kudingxiang (苦丁香) which refers to the pedicel of muskmelon. *Ming Yi Bie Lu* [《名医别录》, *Miscellaneous Records of Famous Physicians*] says it grows in the lakes and swamps of Songgao (嵩高) and can be collected on the seventh of the seventh lunar month and dried in the shade. Now it is one kind of muskmelon and grows everywhere in Beitu (北土) and Zhongzhou (中州) during the favorable season. It is planted in the third lunar month, and spreads vines and grows leaves which are several Cun in size. It blossoms in yellow color in the fifth or sixth lunar month and bears fruits in the sixth or seventh lunar month. The muskmelon has the most various types: In terms of shape, it can be round, long, pointed or flat; in terms of size, it can be as big as one Chi in diameter or as small as a grain. In terms of its appearance, it can be ridged or not ridged; in terms of color, it can be of mixed colors, blue, green, with yellow spots or grits, or with the white pattern or the yellow pattern. Its pulp can be white or red, and its seeds can be yellow, red, white or black. *Wang Zhen Nong Shu* [《王祯农书》, *Agricultural Book of Wangzhen*] says, "There are so many types that they can not be listed all. Based on the shape, it can be called Longgan (龙肝), Huzhang (虎掌), Tutou (兔头), Lishou (狸首), Yangsui (羊髓) and Mitong (蜜筒); based on the color, it can be calld Wugua (乌瓜), Baituan (白团), Huangpian (黄觚), Baipian (白觚), Xiaoqing (小青) and Daban (大斑)." However, all of them have the fragrant and sweet flavor. Lei Xue (雷敩) said, "The white ones should not be used. People should take the blue-green ones whose pedicel falls down on the vines naturally when it is ripe and hang it in the windy place east of the house to dry it."

Nowadays those growing in the middle of Zhejiang (浙江) are muskmelons which are the sweetest among all of the melons, so it is called Tiangua (甜瓜). It is the only one that has fragrance so it is called Xianggua (香瓜). Now people use it to treat jaundice at early stage by burning its pedicel into ashes to preserve its property and sniffing it a little into the nostril. If the yellow water flows out, this disease will be cured for sure. It is very effective.

It grows in lakes and swamps of Songgao (嵩高), sweet in taste, fragrant in smell and yellow in color. It receives the central healthy qi of the heaven and the earth; the melon itself is very sweet but its pedicel is severely bitter. Since it combines the qi transformation of mutual generation between fire and earth, it mainly treats the dropsy of the body and face and four limbs caused by severe edema. It has this effect for it receives the qi of fire and earth and reaches the four limbs, so it can control and transform their dampness. Thus, it can also promote urination. Since earth qi moves around, it can kill parasitic toxin. Bitterness governs discharging, so it can treat the cough with dyspnea and descend adverse-rising qi. Bitterness can upwell and governs discharging, so it can treat the disease in the chest and abdomen caused by eating various fruits and help vomit and defecate them.

Note by Zhang Zhicong（张志聪）：Bitterness is yin, while sweetness is yang. It is trailing grass and its nature is trailing upward. Its severely bitter pedicel bears the extremely sweet melon which goes up from the bottom and changes from yin to yang, so it is used as an emetic formula in *Shang Han Lun*〔《伤寒论》, *Treatise on Cold Pathogenic Diseases*〕and *Jin Gui Yao Lue*〔《金匮要略》, *Synopsis of Golden Chamber*〕.

257．莨菪子

莨菪子 气味苦寒,有毒。主治齿痛出虫,肉痹拘急。久服轻身,使人健行,走及奔马,强志益力,通神见鬼,多食令人狂走。莨,莨浪。菪,音荡。

莨菪子一名天仙子。《别录》曰:生海滨川谷及雍州,今所在皆有之。叶似菘蓝,茎叶皆有细白毛,四月开花紫色,或白色,五月结实有壳,作罂子,状如小石榴,房中子至细,青白色,如粟米粒。

莨菪子气味苦寒,生于海滨,得太阳寒水之气,故治齿痛。太阳上禀寒气,下有标阳,阳能散阴,故能出虫。太阳阳热之气,能温肌腠。又,太阳主筋所生病,故治肉痹拘急。肉痹,肌痹也。拘急,筋不柔和也。久服轻身,使人健行,走及奔马者,太阳本寒标热,少阴本热标寒,太阳合少阴而助跷脉也。盖阳跷者,足太阳之别,起于跟中,出于外踝。阴跷者,足少阴之别,起于跟中,循于内踝。莨菪子禀太阳少阴标本之精,而助跷脉,故轻身健走若是也。禀阴精之气,故强志益力。禀阳热之化,故通神见鬼。下品之药,不宜久服,故又曰:多食令人狂走,戒之也。

257. Langdangzi〔莨菪子, seed of black henbane, Semen Hyoscyami Nigri〕

It is bitter in taste, cold and toxic in property, and it is mainly used to treat the toothache with worms and the muscle impediment with spasm. Long-term taking of it will keep people healthy and make them walk forcefully and as quickly as a galloping horse, strengthen memory, increase the physical strength, enable people to connect with immortals and see ghosts. Excessive taking of it will make people run about wildly. Lang(莨) is pronounced as Lang（浪）; Dang（菪）is pronounced as Dang(荡).

It is also called Tianxianzi（天仙子）. *Ming Yi Bie Lu*［《名医别录》, *Miscellaneous Records of Famous Physicians*］says，"It grew in seashore, valleys and Yongzhou（雍州），and it is everywhere nowadays." Its leaves look like Songlan（菘蓝）and have thin and white hair just like its stems. It blossoms in purple or white color in the fourth lunar month and bears fruits with shells in the fifth lunar month which are used as Yingzi（罌子）with the same shape as the little pomegranate. The seeds in the ovary are very thin and in the color of blue and white, which is just like the grain of Sumi［粟米, millet, Setariae Semen］.

Bitter in taste and cold in property, it grows in seashore and receives the qi of cold water from greater yang, so it can treat toothache. The greater yang receives cold qi upward and has the branch yang downward, and yang can dispel yin, so it can eliminate worms. The yang heat qi of greater yang can warm the interstices of the flesh and greater yang can mainly treat the disease of sinews, so it can treat the muscle impediment with spasm. Muscle impediment refers to the impediment of the flesh. Spasm refers to the inflexibility of sinews. Long-term taking of it will keep people healthy and make them walk forcefully and as quickly as a galloping horse, because the root of greater yang is cold and the branch of it is heat, while the root of lesser yin is heat and the branch of it is cold. The harmony of greater yang and lesser yin assists the springing vessel. The yang springing vessel is different from foot greater yang, which starts from the middle of the foot and comes out of the external ankle. The yin springing vessel is different from foot greater yin, which starts from the middle of the foot and circulates within the internal ankle. It keeps people healthy and makes them walk forcefully and as quickly as a galloping horse because it receives the essence of the root and branch of greater yang and lesser yin to assist the springing vessel. It strengthens memory and increases the physical health because it receives the qi of the yin essence. It enables people to connect with immortals and see ghosts because it receives the transformation from the yang heat. As a medicinal, it is of lower grade, so taking it for a long time is not suitable. Therefore, it is said that excessive taking of it will make people run about wildly, which should be avoided.

258. 夏枯草

夏枯草　气味苦辛寒,无毒。主治寒热,瘰疬鼠瘘,颈疮,破症瘕瘿结气,脚肿,湿痹,轻身。颈,旧作头,讹,今改正。

　　夏枯草《本经》名夕句,又名乃东,处处原野平泽间甚多,冬至后生苗,叶对节生,似旋复花叶,而有细齿,背白,苗高一二尺许,其茎微方,三四月茎端作穗,长一二寸,开花淡紫色,似丹参花,结子每一萼中有细子四粒,夏至后即枯。

夏枯草禀金水之气,故气味苦辛寒,无毒。主治寒热,瘰疬鼠瘘,颈疮者,禀水气而上清其火热也。破症瘕瘿结气者,禀金气而内削其坚积也。脚肿乃水气不行于上,湿痹乃水气不布于外。夏枯草感一阳而生,能使水气上行环转,故治脚气湿痹,而且轻身。

258. Xiakucao [夏枯草, common selfheal spike, Spica Prunellae]

It is bitter and pungent in taste, cold and non-toxic in property, and it is mainly used to treat cold and heat, scrofula and neck sore, break abdominal mass, disperse the goiter caused by the stagnation of qi, resolve the swelling of feet and dampness impediment and keep people healthy. In the past, it was written as head instead of neck, which is wrong.

It is also called Xiju (夕句) and Naidong (乃东) in *Shen Nong Ben Cao Jing* [《神农本草经》, *Shennong's Classic of Materia Medica*], mostly growing in lakes and swamps. It sprouts after the Winter Solstice Day. Its leaves grow opposite to each other from the same position on the stem, similar to the leaves of Xuanfuhua [旋复花, Inula flower, Flos Inula Japonica]. It has thin saw teeth, and its back is white. Its seedling is one or two Chi high and its stem is a little square. It bears ears on the top of the stem in the third or fourth lunar month, which is in the length of one or two Cun. It blossoms with the colour of pale purple, like the flower of Danshen [丹参, salvia, Salviae Miltiorrhizae Radix]. Its fruits have four thin seeds in each calyx. It withers after the Summer Solstice Day.

It receives the qi of metal and water, so it is bitter and pungent in taste, cold and non-toxic in property. It can mainly treat cold and heat, scrofula, and head sore because it receives water qi to go upward and clear fire heat. It breaks abdominal mass and disperses the goiter caused by the stagnation of qi because it receives metal qi to whittle the internal hardness and accumulation. The swelling of feet is caused by the inability of water qi to move upward while dampness impediment is caused by the inability of water qi to evaporate out. Since it grows under the influence of one yang and is able to make water qi go upward and circulate, it can resolve the swelling of feet and dampness impediment, and keep people healthy.

259. 蚤 休

蚤休　气味苦,微寒,有毒。主治惊痫,摇头弄舌,热气在腹中。

　　蚤休《图经》名紫河车,《唐本草》名重楼、金线,后人名三层草,又名七叶一枝花。处处有之,多生深山阴湿之地。一茎独上,高尺余,茎当叶心,叶绿色似芍药,凡二三层,每一层七叶,茎头于夏月开花,一花七瓣,花黄紫色,蕊赤黄色,长三四寸,上有金线垂下,秋结红子,根似肥姜,皮赤肉白。谚云:七叶一枝花,深山是我家,痈疽如迁者,一似手拈拿。又,道家有服食紫河车根法云:可以休粮。

　　一者水之生数也,七者火之成数也,三者一奇二偶,合而为三也。蚤休三层,一层七叶,一七瓣,禀先天水火之精,故主治惊痫,摇头弄舌。惊痫而摇头弄舌,乃小儿胎惊胎痫也。胎惊胎痫,乃热毒之气得于母腹之中,故曰:热气在腹中。

　　愚按:蚤休一名河车,服食此草,又能辟谷,为修炼元真,胎息长生之药,故主治小儿先天受热之病,学者得此义而推展之,则大人小儿后天之病,亦可治也。

　　按《日华本草》言:紫河车治胎风手足搐,故隐菴解:热气在腹中,谓热毒之气得于母腹之中云云,然即谓摇头弄舌,由小儿内热所致,不必作深一层解亦可。苏恭曰:醋磨傅痈肿蛇毒甚效。

259. Zaoxiu〔蚤休, rhizome of multileaf paris, rhizome of pubescent paris, rhizome of narrowleaf paris, Rhizoma Paridis〕

It is bitter in taste, slightly cold and toxic in property, and it is mainly used to treat fright epilepsy, head shivering and waggling tongue, the heat qi in the abdomen.

It is called Ziheche (紫河车) in *Tu Jing*〔《图经》, *Illustrated Classic of Materia Medica*〕, Chonglou (重楼) and Jinxian (金线) in *Tang Ben Cao*〔《唐本草》, *Tang Materia Medica*〕, and Sancengcao (三层草) and Qiye Yizhihua (七叶一枝花) by people later on. It grows everywhere, especially in shady and damp places of remote mountains. The only stem grows straight upward, which is in the height of one Chi and serves as the center of leaves. The leaves are green similar to Shaoyao〔芍药, peony, Radix Paeoniae〕. It usually has two or three layers with seven leaves in each layer. The top of the stem blossoms in the summer month. One flower has seven petals in the color of yellow-purple. Its pistil is red-yellow in color and three or four Cun in length with the golden filament hanging down from above. It bears red seeds in autumn. Its root looks like a big ginger with the red skin and the white flesh. The old saying goes that Qiye Yizhihua (七叶一枝花), growing in the remote mountains, has the striking effect in treating abscess and carbuncle. Those daoists taking the roots of Ziheche (紫河车) said, "It can help them to practise inedia."

One is the number generated by water, seven is the number generated by fire, and three is the number formed by adding the odd number "one" to the even number "two". Zaoxiu (rhizome of multileaf paris, rhizome of pubescent paris, rhizome of narrowleaf paris) has three layers, one layer has seven leaves and one flower has seven petals. It receives the innate essence of water and fire, so it can mainly treat the fright epilepsy with the head shivering and the waggling tongue. Here, fright epilepsy refers to the fetal fright and the fetal epilepsy of children, which is caused by the heat and toxic qi in the mother's abdomen. So it is said that it can the treat heat qi in the abdomen.

Note by Zhang Zhicong（张志聪）：It is called Heche（河车）. Taking it can help people practise the inedia which is the medicinal that can cultivate primordial qi, calm fetus and promote growth. So it can mainly treat the child innate disease caused by heat qi. Doctors get to know this and expand its use to treat the acquired diseases of adults and children after birth.

According to *Ri Hua Ben Cao*［《日华本草》, *Rihuazi's Materia Medica*］, it treats fetal wind and the convulsion of the extremities. So Yin An（隐菴）explained，"The heat qi in the abdomen means the heat and toxic qi is obtained from the mother's abdomen." However, the head shivering and the waggling tongue are caused by the internal heat. So there is no need to explain further. Su Gong（苏恭）said，"Grind and mix it with vinegar, and apply the mixture externally to abscess, swelling and the snake venom. It is very effective in treating these diseases."

260. 白芨根

白芨根 气味苦平,无毒。主治痈肿,恶疮败疽,伤阴死肌,胃中邪气,贼风鬼去,痱缓不收。

白芨近道处处有之,春生苗,叶如生姜、藜芦,三四月抽出一台,开花红紫色,长寸许,中心吐舌,宛若草兰,今浙人谓之箬兰。花后结实,七月中熟,黄黑色,根似菱,黄白色,有三角节,间有毛,可为末作糊,性稠粘难脱。白芨气味苦平,花红根白,得阳明少阴之气化。少阴主藏精,而精汁生于阳明,故主治痈肿疽疮,贼风痱缓诸证。

260. Baijigen［白芨根, bletilla root, Rhizoma Bletillae Radix］

It is bitter in taste, mild and non-toxic in property, and it is mainly used to treat abscess and swelling, severe sore, the carbuncle necrotic muscles caused by the damage to yin, the pathogenic qi in the stomach, the abnormal weather, the ghost attack, and the sequelae difficult to resolve.

It grows everywhere nearby and sprouts in spring. Its leaves are just like those of Shengjiang［生姜, rhizome of common ginger, Rhizoma Zingiberis

Recens] and Lilu [藜芦, root and rhizome of black falsehellebore, Radix et Rhizoma Veratri], growing in the third and fourth lunar months. It blossoms in red-purple color. Its flower, about one Cun long with a bud in the center, is just like that of Liancao (兰草), which is called Ruolan (箬兰) by the people in Zhejiang (浙江) nowadays. It yields fruits after the flower phase in the seventh lunar month, which get ripe in the middle of the seventh lunar month and are yellow-black in color. Its yellow-white roots are like those of water chestnut, having three branches and hair among them. It can be ground into paste, which is sticky.

Bitter in taste and mild in property, its flower being red and its root being white, Baiji [白芨, bletilla, Rhizoma Bletillae] receives the qi transformation of yang brightness and lesser yin. It can mainly treat abscess and swelling, the severe sore, the abnormal weather and sequelae, because lesser yin mainly stores the essence sap while essence comes from yang brightness.

261. 白敛根

白敛根 气味苦平,无毒。主治痈肿疽疮,散结气,止痛除热,目中赤,小儿惊痫,温疟,女子阴中肿痛,带下赤白。

白敛《本经》名白草,近道处处有之,二月生苗,多在林中,蔓延赤茎,叶如小桑,五月开花,七月结实,根如鸡鸭卵而长,三五枚同一窠,皮黑肉白。一种赤敛,皮肉皆赤,而花实功用相同。

敛者,取秋金收敛之义,古时用此药敷敛痈毒,命名盖以此。有赤白二种,赋禀与白芨相同,故主治不甚差别。白芨得阳明少阴之精汁,收藏于下,是以作糊稠粘。白敛乃蔓草,性唯上延,而津液濡上,故兼除热清目,小儿惊痫,及女子阴中肿痛,带下赤白。又,治温疟者,主清下焦之热,其性从下而上也。

261. Bailiangen [白敛根, ampelopsis, Radix Ampelopsis]

It is bitter in taste, mild and non-toxic in property, and it is mainly used to treat abscess, swelling, carbuncle and sore, disperse qi stagnation, relieve pain, clear heat, and treat the red eye, infantile fright epilepsy, warm malaria, the vulva swelling and pain and the leukorrhagia in red and white color.

It is called Baicao（白草）in *Shen Nong Ben Cao Jing*［《神农本草经》, *Shennong's Classic of Materia Medica*］and grows everywhere nearby. It sprouts in the second lunar month and grows mostly in the woods with red stems spreading on the ground. Its leaves are like mulberry leaves. It blossoms in the fifth lunar month and bears fruits in the seventh lunar month. Its root is of the same length as the eggs of chicken and duck and three or five roots stay together with the black skin and the white flesh. There is another kind of it called Chilian（赤敛）, which has the red skin and flesh. But its flowers and fruits have the same effects as those of Bailian（白敛）.

Lian（敛）has the meaning of astringing of the autumn metal. In ancient times, it was applied externally to heal up the abscess toxin, so it got this name. It has two kinds: one is red and the other is white, which have the same properties as those of Baiji［白芨, bletilla, Rhizoma Bletillae］. So they have the similar use in treating diseases. The latter one receives the essence sap of yang brightness and lesser yin and stores it at the bottom, so it is suitable to make the sticky paste while the former one, a kind of trailing grass, has the nature of going upward and makes its fluids moisten upward, so it also can clear heat, improve vision, and treat infantile fright epilepsy, the vulva swelling and pain and leukorrhagia in red and white color. It can treat warm malaria because it has the nature of going upward from the downward and can clear the heat of the lower energizer.

262. 鬼 臼

鬼臼 气味辛温,有毒。主治杀虫毒,鬼疰精物,辟恶气,不祥,逐邪,解百毒。

鬼臼《本经》名九臼,《别录》名天臼。出九真山谷及冤句、荆州、峡州、襄州,近以钱塘余杭径山者为上,生深山岩石之阴。其叶六出或五出,如雁掌,茎端一叶如伞,且对东向,暮则西倾,盖随日出没也。花红紫如荔枝正在叶下,常为叶所蔽,未常见日,故俗名羞天花。一年生一茎,茎枯则作一臼,新根次年另生,则旧根中腐,新陈相易,九年乃作九臼,九臼者有神,根形如苍术及黄精之岐曲,以连生白窍为别也,臼形如马眼,故《本经》又名马眼。

鬼臼以九臼者为良,故名九臼。九,老阳之数也。阳者,天气也。故《别录》名天臼,气味辛温,禀太阳阳热乾金之气,故主杀虫毒鬼痊精物,及恶气不祥,并逐邪解百毒。《金匮》方治伤寒,令愈不复者,助太阳之气也。盖阳气者,若天与日,此花随天日旋转,而又不见天日,犹天德唯藏,不自明也。

262. Guijiu〔鬼臼, common dysosma, Rhizoma Dysosmae Versipellis〕

It is pungent in taste, warm and toxic in property, and it is mainly used to treat the worm toxin, Guizhu〔鬼痊, multiple infixation abscess〕and the strange pathogenic factors, dispel malign and non-auspicious qi and pathogens and resolve various toxins.

It is called Jiujiu(九臼)in *Shen Nong Ben Cao Jing*〔《神农本草经》, *Shennong's Classic of Materia Medica*〕and Tianjiu(天臼)in *Ming Yi Bie Lu*〔《名医别录》, *Miscellaneous Records of Famous Physicians*〕. It grows in the mountain valleys of Jiuzhen(九真)and in Yuanju(冤句), Jingzhou(荆州), Xiazhou(峡州)and Xiangzhou(襄州). Nowadays those on Jing Mountain in Yuhang(余杭), Qiantang(钱塘)are of better quality, growing in the shade of the remote mountain rocks. It has five or six leaves like the palms of wild goose. The leaf on the top of the stem is just like an umbrella facing east at dawn and leaning west at twilight, which changes the directions with the rising and setting of the sun. Its flowers are red-purple similar to the color of lychee, which grows under the leaves. Since they are usually in the shade of leaves without seeing the sunlight very often, they are popularly called Xiutianhua(羞天花). It yields one stem annually. When the stem withers, it becomes a mortar. Its new root will sprout next year and the old root will get rotten inside. The new root will become the old one next year, which repeats year after year. Thus in nine years, there will be nine mortars. Those with nine mortars have spirit. Its root is in the shape of the winding form of Cangshu(苍术)and Huangjing(黄精)with the difference of successive generation of mortars. Because the mortars look like the horse eyes, it is also called Mayan(马眼)in *Shen Nong Ben Cao Jing*〔《神农本草经》, *Shennong's Classic of Materia Medica*〕.

Those with nine mortars are of good quality, so it is called Jiujiu（九臼）. Nine is the number of Laoyang while yang is heaven qi, so it is called Tianjiu（天臼）in *Ming Yi Bie Lu* [《名医别录》, *Miscellaneous Records of Famous Physicians*]. It can mainly treat the worm toxin, multiple infixation abscess and the strange pathogenic factors, dispel malign and non-auspicious qi and pathogens and resolve various toxins because it has the pungent taste, the warm property and receives the fry metal qi of greater yang and the yang heat. Those assisting qi of greater yang are used in the formula in *Jin Gui Yao Lue* [《金匮要略》, *Synopsis of Golden Chamber*] to treat the cold damage and cure it without recurrence. Yang qi is just like the heaven and the sun. Its flowers revolve according to the heaven and the sun but they are sheltered from the sunlight, just as the heaven is characterized by storing, which doesn't become bright by itself but is illuminated by the sun.

263. 梓白皮

梓白皮 气味苦寒,无毒。主治热毒,去三虫。

梓为木中之王,其花色紫,其荚如箸,长近尺,冬后叶落而荚犹在树。李时珍曰:梓木处处有之,有三种,木理白者为梓,赤者为楸、梓之美纹者为椅,楸之小者为榎。

梓楸同类,梓,从辛,楸,从秋,禀金气也。气味苦寒,禀水气也。禀水气,故主治热毒。禀金气,故主杀三虫。阳明篇云:伤寒瘀热在裹,身必发黄,麻黄连轺赤小豆汤主之,内用梓白皮,义可知矣。

263. Zibaipi [梓白皮, root-bark of ovate catalpa, Cortex Catalpae Ovatae Radicis]

It is bitter in taste, cold and non-toxic in property, and it is mainly used to treat heat toxin and eliminate three worms.

Zi [梓, ovate catalpa, Catalpae Ovatae Radicis] is the king of trees. Its flowers are purple in color, and its pods are like chopsticks, with nearly one Chi in length. After winter, its leaves fall while its pods still stay on the tree. Li Shizhen（李时珍）said, "It grows everywhere and has three types. Those with the white texture are called Zi（梓）, and those with the red texture are called Qiu（楸）. Zi（梓）with the beautiful texture is called Yi（椅）and Qiu（楸）of the small size is called Jia（榎）."

Zi（梓）and Qiu（楸）belong to the same category. Zi（梓）is characterized by the pungent taste and Qiu（楸）is characterized by the season of autumn, both of which receive metal qi. Bitter in taste and cold in property, it receives water qi. So it can mainly treat the heat toxin. It receives metal qi, so it can eliminate three worms. *Yang Ming Pian*〔《阳明篇》, *On Yangming*〕says, "Ephedra, Forsythia, and Rice Bean Decoction is mainly used to treat the cold damage in which the stagnated heat in the interior causes the body to turn yellow. Zibaipi（root-bark of ovate catalpa）is used in this decoction, which should be understandable."

264. 柳 花

柳花　气味苦寒,无毒。主治风水、黄疸,面热黑。

　　柳处处有之,有杨有柳,乃一类二种,杨叶圆阔,柳叶细长,杨枝硬而扬起,故曰杨。柳枝弱而垂流,故曰柳。柳有蒲柳、杞柳、柽柳之别,喜生水旁,纵横倒顺,插之皆生。春初生柔荑,即开黄蕊花,是为柳花,至春晚花中结细黑子,蕊落而絮出如白绒,因风飞舞,着于衣物能生虫蛀,入池沼即为浮萍。是为柳絮,盖黄蕊未结子时,为花结于蕊落,即为絮矣。古者春取榆柳之火。《开宝本草》有柽柳一日三起三眠,又名三眠柳。《尔雅》名河柳,即今儿医治痘疹,所谓西河柳是也,乃寒凉通利,下行小便之药,用者以意会之。

柳性柔顺,喜生水旁,受寒水之精,感春生之气,故纵横顺逆,插之皆生。得春气,则能助肝木以平土,故主治风水,黄疸。得水精,则能清热气而资面颜,故治面热黑。

264. Liuhua〔柳花, **flower of babylon weeping willow**, **Flos Salicis Babylonicae**〕

It is bitter in taste, cold and non-toxic in property, and it is mainly used to treat wind edema, jaundice and the black face as if being scorched.

The willow grows everywhere. The poplar and the willow are two species of one genus. The leaves of the poplar are round and broad while those of the willow are thin and long. The twigs of the poplar are hard and go upward, so it is called "poplar" while those of the willow are soft and go downward, so it is called "willow". There are Puliu (蒲柳), Qiliu (杞柳) and Chengliu (柽柳). It prefers to grow by the water and will grow no matter how it is transplanted, vertically, horizontally or upside down. It sprouts at the beginning of spring and then blossoms with the yellow pistil which is Liuhua (flower of babylon weeping willow). It yields thin and black seeds in the flower until the end of the spring. The pistil withers and the white velvet catkins come out which may dance with wind. Once it lands on the clothes, it breeds worms; once it drops into the swamp, it turns into duckweed. The white velvet catkin is Liuxu [柳絮, downy willow seed, Salicis Semen Pilifer]. Those growing before the seeds yielding and after the flower withering are called Xu (絮). The people in ancient times used Yuliu (榆柳) to make fire in spring. According to *Kai Bao Ben Cao* [《开宝本草》, *Kaibao Materia Medica*], Chengliu (柽柳) goes upward and downward three times one day, so it is also called Sanmianliu (三眠柳). In *Er Ya* [《尔雅》, *On Elegance*], it is called Heliu (河柳), which is called Xiheliu (西河柳) used by pediatricians to treat measles nowadays. It is the cold medicinal to dredge and disinhibit urination. Users should have a clear idea about its effects and use it cautiously.

It is supple in nature and likes growing near water. It receives the essence of the cold water and senses the qi of the spring growth, so it will grow no matter how it is transplanted, vertically, horizontally or upside down. It can mainly treat water edema and jaundice because it receives spring qi and assists liver wood to calm earth. It can mainly treat the black face as if being scorched because it receives the water essence and clears heat qi to improve the facial skin.

265. 柳　叶 附

柳叶 附　气味苦寒,无毒。主治恶疥痂疮马疥,煎汁洗之,立愈。又疗心腹内血,止痛。马疥,马鞍热气之疮疥也。《别录》附。

265. Liuye［柳叶, willow leaf, Salicis Folium］*supplement*

It is bitter in taste, cold and non-toxic in property, and it is mainly used to treat malign scabies, crusts, sores and horse scabies. These diseases can be cured quickly by being washed with its decoction. It can also treat the bleeding in the heart and abdomen and relieve pain. Horse scabies are caused by the heat of saddles. Supplemented in *Ming Yi Bie Lu*［《名医别录》, *Miscellaneous Records of Famous Physicians*］.

266. 杨柳枝及根白皮 附

杨柳枝及根白皮 附　气味苦寒,无毒。主治痰热淋疾,可为浴汤,洗风肿瘄,煮酒漱齿痛,近今以屋檐插柳,经风日者,煎汤饮,治小便淋浊痛,通利水道。《唐本草》附。

　　李时珍曰:柳枝去风消肿止痛,其嫩枝削为牙杖,涤齿甚妙。琦按:佛教食后嗽口,必嚼杨枝,毗奈耶云:嚼杨枝有五利,一口不臭,二口不苦,三除风,四除热,五除痰阴,是知杨枝去风、消热、除痰阴,止齿痛诸功,大有益于人也。然削为牙杖,久则枯燥,若以生枝削用,当更见效耳。

266. Yangliuzhi ji Genbaipi［杨柳枝及根白皮, David's poplar twig, willow twig and David's poplar root bark, willow root bark, Populi Davidianae Ramus, Salicis Ramulus, Populi Davidianae Radicis Cortex, Salicis Cortex Radicis］*supplement*

It is bitter in taste, cold and non-toxic in property, and it is mainly used to treat phlegm-heat and stranguria. It can be used as bath water to wash swelling and pruritus due to wind. It can be boiled with liquor and used as gargle to relieve toothache. Nowadays the willow most grows next to the roof. Those exposed to wind and sunlight can be decocted to drink, which can treat dribbling, turbid and painful urine and dredge, and promote the water passage. Supplemented in *Tang Ben Cao*［《唐本草》, *Tang Materia Medica*）].

　　Li Shizhen（李时珍）said, "Liuzhi［柳枝, willow twig, Salicis Ramulus］dispells wind, disperses swelling and relieves pain. Its twig can be whittled into toothpicks which are very good for cleansing teeth. " Qi（琦）noted：The buddhists always chew some Yangzhi［杨枝, David's poplar twig, Populi Davidianae Ramus］when gargling after meal. Vinaya stated：There are five benefits in chewing it. Firstly, it can eliminate the fetid mouth odor. Secondly, it can clear bitter taste in mouth. Thirdly, it can expel wind. Fourth, it can clear heat. Fifth, it can eliminate the phlegm yin. According to Vinaya, people know that it has the functions of expelling wind, clearing heat, eliminating the phlegm yin and relieving toothache, which benefits people a lot. Those toothpicks whittled by it will be dry if stored for a long time, so using its fresh twigs will be more effective.

267. 郁李仁

郁李仁 气味酸平,无毒。主治大腹水肿,面目四肢浮肿,利小便水道。

郁李山野处处有之,树高五六尺,花叶枝干并似李子,如小李,生青熟红,味甘酸,可啖,花实俱香,《尔雅》所称棠棣,即是此树。

李乃肝之果,其仁当治脾。郁李花实俱青,其味酸甘,其气芳香,甲已合而化土也。土气化,则大腹水肿,面目四肢浮肿自消,小便水道自利。

267. Yuliren［郁李仁, seed of dwarf flowering cherry, Semen Pruni］

It is sour in taste and mild in property, and it is mainly used to treat the enlarged abdomen with edema, the dropsy of the face, eyes and the four limbs, and disinhibit urination and the water passage.

Yuli［郁李, dwarf flowering cherry, Pruni］grows everywhere in mountains and hills. Its trees are five or six Chi in height, and its leaves, flowers and stems are similar to those of Lizi［李子, plum, Pruni Salicinae Fructus］. Just like the small plums, it is green when fresh and red when ripe. Sweet and sour in taste, it is edible and its flowers and fruits have fragrant aroma. It is also called Tangdi（棠棣）in *Er Ya*［《尔雅》, *On Elegance*］.

The plum is good for the liver, and its seed can benefit the spleen. The flowers and fruits of Yuli（dwarf flowering cherry）are green in color with sweet and sour taste and fragrant aroma. These two factors harmonizing together makes spleen qi transport and transform. Therefore, taking it can treat naturally the enlarged abdomen with edema, the dropsy of the face, eyes and the four limbs, and promote urination and the water passage.

268. 巴 豆

巴豆 气味辛温,有毒。主治伤寒温疟寒热,破症瘕结聚,坚积留饮,痰澼,大腹,荡练五脏六腑,开通闭塞,利水谷道,去恶肉,除鬼毒蛊疰邪物,杀虫鱼。

巴豆出巴郡川谷,今嘉州、眉州、戎州皆有之。木高一二丈,叶似樱桃而厚大,初生青色,后渐黄赤,至十二月叶渐凋,二月复渐生,四月旧叶落尽,新叶齐生,即花发成穗,微黄色,五六月结实作房青色,七八月成熟而黄,类白豆蔻,渐渐自落乃收之,一窠有三子,子仍有壳,用之去壳。戎州出者,壳上有纵纹隐起如线,或一道,或二道,或三道,土人呼为金线巴豆,最为上品。

巴豆生于巴蜀,气味辛温,花实黄赤,大热有毒。其性慓悍,主治伤寒温疟寒热者,辛以散之,从经脉而外出于肌表也。破症瘕结聚,坚积留饮,痰澼,大腹者,温以行之,从中土而下泄于肠胃也。用之合宜,有斩关夺门之功,故荡练五脏六腑,开通闭塞,闭塞开通,则水谷二道自利矣。其性慓悍,故去恶肉。气合阳明,故除鬼毒蛊疰邪物,杀虫鱼。《经》云:两火合并是为阳明。巴豆味极辛,性大温,具两火之性,气合阳明,故其主治如此。

愚按:凡服巴霜,即从胸胁大热,达于四肢,出于皮毛,然后复从肠胃而出。《伤寒论》有白散方,治伤寒寒实结胸用此。古人称为斩关夺门之将,用之若当,真瞑眩瘳疾之药,用之不当,非徒无益而反害矣。

268. Badou [巴豆, croton, Fructus Crotonis]

It is pungent in taste, warm and toxic in property, and it is mainly used to treat cold damage, warm malaria and chills and fever, break abdominal mass, accumulation binding, hypochondriac lump and persistent fluid retention, treat phlegm afflux and enlarged abdomen, scour the five zang-organs and the six fu-organs, open and dredge block and closure, promote urination and defecation, remove the necrotic muscles, eliminate vicious toxin like ghost and the accumulation of worms and the pathogenic factors, and kill worms and fish.

Originally growing in the mountain valleys of Bajun (巴郡), now it grows in Jiazhou (嘉州), Meizhou (眉州) and Rongzhou (戎州). Its stem is one or two Zhang in height, and its leaves are thick and big just like those of the cherry tree. The leaves are green when fresh, then change to yellow-red color, wither in the twelfth lunar month, re-generate in the second lunar month of next year and fall in the fourth lunar month. After that, new leaves grow densely and flowers grow into ears with the color of slightly yellow. It bears green fruits and ovary in the fifth or sixth lunar month which become ripe and yellow in the seventh or eighth lunar month. It is similar to Baidoukou [白豆蔻, cardamom, Amomi Fructus Rotundus], which falls by itself before it is collected. There are three seeds in one pod and there is shuck covering each seed which should be removed when the seeds are used. Those growing in Rongzhou (戎州) have the thread-like vertical grains, and there may be only one grain, or two or three. The local people call it the gold-thread Badou (金线巴豆) which is ranked in the top grade.

Growing in Bashu (巴蜀), it is pungent in taste and warm in property. Its flowers and fruits are yellow-red, severely hot and toxic in property. It mainly treats cold damage, warm malaria and cold and heat, because it has the wild and strong property and its pungent taste can dispel the cold and heat in the collaterals out to the fleshy exterior. It breaks abdominal mass, accumulation binding, hypochondriac lump and persistent fluid retention and treats phlegm afflux and the enlarged abdomen, because its warm property moves in the body and makes the diseases drain from the spleen to the stomach and intestines. Using it properly may have the great effect of discharging. So it can scour the five zang-organs and the six fu-organs, open and dredge block and closure. Since the block and closure are unobstructed, urination and defecation will be promoted naturally. It removes the necrotic muscles because of its wild and strong property. It eliminates the vicious toxin like ghost and the accumulation of worms and the pathogenic factors, and kill worms and fish, because its qi is characterized by yang brightness. *Huang Di Nei Jing* [《黄帝内经》, *Huangdi's Internal Classic*] says, "The double fire combining together forms yang brightness." Its severely pungent taste and severely warm property feature double fire, so its qi is characterized by yang brightness. So it can treat all diseases listed above.

Note by Zhang Zhicong（张志聪）: Once taking Bashuang（巴霜）, the severe heat will start from the chest and rib-side, run to the limbs, emerge from the skin and hair, and it is drained out from the stomach and intestines again. There is White Powder Prescription in *Shang Han Lun*［《伤寒论》, *Treatise on Cold Pathogenic Diseases*］which uses it to treat cold damage and cold repletion chest bind. The ancient people referred to it as the effective and decisive factor. If used properly, it is the real medicinal that can cure diseases; if used improperly, it will cause damage instead of benefits.

269. 雷 丸

雷丸 气味苦寒,有小毒。主杀三虫,逐毒气,胃中热,利丈夫,不利女子。

雷丸出汉中、建平、宜都及房州、金州诸处,生竹林土中,乃竹之余气所结,故一名竹苓。上无苗蔓,大小如栗,状似猪苓而圆,皮黑而微赤,肉白甚坚实。

雷丸是竹之余气,感雷震而生,竹茎叶青翠,具东方生发之义。震为雷,乃阳动于下,雷丸气味苦寒,禀冬令寒水之精,得东方震动之气,故杀阴类之三虫,而逐邪毒之气,得寒水之精,故清胃中热。震为雷,为长男,故利丈夫,不利女子。

按:《别录》云:雷丸久服令人阴痿,当是气味苦寒,久服则精寒故耳。男子多服阴痿,则女子久服子宫寒冷,不能受孕,其不利可知。《本经》乃两分之曰:利丈夫,不利女子,未审何义。马志云:疏利男子元气,不疏利女子脏气。隐庵以震为雷,为长男为解,均未得当,尚当另参。

269. Leiwan［雷丸, omphalia, Omphalia］

It is bitter in taste, cold and slightly toxic in property, and it is mainly used to kill three worms, expel toxin qi, clear the heat in the stomach, which is effective in treating men, but ineffective with women.

It grows in Hanzhong（汉中）, Jianping（建平）, Fangzhou（房州）and Jinzhou（金州）. Since it grows in the soil of bamboo forests, it is the accumulation of the bamboo's residual qi, and also called Zhuling（竹苓）. Without sprouts on the top, it is in the size of chestnut and in the round shape of Zhuling（猪苓）. Its skin is black and slightly red, and its flesh is white and solid.

It is the bamboo's residual qi and was born under the influence of thunder quake. The bamboo's stem and leaves are fresh and green which indicates springing in the east. The quake relates to thunder, which means yang moving below the surface. It can kill three worms, expel toxin qi and clear the heat in the stomach because it is bitter in taste and cold in property and receives the essence of the cold water in winter and quake the qi in the east. The quake means thunder, which refers to the eldest son, so it is favorable to men not women.

Note by Gao Shishi（高世栻）: *Ming Yi Bie Lu*［《名医别录》, *Miscellaneous Records of Famous Physicians*］says, "Long-term taking of it may cause impotence because its pungent taste and cold property can cold the semen if taken for a long time. The men who take it too much may get impotence while women may have the uterine cold and fail to conceive. Accordingly its harm goes without saying." *Shen Nong Ben Cao Jing*［《神农本草经》, *Shennong's Classic of Materia Medica*］just respectively says, "It is favorable to men but not women." However, this conclusion is not investigated for sure. Ma Zhiyun（马志云）said, "It is effective to sooth and promote the men's original qi but not the women's visceral qi." Yin An（隐庵）considered quake as thunder and explained it as the eldest son, both of these two conclusions may be not proper and need more textual research.

270. 代赭石

代赭石　气味苦寒,无毒。主治鬼疰,贼风,蛊毒,杀精物恶鬼,腹中毒邪气,女子赤沃漏下。

代赭石《本经》名须丸,《别录》名血师,研之作朱色,可以点书,故俗名土朱,又名铁朱。管子曰:山上有赭,其下有铁。《北山经》曰:少阳之山中多美赭。《西山经》曰：石脆之山灌水出焉，中有流赭皆谓此石。《别录》曰：代赭生齐国山谷，赤红青色，如鸡冠有泽，梁爪甲不渝者良。今代州，河东、江东处处山中有之，以西北出者为良。

赭石，铁之精也，其色青赤，气味苦寒，禀水石之精，而得木火之化。主治鬼疰贼风蛊毒者，色赤属火，得少阳火热之气，则鬼疰自消也。石性镇重，色青属木，木得厥阴风木之气，故治贼风蛊毒也。杀精物恶鬼，所以治鬼疰也。腹中毒，所以治蛊毒也。邪气，所以治贼风也。赭石，一名血师，能治冲任之血，故治女子赤沃漏下。

270. Daizheshi［代赭石，hematite，Haematitum］

It is bitter in taste, cold and non-toxic in property, and it is mainly used to treat Guizhu［鬼疰，multiple infixation abscess］, the abnormal weather and the parasitic toxin, kills the strange pathogenic factors like ghosts, eliminate toxin and the pathogenic qi in the abdomen, and treat the constant stranguria during flooding and spotting in women.

It is called Xuwan（须丸）in *Shen Nong Ben Cao Jing*［《神农本草经》，*Shennong's Classic of Materia Medica*］and Xueshi（血师）in *Ming Yi Bie Lu*［《名医别录》，*Miscellaneous Records of Famous Physicians*］. The red powder ground from it can be used to mark the book, so it is popularly called Tuzhu（土朱）or Tiezhu（铁朱）. Guanzi（管子）said, "If there is Daizheshi（hematite）on the mountain, there must be iron under it." *Bei Shan Jing*［《北山经》，*Beishan Canon*］says, "The one on Shaoyang Mountain（少阳山）is the most beautiful." *Xi Shan Jing*［《西山经》，*Xishan Canon*）］says, "Pour water into the hill of brittle stones and almost all the brown stones flowing out are Daizheshi（hematite）." *Ming Yi Bie Lu*［《名医别录》，*Miscellaneous Records of Famous Physicians*］says, "It exists in valleys in the State of Qi（齐）and is reddish-cyan in color, shining like cockscombs. The one touched by paws or nails without color fading is good." Now it can be collected in the mountains of Daizhou（代州）, Hedong（河东）and Jiangdong（江东）. Those collected in the northwest are of good quality.

It is the essence of iron with blue-red color. Bitter in taste and cold in property, it receives the essence of water and stones and the transformation of wood and fire. It can mainly treat Guizhu〔鬼疰，multiple infixation abscess〕, the abnormal weather and the parasitic toxin because its red color pertains to fire and it receives fire and the heat qi of lesser yang. It mainly treats the abnormal weather and the parasite toxin because it is calm in nature and its cyan color pertains to wood which receives the wind-wood qi of reverting yin. It can kill the strange pathogenic factors like ghosts, so it can naturally treat Guizhu〔鬼疰，multiple infixation abscess〕. Eliminating the toxin in the abdomen means it can eliminate the parasite toxin. It can expel pathogenic qi, so it can treat the abnormal weather. It can treat the constant stranguria during flooding and spotting in women because it, also called Xueshi（血师）, can treat the blood of thoroughfare and conception vessels.

271. 铅 丹

铅丹 气味辛，微寒，无毒。主治吐逆反胃，惊痫，癫疾，除热，下气，炼化还成九光。久服通神明。

铅丹一名丹粉，今炼铅所作黄丹也。铅名黑锡，又名水中金，五金中之属水者也，有银坑处皆有之。

铅丹木金水之精，得火化而变赤，气味辛微寒，盖禀金质而得水火之气化。主治吐逆反胃者，火温其土也。治惊痫者，水济其火也。治癫疾者，火济其水也。气味辛寒，寒能除热，辛能下气也。炼化还成九光者，炼九转而其色光亮，还成黑铅也。炼化还光而久服，则金水相生，水火相济，故通神明。

愚按：铅有毒，炼铅成丹，则无毒。铅丹下品，不堪久服，炼铅丹而成九光，则可久服，学者所当意会者也。

271. Qiandan〔铅丹, red lead, Plumbum Preparatium〕

It is pungent in taste, slightly cold and non-toxic in property, and it is mainly used to treat vomiting, stomach reflux, fright epilepsy and madness, clear heat and descend qi. When burnt and refined, it will restore the nine sorts of brightness. Long-term taking of it will invigorate spirit and mentality.

It is also called Danfen（丹粉）, which is actually the yellow elixir from refining lead nowadays. Qian（铅）is called Heixi（黑锡）and also known as Shuizhongjin（水中金）, which pertains to water among the five metals and exists in the silver pits.

It receives the essence of wood, metal and water and becomes red by the fire transformation. It has pungent taste and slightly cold property, because it is characterized with metal quality and receives the qi transformation of water and fire. It can mainly treat vomiting and stomach reflux because fire warms stomach earth, treat fright epilepsy because kidney water helps the heart fire, and treat madness because the heart fire helps kidney water. Its cold property can clear heat, and its pungent taste can descend qi. The one that restores the nine sorts of brightness after burning and refining will shine brightly after being refined nine times and then turns into black color. Long-term taking of it will invigorate spirit and mentality because of the mutual generation between metal and water and the mutual help between water and fire.

Note by Zhang Zhicong（张志聪）：The lead is toxic, but refining it into elixir can eliminate toxin. Qiandan（red lead）is of lower grade and should not be taken for a long time. If it can restore the nine sorts of brightness after refinement, it can be taken for a long term. Scholars speculate that it has these effects based on their understanding of it.

272. 铅　粉

铅粉　气味辛寒，无毒。主治伏尸，毒螫，杀三虫。

因化铅而成粉，故名铅粉。《本经》名粉锡，《别录》名胡粉，今名水粉。李时珍曰：铅锡一类也，古人名铅为黑锡，故名粉锡。

伏尸者，伏于泉下之尸，相瘵而为传尸鬼疰之病。铅粉从黑变白，从阴出阳，故主治伏尸。禀水气而性寒，故消螫毒。禀金气而味辛，故杀三虫。

愚按：黄丹、铅粉皆本黑锡所成，而变化少有不同。变白者，得金水之气而走气分。变赤者，得火土之气而走血分。黄丹禀火土之气，故入膏丹，主痈疽恶疮之用。今时则用铅粉收膏药。以代黄丹。

272. Qianfen〔铅粉, processed galenite, Galenitum Praeparatum〕

It is pungent in taste and cold in property, and it is mainly used to treat Fushi 〔伏尸, serious diseases caused by overstrain〕 and the venomous sting and kill three worms.

It is the powder from processing Qian〔铅, galenite, Galenitum〕, so it called Qianfen (processed galenite). It is called Fenxi (粉锡) in *Shen Nong Ben Cao Jing*〔《神农本草经》, *Shennong's Classic of Materia Medica*〕, Hufen (胡粉) in *Ming Yi Bie Lu*〔《名医别录》, *Miscellaneous Records of Famous Physicians*〕 and Shuifen (水粉) nowadays. Li Shizhen (李时珍) said,"Qian (galenite) and Xi (锡) are of the same category. The ancient people called Qian (galenite) as Heixi (黑锡), so Qian (galenite) is also called Fenxi (粉锡)."

Since the corpse is lying in the nether world, it is the disease of Chuanshi〔传尸, infectious consumptive diseases〕 and Guizhu〔鬼疰, multiple infixation abscess〕. Qianfen (processed galenite), changing from black to white similar to the process of transforming yin into yang, can mainly treat the serious diseases caused by overstrain. It can eliminate the venomous sting because it receives water qi and has cold property. It can kill three worms because it receives metal qi and has the pungent taste.

Note by Zhang Zhicong (张志聪): Huangdan〔黄丹, minium, Minium〕 and Qianfen (processed galenite) are both made of Heixi (黑锡) with almost no difference. Those turning white receive the metal and water qi and belong to the qi aspect while those turning red receive the fire and earth qi and belong to the blood aspect. Huangdan (minium), receiving the fire and earth qi and used in paste and pellet can the mainly treat carbuncle and malign sore. Now it is replaced by Qianfen (processed galenite) in paste.

273. 戎 盐

戎盐 气味咸寒,无毒。主明目目痛,益气,坚肌骨,去毒蛊。

戎盐产自西戎,故名戎盐。生酒泉福禄城东南之海中,相传出于北海者青,出于南海者赤,此由海中潮水溅渍山石,经久则凝结为盐,不假人力而成。所谓南海、北海,乃西海之南北,非南方之海也。青红二种,皆名戎盐。今医方但用青盐,不用红盐。

戎盐由海中咸水,凝结于石土中而成,色分青赤,是禀天一之精,化生地之五行,故主助心神而明目,补肝血而治目痛,资肺金而益气,助脾肾而坚肌骨。五脏三阴之气,交会于坤土,故去蛊毒。

273. Rongyan〔戎盐, halite, Halitum〕

It is salty in taste, cold and non-toxic in property, and it is mainly used to improve vision, relieve the eye pain, replenish qi, strengthen muscles and bones, and eliminate the parasitic toxin.

It gets its name because it comes from Xirong（西戎）. It exists in the sea located to the southeast of Fulu（福禄）city of Jiuquan（酒泉）. Tradition has it that the one growing in the north sea is green and the one growing in the south sea is red and that it is solidified without manpower from the process of seawater splashing and soaking the mountain rocks for a long time. The so-called south sea and north sea refer to the south and north of Qinghai（青海）Lake rather than the sea in the south. Both the green one and the red one are called Rongyan（halite）. However, it is the green one rather than the red one that is used in the medicinal formula.

It is generated from the salty seawater congealed in rock soil, with the two colors of green and red. It receives the essence of water, transforms and generates the five elements of the earth, so it can aid the heart spirit to improve vision; it can tonify the liver blood to relieve the eye pain; it can promote the lung metal to replenish qi; and it can assist the spleen and the kidney to strengthen muscles and bones. It can eliminate the worm toxin because the qi of the five zang-organs and three yin join at Kun-Earth.

274. 石 灰

石灰　气味辛温,有毒。主治疽疡疥瘙,热气恶疮,癞疾,死肌,堕眉,杀痔虫,去黑子息肉。

　　石灰一名石垩,又名石锻,山中人烧青石为之,作一土窑,下用柴或煤炭作一层,上累青石作一层,如是相间,作数层,自下发火,层层自焚,一昼夜则石成灰矣。化法有风化,水化二种,入药宜用风化,且陈年者。

　　石者土之骨,以火煅石成灰,色白味辛性燥,乃禀火土之气,而成燥金之质,遇风即化,土畏木也。遇水即化,火畏水也。禀金气而祛风,故治疽疡疥瘙。禀土气而滋阴,故治热气恶疮癞疾死肌。禀性燥烈,服食少而涂抹多,涂抹则堕眉,杀痔虫,去黑子息肉。

　　苏颂曰:古方多用石灰合百草团末,治金疮殊胜。李时珍曰:石灰止血神品也,但不可著水,著水则肉烂。今时以石灰同韭菜捣成饼,粘贴壁上,阴干细研成末,治跌打损伤,皮肉破处止血如神。

274. Shihui [石灰, lime, Limestonum seu Calx]

It is pungent in taste, warm and toxic in property, and it is mainly used to treat carbuncle, ulcer, scabies and itching, the malign sore caused by heat qi, leprosy, the necrotic muscles and the loss of eyebrows, eliminate hemorrhoids, kill worms and remove the black spots and polypus.

It is also known as Shie (石垩) and Shiduan (石锻). The people in the mountain burn blue stones to make it. They set up an earth kiln, use the firewood or coal as the basement, put a layer of blue stones on the top of it and then alternate them one after another to make several layers of this construction and set fire from the bottom. Each layer burns one after another for one night, and the blue stones are burnt into lime over one night. There are two kinds of transformation: wind transformation and water transformation. The one transformed through wind and stored for a long time is suitable to be used as medicinal.

The stone is the bone of earth. The lime, generated from burning stones, white in color, pungent in taste and dry in property, receives the qi of fire and earth and has the quality of dry metal. It will be transformed immediately when meeting wind because earth is restricted by wood and will be transformed immediately when meeting water because fire is restricted by water. It can treat carbuncle, ulcer, scabies and itching because it receives metal qi to dispel wind. It can treat the malign sore caused by heat qi, leprosy and the necrotic muscles because it receives earth qi to tonify yin. People usually apply it externally instead of taking it as it is dry but not drastic in property. Applying it externally can treat the loss of eyebrows, eliminate hemorrhoids, kill worms and remove the black spots and polypus.

Su Song（苏颂）said, "In the ancient formula, it was usually used with the herb powder to treat the incised wounds and the effect was especially good. " Li Shizhen（李时珍）said, "It is the best drug to stop bleeding, but the wound should avoid water otherwise the flesh will putrefy. " Nowadays it is pounded into the flat cake with Jiucai［韭菜, Chinese leek, Allii Tuberosi Folium］. Pasted to the wall, dried in the shade and ground into powder, it has amazing effects in treating knocks and falls and stopping the bleeding of wounds of the flesh and the skin.

275. 天鼠屎

天鼠屎 气味辛寒,无毒,主治面痈肿,皮肤洗洗时痛,腹中血气,破寒热积聚,除惊悸。

天鼠《本经》名伏翼,列于上品,即蝙蝠也。天鼠屎《日华本草》名夜明砂。天鼠罕用,夜明砂常用,故录之。天鼠冬蛰夏出,昼伏夜飞,多处深山崖穴中及人家旧屋内,食蚊蚋乳石精汁。李时珍曰:凡采得以水淘去灰土恶气,取细砂晒干焙用,其砂即蚊蚋眼也。

蝙蝠形极类鼠而飞翔空中,故曰:天鼠。身有翼而昼伏,故曰伏翼。屎乃蚊蚋乳石之余精,气味辛寒,感阳明太阳金水之化。主治面痈肿者,面属阳明也。皮肤洗洗时痛者,皮肤属太阳也。痈肿则血气不和,阳明行身之前,而治面之痈肿,则腹中血气之病,亦可治也。皮肤洗洗,则身发寒热。皮肤时痛,则寒热积聚,太阳主通体之皮肤,而治皮肤洗洗之时痛,则自发寒热而邪积凝聚者,亦可破也。肝病则惊,心病则悸,除惊悸者,禀阳明金气,而除风木之惊,禀太阳水气,而除火热之悸也。

275. Tianshushi〔天鼠屎，bat's droppings，Faeces Vespertilionis〕

It is pungent in taste, cold and non-toxic in property, and it is mainly used to treat the facial abscess and swelling, the chilliness and shivering of the skin with the occasional pain and the disharmony of blood and qi in the abdomen, break cold and heat accumulation and eliminate the palpitation due to fright.

Tianshu（天鼠）is called Fuyi〔伏翼，bat，Vespertilio〕in *Shen Nong Ben Cao Jing*〔《神农本草经，*Shennong's Classic of Materia Medica*〕and listed as the upper grade. Tianshushi（bat dung）is called Yemingsha（夜明砂）in *Ri Hua Ben Cao*〔《日华本草，*Rihuazi's Materia Medica*〕. Tianshushi（bat's droppings）is seldom used while Yemingsha（夜明砂）is usually used. So the latter one is recorded. Tianshu（bat）hibernates in caves in winter and comes out in summer, sleeps in daytime and flies out at night. It usually hides in the cliff caves of remote mountains or in old houses, eats mosquitoes and drinks the essence juice of stalactite. Li Shizhen（李时珍）said, "Once collected, people can use water to wash away dust and pathogenic qi and dry it with fine sand in the sun for the baking use. The sand is the eyes of the mosquitoes."

The bat looks like a rat in appearance and flies in the sky, so it is called Tianshu（天鼠）. It has wings and sleeps in daytime, so it is also called Fuyi（伏翼）. Its dung is the surplus essence of mosquitoes and stalactite, so it has the pungent taste and the cold property, which is the transformation from metal and water from yang brightness and greater yang. It can treat the facial abscess and swelling because the face pertains to yang brightness. It can treat the chilliness and shivering of the skin with the occasional pain because skin pertains to greater yang. The facial abscess and swelling is the manifestation of the disharmony of blood and qi. Yang brightness runs through the exterior part of the body. Since it can treat the facial abscess and swelling, it can also treat the disharmony of blood and qi in the abdomen. The chilliness and shivering of the skin is the manifestation of cold and heat of the body and the occasional pain is the manifestation of cold and heat accumulation. Greater yang dominates the whole body's skin. Since it can treat the chilliness and shivering of the skin with the occasional pain, it can also break the cold-heat accumulation. Those who have liver diseases are easy to be frightened and those who have heart diseases are easy to palpitate. It can eliminate the fright of wind and wood, because it receives the metal qi of yang brightness; it can eliminate the palpitation of fire and heat because it receives the water qi of greater yang.

276. 虾 蟆

虾蟆 气味辛寒,有毒。主治邪气,破癥坚血,痈肿阴疮。服之不患热病。

《本经》下品有虾蟆,《别录》下品有蟾蜍,乃一类二种也。虾蟆生陂泽中,背有黑点,身小能跳,作呷呷声。举动极急。蟾蜍在人家湿处,身大黑,无点多痱癗,不能跳,不解作声,行动迟缓,功用大同小异。李时珍曰:古方多用虾蟆,今方多用蟾蜍,考二物功用亦不甚远,今人只用蟾蜍有效,而虾蟆不复入药,疑古人所用者,亦多是蟾蜍,盖古时通称蟾蜍为虾蟆耳。《王荆公字说》云:俗言虾蟆怀土取置远处,一夕复还其所,虽或遏之,常慕而返,故名虾蟆。今俗传其能作土遁,盖亦有所本云。

虾蟆生于阴湿陂泽,能作土遁,其色黄黑,气味辛寒,盖禀土金水之气化所生。主治邪气者,辛以散之也。禀金气,故破癥坚血。禀土气,故治痈肿阴疮。禀水气,故服之不患热病。

276. Xiamo [虾蟆, rice-paddy frog, Rana Limnocharis]

It is pungent in taste, cold and toxic in property, and it is mainly used to expel pathogenic qi, break movable abdominal mass, hardness, stop bleeding and treat swollen welling-abscesses and pudendal sore. Taking it can make people not contract the heat disease.

There are Xiamo (rice-paddy frog) of the lower grade in *Shen Nong Ben Cao Jing* [《神农本草经》, *Shennong's Classic of Materia Medica*] and Chanchu [蟾蜍, dried toad, Bufo Siccus] of the lower grade in *Ming Yi Bie Lu* [《名医别录》, *Miscellaneous Records of Famous Physicians*]. They are two species of one group. The former one lives in lakes and swamps with the black spots on its back. With the small body, it can jump, make the sound of gaga and move fast. The latter one exists in damp places in people's home, darker in color, having dormant papules rather than spots. It can not jump and make the sound and moves slowly, with the same effect as that of the former. Li Shizhen（李时珍）said, "The former one is mostly used in the ancient formula while the latter one is mostly used in the current formula." Study shows that they both have the similar effects. However, the modern people usually use Chanchu（dried toad）instead of Xiamo（rice-paddy frog）because what the ancient people used is mostly Chanchu（dried toad）and Chanchu（dried toad）was generally called Xiamo（rice-paddy frog）in ancient times. *Wang Jin Gong Zi Shuo* [《王荆公字说》, *Wangjinggong's Annalysis of Chinese Characters*] says, "As the saying goes, if Xiamo（rice-paddy frog）removes to a faraway place with some soil of its original living environment, it will return to its place one night later. Even if it is far away, Xiamo（rice-paddy frog）will return occasionally due to its attachment to the previous place, so it is called Xiamo（rice-paddy frog）." Now it is popularly said that it can become invisible under the soil which is also based on the saying above.

Xiamo（rice-paddy frog）lives in damp and shady lakes and swamps and can become invisible under the help of soil. It is black-yellow in color and has pungent taste and cold property, as it is born from the qi transformation of earth, metal and water. It can mainly expel pathogenic qi because its pungent taste can expel pathogenic qi. It can break movable abdominal mass, hardness and stop bleeding because it receives metal qi. It can treat swollen welling-abscesses and pudendal sore because it receives earth qi. Taking it will not contract the heat disease because it receives water qi.

277. 蜈　蚣

蜈蚣　气味辛温,有毒。主治鬼疰蛊毒敢,诸蛇虫鱼毒,杀鬼物老精,温疟,去三虫。

蜈蚣江以南处处有之,春出冬蛰,节节有足,双须岐尾,头上有毒钳。入以头足赤者为良。蜈蚣一名天龙,能制龙蛇蜥蜴,畏虾蟆、蛞蝓、蜘蛛、雄鸡。《庄子》所谓:物畏其天。《阴符经》所谓:禽之制在气也。

蜈蚣色赤性温,双钳两尾,头尾咸红。生于南方,禀火毒之性,故《本经》主治皆是以火毒而攻阴毒之用也。

愚按:蛇属金,蜈蚣属火,故能制之。鸡应昴宿,是又太阳出而爝火灭之义矣。

277. Wugong［蜈蚣, centipede, Scolopendra］

It is pungent in taste, warm and toxic in property, and it is mainly used to treat Guizhu［鬼疰, multiple infixation abscess］and the worm toxin, eliminate various toxins of snakes, worms and fish, perish the ghost-like vicious factors, treat warm malaria and expel three worms.

Wugong (centipede), existing everywhere in the south of the Yangtze River, comes out in spring and hibernates in winter. It has feet on each segment of the body, double cirrus, the branching tail and poisonous clamps on its head. Those with the red head and feet are good to be used as medicinal. Also called as Tianlong (天龙), it can control dragons, snakes and lizards, while it is afraid of the rice-paddy frog slug, spider and rooster. *Zhuang Zi* ［《庄子》, *Chuang Tzu*］says that animals are afraid of their natural enemies. *Yin Fu Jing*［《阴符经》, *Yin Fu Canon*］says the reason why birds can fly freely in the air is that they can control the airflow around them.

Wugong (centipede), red in color and mild in property, has double clamps and tails in deep red color. Found everywhere in southern China, it is characterized with the fire toxin in property, so it can mainly attack the yin toxin by the fire toxin in *Shen Nong Ben Cao Jing*［《神农本草经》, *Shennong's Classic of Materia Medica*］.

Note by Zhang Zhicong (张志聪): The snake pertains to metal, while Wugong (centipede) pertains to fire, so Wugong (centipede) can control the snake. The rooster responds to Pleiades (昴宿), so the greater yang of rooster can control the low fire of Wugong (centipede).

278. 蚯 蚓

蚯蚓 气味咸寒,无毒。主治蛇瘕,去三虫,伏尸鬼疰,蛊毒,杀长虫。

蚯蚓生湿土中，凡平泽膏壤地中皆有之，孟夏始出，仲冬蛰藏，雨则先出，晴则夜鸣，其土娄如丘，其行也引而后伸，故名蚯蚓。能穿地穴，故又名地龙。入药宜大而白颈，是其老者有力。日华子曰：路上踏杀者，名千人踏，入药更良。

蚯蚓冬藏夏出，屈而后伸，上食稿壤，下饮黄泉，气味咸寒，宿应轸水，禀水土之气化。主治尸疰虫蛊，盖以泉下之水气上升，地中之土气上达，则阴类皆从之而消灭矣。蜈蚣属火，名曰天龙。蚯蚓属水，名曰地龙。皆治鬼疰，蛊毒，蛇虫毒者，天地相交，则水火相济，故禀性虽有不同，而主治乃不相殊。

278. Qiuyin［蚯蚓，earthworm，Pheretima］

It is salty in taste, cold and non-toxic in property, and it is mainly used to resolve the snake-shaped movable abdominal mass, eliminate three worms, treat Fushi［伏尸，serious diseases caused by overstrain］and Guizhu［鬼疰，multiple infixation abscess］, resolve the parasitic toxin and kill long worms.

Qiuyin (earthworm) lives in wet soil and can be found everywhere in swamps and the fertile soil. It comes out in the first month of summer and hibernates in midwinter. It comes out when it is going to rain, and makes noise on clear nights. Its nest looks like the small mound and it moves forward by shrinking first then stretching, so it is named Qiuyin (earthworm). It can move underground, so it is also named Dilong (地龙). Those big in size and having white necks are proper to be used as medicinal for the old is strong. Ri Huazi (日华子) said that those trodden by passers-by on road are called Qianrenta (千人踏) which are better to be used as medicinal.

Qiuyin (earthworm) hibernates in winter and comes out in summer, shrinks first and stretches after, and feeds on the dry soil and spring water underground. Salty in taste, cold and non-toxic in property, responding to Zhenshuiyin (轸水蚓) Star, it receives the qi transformation of water and earth. It can mainly treat the latent disease and the fatal tuberculosis as the qi of the spring water underground moves upward and earth qi in soil rises, and thus the yin aspect is expelled. Wugong (centipede) pertains to fire, so it is named Tianlong (天龙). It pertains to water, so it is named Dilong (地龙). Both of them can treat Guizhu

［鬼疰，multiple infixation abscess］and resolve the parasitic toxin. The connection between these two is the communication of heaven qi and earth qi which promotes the coordination of water and fire. Despite they have different natures, they have similar effects.

279. 蛇 蜕

蛇蜕　气味咸甘平，无毒。主治小儿百二十种惊痫，蛇痫，癫疾，瘛疭，弄舌摇头，寒热肠痔，蛊毒。

蛇蜕人家墙屋木石间多有之，其蜕无时，但着不净则蜕，或大饱亦蜕。凡青黄苍色者勿用，须白色如银者良，于五月五日蜕者更佳。又，蕲州之白花蛇，龙头虎口黑质，白花者，其蜕尤佳。

蛇蜕色白如银，至洁至净，气味咸平，禀金水之气化，金能制风，故主治小儿百二十种惊痫，蛇痫之证。癫疾瘛疭，惊痫病也。弄舌摇头，蛇痫病也。水能清热解毒，故主治大人寒热肠痔蛊毒。寒热者，肠痔蛊毒之寒热也。

愚按：痫证唯一，即曰：惊痫。复曰：蛇痫，则痫证不止一端，若以内之七情，外之形象求之，不啻百二十种，先圣立言，当意会也。

279. Shetui［蛇蜕，snake slough，Periostracum Serpentis］

It is salty and sweet in taste, mild and non-toxic in property, and it is mainly used to treat one hundred and twenty kinds of infantile fright epilepsy, the snake-like epilepsy, the epileptic disease, the clonic convulsion, the frequent protrusion of tongue and the shaking of head, cold and heat, the anal abscess and the parasitic toxin.

The snake usually sloughs under walls and among woods and stones, but the time is uncertain. Sloughing happens when the snake has something dirty on, or gets full enough. The green, yellow and ashy slough is forbidden to be used as medicinal. The slough, as white as silver, is good to be used as medicinal. The slough got on the fifth day of the fifth lunar month is better. What's more, the slough of the long-nosed pit viper（白花蛇）in Qizhou（蕲州），which has a big head and mouth, the black body and white dapples, is best.

Shetui (snake slough), as white as silver, clean and pure, salty in taste and mild in property, receives the qi transformation of metal and water. Metal can control wind, so it can mainly treat one hundred and twenty kinds of infantile fright epilepsy and the snake-like epilepsy. The fright epilepsy is manifested as the epileptic disease and the clonic convulsion. The snake epilepsy is manifested as the frequent protrusion of tongue and the shaking of head. Water can clear heat and remove toxin, so it can treat the adult cold and heat, the anal abscess and the parasitic toxin. Cold and heat is manifested as hemorrhoids and the worm toxin.

Note by Zhang Zhicong (张志聪): If the epilepsy is manifested as one symptom, it refers to the fright epilepsy. It is also said that the snake-like epilepsy is manifested as more than one symptom. In consideration of seven emotions (joy, anger, anxiety, thought, sorrow, fear, and fright) and the manifested symptoms, there are one hundred and twenty kinds of epilepsy. What sages have said should be understood by insight.

280. 斑 蝥

斑蝥 气味辛寒,有毒。主治寒热鬼疰蛊毒,鼠瘘恶疮,疽蚀,死肌,破石癃。

> 斑蝥甲虫也,斑言其色,言蝥其毒,如矛刺也。所在有之,七八月在大豆叶上,长五六分,大者寸许,黄黑斑纹,乌腹尖喙。《太平御览》引《神农本草经》云:春食芫花为芫青,夏食葛花为亭长,秋食豆花为斑蝥。冬入地中为地胆,其斑蝥甲上有黄黑斑点。芫青青绿色,亭长黑身赤头,地胆黑头赤尾,色虽不同,功亦相近。
>
> 斑蝥感秋气,食豆花,气味辛寒,色兼黄黑,盖禀金水之化而为毒虫,故主散恶毒,消恶疮,攻死肌,破石癃,乃以毒而攻毒也。

280. Banmao [斑蝥, blister beetle, Mylabris]

It is pungent in taste, cold and non-toxic in property, and it is mainly used to treat cold and heat, Guizhu [鬼疰, multiple infixation abscess], the parasitic toxin, mouse fistula, malign sore, carbuncle and corrosion, necrotic muscles and stony ischuria.

Banmao（blister beetle）is a kind of beetle. Ban（斑）refers to the colorful spots on its body, and Mao（螯）means that it is toxic and sharp as the spear. It lives everywhere and exists on the soybean leaves in the sixth and seventh lunar months. Generally, it is five or six Fen in length and the bigger ones are about one Cun in length with the yellow-black strips on its body, the black abdomen and the pointed mouth. *Tai Ping Yu Lan*［《太平御览》，*A Reference Book Written during the Reign of the Emperor Taizong of Song*］quotes *Shen Nong Ben Cao Jing*［《神农本草经》，*Shennong's Classic of Materia Medica*］saying that those feeding on Yuanhua［芫花，genkwa, Genkwa Flos］in spring are Yuanqing［芫青，lytta, Lytta］, those feeding on Gehua［葛花，pueraria flower, Puerariae Flos］in summer are Tingchang［亭长，epicauta, Epicauta］, those with the yellow and black spots on its back and feeding on bean flowers in autumn are Banmao（blister beetle）, and those existing under the ground in winter are Didan［地胆，oil beetles, Meloe coarctatus］with the yellow-black spots on the shell. Yuanqing（lytta）is turquoise in color, Tingchang（epicauta）has the black body and the red head, Didan（oil beetles）has the black head and the red tail. In spite of different colors, they have similar effects.

Sensing the coming of autumn and feeding on bean flowers, pungent in taste, cold in property, and yellow and black in color, it receives the transformation of metal and water, so it is toxic and can mainly resolve the severe toxin, eliminate malign sore and treat the necrotic muscles and the stony dysuria, which is the result of attacking toxin with toxin.

281. 蜣 螂

蜣螂 气味咸寒,有毒。主治小儿惊痫瘈疭,腹胀寒热,大人癫疾狂阳。

蜣螂所在有之,有大小二种,小者身黑而暗,不堪入药。大者身黑而光,名胡蜣螂。腹翼下有小黄子,附母而飞,见灯光则来,宜入药用。蜣螂以土包粪,转而成丸,雄曳雌推,置于坝中覆之而去,数日有小蜣螂出,盖孚乳于中也,故一名推丸,又名推车客。深目高鼻,状如羌胡,背负黑甲,状如武士,故一名铁甲将军,昼伏夜出,故又名夜游将军。

蜣螂甲虫也,出于池泽,以土包转而成生育。气味咸寒,是甲虫而禀水土之气化。甲虫属金,金能制风,故主治小儿惊痫瘈疭。禀土气,故治腹胀之寒热。禀水气,故治大人癫疾之狂阳。

281. Qianglang〔蜣螂, dung beetle, Catharsius〕

It is salty in taste, cold and toxic in property, and it is mainly used to treat the infantile fright epilepsy, the clonic convulsion, the abdominal distension, cold and heat, the epilepsy and mania in adults.

It lives everywhere and has two kinds. The smaller one with the dark black body can not be used as medicinal, while the bigger one with the bright black body is named Huqianglang（胡蜣螂）, which has small yellow larva under the wings on its belly. The larva flies with the mother Huqianglang（胡蜣螂）, chasing the light. The bigger one is proper to be used as medicinal. Qianglang（dung beetle）covers the excrement with earth and makes it into a ball. The male pulls and the female pushes the ball into the dam, the female lays eggs in the excrement ball and then covers it. Some days later, the larvae are born. Therefore, it is also known as Tuiwan（推丸）or Tuicheke（推车客）. With deep eyes and a high nose, it looks like Qianghu（羌胡）. With the black shell, it is as strong as a warrior, so it is also called as Tiejia Jiangjun（铁甲将军）. It hides in daytime and comes out at night, so it is also called as Yeyou Jiangjun（夜游将军）.

Qianglang（dung beetle）is a kind of beetle. Existing in lakes and pools, it was born by covering excrement with earth. Receiving the qi transformation of water and earth, it is salty in taste and cold in property. Beetle pertains to metal and metal can control wind, so it can mainly treat the infantile fright epilepsy and the clonic convulsion. It receives earth qi, so it can treat the abdominal distension and cold and heat. It receives water qi, so it can be used to treat the epilepsy and mania in adults.

282. 鼠 妇

鼠妇 气味酸温,无毒。主治气癃,不得小便,妇人月闭血瘕,痫痉寒热,利水道,堕胎。

鼠妇处处有之,多在人家地上下湿处,凡瓷器底及土坎中更多,形似衣鱼,稍大,灰色,多足,背有横纹蹙起,《诗经》所谓蚰蟒在室,即此虫也。

鼠妇感阴湿而生,气味酸温,禀太阳寒水厥阴风木之化。太阳水气行于肤表,则气癃而不得小便者可治也。厥阴木气上行外达,则妇人月闭而为血瘕者可治也。膀胱气癃,在内则不得小便,在外则有痫痉寒热之病。鼠妇治气癃,则痫痉之寒热亦可治也。不得小便,则水道不利,鼠妇治不得小便,则水道亦可利也。妇人恶血内闭,则为血瘕。新血内聚,则为妊娠。鼠妇治妇人月闭血瘕,则堕胎亦其验矣。

282. Shufu［鼠妇, pillbug, Armadillidium］

It is sour in taste and warm in property, and it is mainly used to treat qi ischuria, dysuria, the amenorrhea with the blood conglomeration in women, epilepsy and cold and heat. It can promote the water passage and induce abortion.

Shufu (pillbug) can be easily found everywhere, mainly in the wet places in people's houses, especially at the bottom of urns and in the mound. It is similar to the silverfish in shape but a little bigger in size. It is grey in color and has many feet. It has a rough back with horizontal dapples. *Shi Jing*［《诗经》, *The Book of Songs*］says there is Yiwei (蚰蟒) in the house. Here Yiwei (蚰蟒) refers to Shufu (pillbug).

Shufu (pillbug), generated through sensing dampness, is sour in taste and warm in property. It receives the transformation of the cold water from greater yang and the wind wood of reverting yin. The water qi of greater yang moves on the skin surface, so the qi ischuria and dysuria can be treated. The wood qi of reverting yin reaches upward and outward, so amenorrhea with the blood conglomeration in women can be treated. The qi ischuria of the bladder causes dysuria inside and epilepsy and cold and heat outside. Shufu (pillbug) can treat the qi ischuria so that the cold and heat disease and epilepsy can be treated. Dysuria means the water passage is blocked. Shufu (pillbug) can treat dysuria, so the water passage can be promoted. The malign blood blocked and conglomerated inside is called the blood conglomeration. The new blood produced and gathered inside is pregnancy. Shufu (pillbug) can treat amenorrhea with the blood conglomeration in women, so it can also induce abortion.

283. 水 蛭

水蛭 气味咸苦平,有毒。主逐恶血瘀血,月闭,破血症积聚,无子,利水道。

水蛭处处河池有之,种类不一,在山野中者,名山蜞,在草中者,名草蛭,在泥水中者,名水蛭,大者谓之马蜞,今名马蟥。

水蛭乃水中动物,气味咸苦,阴中之阳也。咸苦走血,故主逐恶血瘀血,通月闭。咸软坚,苦下泄,故破血症积聚及经闭无子。感水中生动之气,故利水道。仲祖《伤寒论》治太阳随经瘀热在里,有抵当汤,内用水蛭,下瘀血也。

283. Shuizhi〔水蛭, leech, Hirudo〕

It is salty and bitter in taste, mild and toxic in property, and it is mainly used to eliminate the malign blood and the static blood, treat amenorrhea, break the accumulation-gathering of the blood stasis, treat infertility, and promote the water passage.

It can be easily found in lakes and pools. There are many different kinds of Shuizhi (leech). That living in the remote mountains is called Shanqi (山蜞). That living in the grass is called Caozhi (草蛭). That living in the muddy water is called Shuizhi (水蛭), of which the bigger one is called Maqi (马蜞) and called as Mahuang (马蟥) nowadays.

Shuizhi (leech), living in water, salty and bitter in taste, pertains to yang within yin. The salty and bitter taste mobilizes blood, so it can eliminate the malign and static blood and treat amenorrhea. Saltiness can soften hardness and bitterness is purgative, so it can break the accumulation-gathering of the blood stasis and treat amenorrhea and infertility. It senses the moving qi in water, so it can promote the water passage. *Shang Han Lun*〔《伤寒论》, *Treatise on Febrile Diseases*〕, written by Zhang Zhongjing (张仲景), says that Dead-On Decoction (抵当汤) is effective in treating the disease of greater yang following meridian and the pathognic heat intruding into the interior, in which Shuizhi (leech) is used to eliminate the static blood.

284. 雀瓮

雀瓮 气味甘平,无毒。主治寒热结气,蛊毒,鬼疰,小儿惊痫。

雀瓮《本经》谓之躁舍,后人谓之蛄蟖房,乃刺毛虫所作窠也。其形如瓮,雀好啄其瓮中之蛹,故名雀瓮,又谓之雀儿饭瓮。刺毛虫一名蛄蟖,俗名杨瘌子,因其背上毛有毒,能螫人作痛也。生树枝间,如蚕而小,背上有五色斑毛。将老者,口中吐白汁,作茧自裹,凝聚渐硬,正如雀卵,紫白裯斑,其虫在中成蛹,如蚕之在茧也。夏月羽化而出作蛾,放子于叶间,如蚕子。处处树上有之,牡丹上尤多,入药唯取石榴树上及棘上房内有蛹者,正如螵蛸诸树皆有,入药唯取桑上者耳,故《图经》有天浆子之称。《衍义》有棘刚子之号。天浆乃甜榴之名也。

雀瓮多生榴棘树上,夏月羽化而出,毛虫有毒,雀瓮则无毒矣,气味甘平,感木火土之气化,土气和于内外,则寒热结气可治矣。木气条达,则土气苏通,而蛊毒可治矣。火气光明,则鬼疰及小儿惊痫皆可治矣。

284. Queweng [雀瓮, cocoon of oriental moth, Incunabulum Cnidocampae Flavescentis]

It is sweet in taste, mild and non-toxic in property, and it is mainly used to treat the qi stagnation caused by cold and heat, the parasitic toxin, Guizhu [鬼疰, multiple infixation abscess] and the infantile fright epilepsy.

It is called Zaoshe (躁舍) in *Shen Nong Ben Cao Jing* [《神农本草经》, *Shennong's Classic of Materia Medica*] and people later on call it Gusifang (蛄蟖房) which is the cocoon of the eucleid caterpillar. It looks like an urn in which sparrows peck the chrysalis, so it is called Queweng (cocoon of oriental moth) or Que'er Fanweng (雀儿饭瓮). The eucleid caterpillar, also called Gusi (蛄蟖), is popularly called as Yanglazi (杨瘌子) as it can sting others with the toxic setae on its back. The eucleid caterpillar grows among the twigs and branches of trees, in the size of silkworms, with the colorful setae on its back.

When it grows mature, it disgorges the white liquid from the mouth and wraps itself in cocoons. Then it is agglomerated and becomes the hard cocoon, looking like the sparrow egg, with the alternate purple and white stripes, in which it metamorphoses into chrysalis like silkworms in the cocoon. It flies out and becomes a moth in summer and lays eggs on the leaves which look like the silkworm eggs. It exists everywhere on all kinds of trees, especially on the peony. Only those with chrysalis inside the cocoon which exist in pomegranate trees and sour jujube trees can be used as medicinal, just as Piaoxiao [螵蛸, mantis egg-case, Mantidis Ootheca] exists on all kinds of trees but only those on mulberry trees can be used as medicinal, so it is called Tianjiangzi (天浆子) in *Ben Cao Tu Jing* [《本草图经》, *Commentaries on the Illustrations*]. *Ben Cao Yan Yi* [《本草衍义》, *Explanation and Analysis of Materia Medica*] calls it Jigangzi (棘刚子). Tianjiang [天浆, sweet pomegranate, Granati Fructus Dulcis] is the name of the sweet pomegranate.

Queweng (cocoon of oriental moth) mainly exists in the pomegranate trees and the sour jujube trees and ecloses in summer. The eucleid caterpillar is toxic in property, but Queweng (cocoon of oriental moth) is non-toxic in property. It is sweet in taste, mild in property and senses the qi transformation of wood, fire and earth. Earth qi can harmonize the interior and exterior, so it can treat the qi stagnation caused by heat and cold. When wood qi is in the free activity, earth qi can move smoothly, so it can treat the parasitic toxin. Fire qi is clear and bright, so it can treat Guizhu [鬼疰, multiple infixation abscess] and the infantile fright epilepsy.

285. 萤 火

萤火 气味辛,微温,无毒。主明目。

萤火《本经》名夜光,《别录》云萤火,生阶地池泽,七月七日取阴干。萤有三种,一种小而宵飞,腹下光明,乃茅根所化。《吕氏月令》所谓:腐草化为萤者是也。一种长如蛆蠋,尾后有光,无翼不飞,乃竹根所化,其名曰蠲。《明堂月令》所谓:腐草化为蠲者是也。一种水萤,居水中。唐李子卿《水萤赋》所谓:彼何为而草化,此何为而居泉是也。入药用飞萤。

润下作咸,其臭腐,腐草为萤,禀水气也。萤为火宿,名曰萤火,禀火气也。生于七月,其时大火西流,故气味辛温。水之精,火之神,共凑于目,故《本经》主明目,而《别录》又云:通神精。

285. Yinghuo〔萤火, firefly, Luciola〕

It is pungent in taste, slightly warm and non-toxic in property, and it is mainly used to improve vision.

Yinghuo (firefly) is also called Yeguang (夜光) in *Shen Nong Ben Cao Jing* 〔《神农本草经》, *Shennong's Classic of Materia Medica*〕and Yinghuo (萤火) in *Ming Yi Bie Lu* 〔《名医别录》, *Miscellaneous Records of Famous Physicians*〕. It exists in the lakes and the pools of terrace, and it is collected on the 7th of the seventh lunar month and dried in shade. There are three kinds of fireflies. One is small in size and glows under the belly while flying at night, which is said to eclose from the grass roots. *Lü Shi Yue Ling* 〔《吕氏月令》, *Lü's Monthly Order*〕says that the firefly ecloses from the rotten grass. Another kind, called Juan (蠲), looks like the maggot with a gleamy tail. Without wings, it cannot fly and it is said to eclose from the bamboo roots. *Ming Tang Yue Ling* 〔《名堂月令》, *Ming Tang Monthly Order*〕says Juan (蠲) ecloses from the rotten grass roots. The other kind, called Shuiying (水萤), lives in water. *Shui Ying Fu* 〔《水萤赋》, *Ode to Water Firefly*〕, composed by Li Ziqing (李子卿) of the Tang Dynasty, says that some fireflies eclose from grass while some live in water. The flying fireflies can be used as medicinal.

Water flows downwards and salty taste is produced. It smells foul. The firefly ecloses from the rotten grass and receives water qi. Ying (萤) pertians to fire and recevies fire qi, so it is called Yinghuo (firefly). The firefly is born in the seventh lunar month when Dahuo (大火) is moving towards the horizon, so it is pungent in taste and slightly warm in property. Yinghuo (firefly), with the water essence and the fire spirit, takes effect on the vision. So *Shen Nong Ben Cao Jing* 〔《神农本草经》, *Shennong's Classic of Materia Medica*〕says that it can improve vision, and *Ming Yi Bie Lu* 〔《名医别录》, *Miscellaneous Records of Famous Physicians*〕says that it can invigorate the spirit.

286. 衣 鱼

衣鱼 气味咸温,无毒。主治妇人疝瘕,小便不利,小儿中风,项强背起,摩之。

衣鱼一名白鱼,即蠹鱼也,生衣帛及书纸中,故名衣鱼,形略似鱼身有白粉,其色光亮如银,故又名白鱼。俗传衣鱼入道经中,食神仙字,则身有五色,人得吞之,可至神仙,此方士谬传,不可信也。

衣鱼色白,碎之如银,禀金气也。命名曰鱼,气味咸温,禀水气也。水能生木,故治妇人之疝瘕。妇人疝瘕,肝木病也。金能生水,故治小便之不利。小便不利,水不行也。小儿经脉未充,若中于风,日久不愈,则项强背起,乃督脉为病,督脉合肝部,属太阳。衣鱼禀金水之化,故当用以摩之。

286. Yiyu〔衣鱼, silverfish, Lepisma Saccharina〕

It is salty in taste, warm and non-toxic in property, and it is mainly used to treat hernia and movable abdominal mass in women, dysuria, infantile stroke and the neck rigidity involving the back by rubbing manipulation.

Yiyu (silverfish) is also called as Baiyu (白鱼) or Duyu (蠹鱼). It exists in silk clothes, books and papers, so it is called Yiyu (衣鱼). Similar to fish in shape and silvery in color with white powder on its body, it is also called Baiyu (白鱼). It's popularly said that Yiyu (silverfish) eats the characters of the immortals in Taoist Scriptures, so its body has five colors. People could become immortals after eating it, which is a false description by alchemists and unbelievable.

Yiyu (silverfish), white in color and like silver after grinding, receives metal qi. It is called Yu (鱼), salty in taste and warm in property, as it receives water qi. Water generates wood, so it can treat hernia and the movable abdominal mass in women which is the disease with the liver. Metal generates water, so it can treat dysuria which is caused by the inhibited water passage. For the infants with fragile channels in body, if they get the wind invasion and cannot be healed for a long time, their neck involving the back will become rigid, which is the dysfunction of the governor vessel that is related to the liver and pertains to greater yang. Yiyu(silverfish) receives the transformation of metal and water, so it can be used in rubbing manipulation.